Introduction to Mental Health Nursing

Introduction to Mental Health Nursing

Edited by Nick Wrycraft

 McGraw Hill

Open University Press

Open University Press
McGraw-Hill Education
McGraw-Hill House
Shoppenhangers Road
Maidenhead
Berkshire
England
SL6 2QL

email: enquiries@openup.co.uk
world wide web: www.openup.co.uk

and Two Penn Plaza, New York, NY 10121-2289, USA

First published 2009, Reprinted 2010

A catalogue record of this book is available from the British Library

ISBN-13: 9780335233588 (pb) 9780335233571 (hb)
ISBN-10: 0335233589 (pb) 0335233570 (hb)

Library of Congress Cataloging-in-Publication Data
CIP data applied for

Typeset by YHT Ltd, London
Printed in the Britain by CPI Antony Rowe, Chippenham, Wiltshire SN14 6LH

The McGraw·Hill Companies

Contents

Contents

The editor and contributors

Geoffrey Amoateng is a senior lecturer in mental health at Anglia Ruskin University, and previously worked in both acute admission and psychiatric intensive care units in a medium secure setting and as a forensic community mental health nurse. His areas of interest include the development of nursing within secure mental health care, pre- and post-registration nursing, and the role of culture in understanding mental illness.

Amanda Blackhall currently teaches on pre-registration nursing programmes and continuing professional development courses related to the mental health of older adults, including caring for people with dementia. She has an interest in the mental health and well-being of people with long-term medical conditions, and in the specialism of liaison psychiatry.

Alyson Buck is a senior lecturer and Pathway leader for pre-registration mental health nursing at Anglia Ruskin University. Alyson has an interest in perinatal mental health and the physical care issues of people with mental illness.

David A. Hingley is a senior lecturer in mental health at Anglia Ruskin University and a pre-registration nurse training facilitator. He has a particular interest in the concept of recovery and currently leads a post-registration module in the management of violence and aggression.

Richard Khoo currently works as an independent adviser and consultant in mental health legislation and medical law. He also works part-time on the Investigating Committee, Fitness to Practise at the NMC and on the Mental Health Review Tribunal. Prior to this he was principal lecturer at Anglia Ruskin University and led the LLM in medical law.

Mark McGrath has over 25 years' experience working within secure mental health care settings, both low and medium. He presently works for St Andrew's Healthcare as a training lead and as a senior lecturer for Anglia Ruskin University. His area of interest is staff development within secure care settings and pre-postgraduate training.

Mary Northrop is a senior lecturer at Anglia Ruskin University. She has worked in higher education for the last 20 years in areas including pre- and post-registration nursing and has helped to develop the foundation degree for health care support workers. She is a registered mental health and adult nurse, and has worked in acute mental health care, elderly care and medical settings. She has an interest in how skills from both medical and mental health disciplines can be applied to any health care setting.

Lyn Parsons has worked in mental health since 2002, specifically with mentally disordered offenders in prison and hospital settings. Latterly, this was within the Dangerous and Severe Personality Disorder Service. She now works as a self-employed cognitive behaviour therapist at the CBT Partnership in Hertford and lectures on the IAPT postgraduate diploma course at the University of Hertfordshire.

Tim Schafer is an experienced mental health nurse, lecturer and researcher who has developed a strong commitment to mental health promotion and promoting user and carer involvement in research, service evaluation and monitoring. He is currently working as a lecturer and researcher and teaches mental health promotion to mental health workers and to a range of other primary care-based practitioners at Anglia Ruskin University.

Allen Senivassen is a senior lecturer for pre-registration mental health nursing at Anglia Ruskin University and a pre-registration nurse training facilitator. Allen has a particular interest in principles-based practice, group dynamics and leadership within health care. Currently he has a leading role in implementing *The Ten Essential Shared Capabilities* and inclusive practice in mental health nursing, and in involving service users in curriculum design and delivery at Anglia Ruskin.

Julie Teatheredge is a registered mental health nurse and specialist practitioner as well as a senior lecturer in mental health at Anglia Ruskin University. Julie's specialist interest is in human development. Currently she is carrying out training for practice mentors and undertaking research towards her doctoral thesis which is a longitudinal study into mentorship in mental health nursing practice.

James Trueman is a senior lecturer at Anglia Ruskin University, and a pre-registration nurse training facilitator. His specialist area of interest is mental health legislation.

Henck van Bilsen is a consultant clinical psychologist working as director of the CBT-Partnership (a leading provider of cognitive behaviour therapies in Hertfordshire and London). He is also a co-director of the IAPT programmes of the University of Hertfordshire, where he directs the postgraduate diploma and masters programme in cognitive behaviour therapies.

Steven Walker is theme leader for advanced studies in child and adolescent mental health at Anglia Ruskin University. He trained in social work and social policy at the LSE and has worked in child protection and specialist CAMH services in London and Essex. He is widely published in this specialist area. He is a fellow of the Higher Education Academy and a registered systemic psychotherapist (UKCP). His research interests are in service evaluation, children's rights and cultural competence.

Steve Wood is head of the Department of Mental Health & Learning Disabilities at Anglia Ruskin University. His clinical interests include community mental health care, clinical leadership and innovation, early intervention in, and personal experiences of, dementia, and new applications of psychological therapies. Steve's research and publications include the experiences of mental health nursing students, the change process as perceived by community psychiatric nurses and specialist papers relevant to caring for the older adult.

Nick Wrycraft is a senior lecturer at Anglia Ruskin University, module tutor for Module 1 of the pre-registration nurse training programme and admissions tutor for pre-registration mental health nursing. He has a particular interest in the changing role of mental health nursing, mental health services in primary care and service design.

Acknowledgements

I would like to thank the following students for providing the quotes and insights that have been used throughout the book: Jess Bradley, Spencer Dînnage, Evelyn Dudra, Tracy McLane, Lucy Newman, Alex Orrock and Marcin Prochnicki.

In addition, I would like to thank Catherine Amongi, Kevin Clarke, Youssouf Dickreeah, Ezekiel Onifade and Casey Rogers for the quotes and insights used in Chapter 1.

Finally, I'd like to say thanks to my wife Alex without whose help and support this would not have been possible, and our two children, Emily and Hamish.

Introduction

Mental health nursing is grounded in human experience, and this book aims to provide a 'student's eye' perspective of pre-registration training. The idea for the book developed from discussions with students and colleagues involved in a pre-registration mental health nursing course. Four strands of thought emerged.

Firstly, there was a need for an easy to read text written at an accessible level. This book is intended for people who have never before worked in mental health nursing but have always been curious about the work mental health nurses carry out. It also provides a background for people considering applying to train as a mental health nurse. At the same time it will be a useful introduction for students during the early stages of pre-registration training, helping you to identify what it is important to know, and assisting you to begin to develop an understanding of the role of the mental health nurse.

Secondly, the work of mental health nursing is not well understood and is often the subject of myth and misconception. In spite of care in the community having been established for decades, many people still think mental health nursing only happens within the walls of large institutions. Unfortunately, due to the low-key profile of mental health nursing and an often negative public view of mental health, many people with suitable skills and disposition never consider entering this exciting and rewarding area of the profession. This book aims to provide a realistic and balanced understanding of mental health nursing that redresses the balance.

Thirdly, the book provides a range of useful knowledge on all aspects of modern mental health nursing practice and skills. The majority of the contributing authors all work with pre-registration mental health nurses and careful thought has been given to the information which has been included. In addition, we have also chosen to write about themes and issues which will be useful to students new to nursing and the practice setting.

Fourthly, health and social care is increasingly being delivered by mental health nurses jointly with staff from other health care disciplines in community settings. These changes have led to some people experiencing doubts about what it is that mental health nurses do, and undoubtedly the work of mental health nursing has changed. This book brings together a number of aspects of this new role which have emerged in recent years, yet we also challenge students to question their practice. Through gaining an understanding of our unique contribution to the care of people with mental health problems we will arrive at a new and more definite understanding of mental health nursing.

While the work of mental health nursing is often highly rewarding because it offers the opportunity to help people bring about positive change in their lives, it would be naïve to suggest there are only benefits. Coping with difficult and stressful circumstances is a reality and training requires that we become aware of our personal values and coping resources. An important part of preparing for professional practice is to develop skills in dealing with adverse circumstances, managing problems and difficulties, and learning from experience.

Becoming a self-knowing and reflective practitioner does not happen by accident. In order to help you to develop these skills, throughout the book there are practice-focused scenarios to provide a close connection with the clinical setting. There are also a number of exercises intended to actively engage you in reflecting on your own personal and professional experience, views and attitudes. These will help you to develop your own understanding of practice and allow you to recognize your growing competence and developing professional knowledge.

Structure of the book

This book is written in three sections. In the first we discuss the *essential information* you will need for the pre-registration nursing course. In the second section we consider *mental health and illness at different stages of the lifespan*, while in the final section we look at *therapeutic and theoretical perspectives*.

The reason the book is organized in this way is that the work of mental health nursing involves a highly specific body of knowledge concerning *legislation*, the *Care Programme Approach* (CPA) and *risk assessment*. It is necessary to understand these fundamental aspects in order to be able to practise. *Mental health promotion* is also a concept which has gained momentum in recent years; there are a wide variety of ways in which mental health can be promoted and mental health nurses need to incorporate this into the basis of their practice.

At the same time we need to regard the person with a mental health problem as a unique individual. Their age, socioeconomic circumstances and support network are all important considerations with regard to how the person experiences a mental health problem, and the possible interventions which may be appropriate and effective at different times of a person's life. The work in which mental health nurses engage will vary from person to person depending on the age of the patient, their environment or the clinical setting. Further, mental health nursing involves a wide range of interventions which might often appear outside the expectations of a nursing role. For example, one student mental health nurse provided the following account:

> I really enjoyed spending time taking part in outside activities like visiting drop-in centres and taking service users swimming. The swimming was great, because we were all down to basics, no ID badges, no make up or fancy hair dos, just a small group people enjoying the pool, and ... I got the chance to chat to service users and find out what's really been going on in their lives.

In order to know that we are not simply acting randomly but working therapeutically with people, we require a deeper understanding to support our practice. To meet this need, mental health nursing is supported by therapeutic models, theory and principles. Throughout the book we repeatedly focus on *The Ten Essential Shared Capabilities* (DoH 2004). These are useful to consider as they provide a set of principles and values to guide mental health nursing. In the third section of the book we consider various therapeutic and theoretical approaches in more depth.

We begin Section 3 by considering physical assessment skills in mental health settings. This may seem surprising, and you might expect to see this chapter in Section 1, however, they are included at this point for several reasons.

Mental health nurses and students often lack confidence in assessing physical health but these skills are as important as the psychological theories and approaches we discuss later in Section 3. As future nurses and in accordance with the code of professional conduct you are responsible for caring for the *whole person*, which includes their physical as well as mental health (NMC 2008). Each chapter in this section adopts a particular perspective on the person and the physical functioning of the person is one of these perspectives. These perspectives or models all rest on a number of specific assumptions about how people function and adopting a single approach excludes all of the others. Since people are all different and have widely varying problems, in order to be able to address all of these issues effectively we need to have access to, and use, a wide and varied range of knowledge in our practice. Therefore we suggest you read all of these chapters with a view to incorporating these theories, approaches, interventions and principles within your practice in various ways.

Mental health nursing offers a challenging but rewarding career. In order to be effective in practice we need to use our skills as people but also involve principles and theories to provide rationales for our interventions. Training to be a mental health nurse not only involves gaining knowledge of facts and information but also requires us to develop our attitudes, examine our principles and cultivate a sense of self-awareness and reflection so that we are best able to learn from our experiences. This book will help you begin to set these foundations in place and establish a worth-while and rewarding career in mental health nursing.

References

DoH (Department of Health) (2004) *The Ten Essential Shared Capabilities: A Framework for the Whole of the Mental Health Workforce.* London: DoH.

NMC (Nursing and Midwifery Council) (2008) *Standards of Conduct, Performance and Ethics for Nurses and Midwives.* London: NMC.

Section 1
Essential information

Learning on practice placements

Nick Wrycraft

1

Learning objectives

By the end of this chapter you will have:

- Gained an understanding of how adults learn using different styles.
- An insight into the expectations and demands of the placement setting.
- Developed an understanding of a range of learning tools in the practice setting, including learning contracts, practice documents, formative and summative assessment, reflection and reflective journals and the importance of professional portfolios for long-term learning and professional development.
- Developed an insight into the relationship between practice and theory in the process of learning nursing.

Introduction

In this chapter we will discuss how to prepare for, and gain the most benefit from, your practice placements in the mental health setting.

We begin by discussing what adult learning is, and different learning styles, before considering how to prepare for placements in either community or inpatient settings. The chapter will then focus on tools which provide a framework for your learning in practice, and which will generate evidence of your development as a student mental health nurse. These comprise both conceptual approaches and practical methods for documenting and providing evidence of your accumulated learning, and include learning contracts, the practice document, formative and summative assessment, reflection and reflective journals and the professional portfolio. Finally the chapter considers the concepts of practice and theory, and how these can be integrated into your developing understanding of mental health nursing.

In conclusion we will reflect on the issues discussed in the chapter. From these beginnings you can start to develop methods of guiding and planning your learning in the practice setting, consistent with your role as an adult learner.

Scenarios and examples will be presented throughout the chapter to illustrate the clinical and professional complexities involved. Several exercises will help you identify areas of practice which can be developed through further reading and reflection on practice, together with discussions with your practice supervisor, other students and lecturers, to facilitate further lifelong learning.

Before we start, here are two students' insights into practice placements.

A mental health student says ...

Seek out your own learning experiences and prepare yourself for an emotional rollercoaster that will see you burst with pride and cry from despair. The highs and lows of nursing will change you forever.

A mental health student says ...

If I had one bit of advice for a new student, it would be that offering to make the tea says a lot about your enthusiasm and should not be seen as an insignificant job!

Preparing for placement

This section will discuss how to prepare for and gain maximum benefit from your practice placement. However, to begin with, it is helpful to identify how adults learn in order to identify skills and the areas in which we need to develop.

What is learning?

Learning appears straightforward and we all do it all the time, yet in fact it is a complex multifaceted process.

For many of us our most familiar experience of learning is from the classroom at school when we were children. However, in adult learning we process information and learn very differently, and need to be taught using other methods (Knowles 1984).

Differences between child and adult learners

- Children accept information without question whereas adults require the importance of the information and relevance of the learning to be made clear (Knowles 1984).
- Adults approach education with a broad and diverse background of life experience which varies enormously between people. The process of learning as an adult involves evaluating whether the new knowledge is consistent with previous understanding or adds a fresh perspective (Bloom 1964; Nicklin and Kenworthy 2000).
- Adult learners are mentally and emotionally mature whereas children are at various stages of psychological growth and impressionability.
- Adults involve their feelings in their learning and assimilate new information and experience not only on an intellectual level but with regard to their values, beliefs and attitudes (Bloom 1964; Nicklin and Kenworthy 2000).

It has been suggested there are three elements to adult learning: the *cognitive* aspect refers to factual and empirical knowledge; the *affective* component concerns emotions and feelings; and *psychomotor* learning concerns actions or practical tasks (Bloom 1964; Nicklin and Kenworthy 2000). Yet most important of all is the capacity to understand, interpret and apply this information effectively in the practice setting in the care of service users. Nursing is a mix of cognitive, psychomotor and affective learning which involves the use of a wide range of different skills. As learning is a complex process it is not surprising that people learn in markedly different ways and it is helpful to know how we as individuals learn most effectively. Honey and Mumford's (1992) learning styles inventory questionnaire, which is available online, identifies four different learning styles: activists, reflectors, theorists and experimental learners. These are outlined in more detail in the next panel.

Honey and Mumford's (1992) taxonomy of learning styles

- *Activists* are keen to volunteer, meet new people and engage in different experiences. Activist learners prefer *doing*, and will *get on with the job* before receiving all of the instructions. While being adventurous and learning through their experiences they are prone to spontaneity and need to be wary of not finishing what they have started.
- *Reflective learners* watch and observe others complete a task before trying it out for themselves. When making a decision, reflective learners consider all of the consequences and want to know all the information available. However, they can be indecisive and reluctant to try new experiences.
- *Theorists* consider problems logically in sequential stages and seek to understand the broad overview or *bigger picture*. However, they can find individual cases which do not conform to a pattern confusing, and often lack the skills of being able to respond inventively in crisis situations and improvise.

- *Experimental learners* are keen to apply new ideas or learning in practice and are enthusiastic about solving problems, yet become frustrated if the change takes a long time to implement, or there are barriers requiring detailed problem-solving.

People rarely completely embody one learning style. Instead it is advisable to be a balanced or *multimodal* learner, and in order to achieve this you need to work at areas where you have weaknesses in order to achieve a balanced learning style. Developing a repertoire of different skills and capabilities on which to draw will better equip you for the variety of different situations and challenges you will experience in nursing practice.

Over time our individual profile of learning style can change, depending on study habits, the work environment, the influence of other people with whom we come into contact and our personal goals. It is worth repeating the learning styles questionnaire at regular intervals during your course to monitor how you have changed and developed as a learner.

To illustrate how knowing our preferred learning styles can be useful, two scenarios involving mental health nursing students are provided in the next section.

Scenario: Julie

Julie is 37 and has just started the training course. She previously worked as a health care assistant on a general medical ward for a number of years after having two children. She has not studied since leaving school when she was 18.

Julie completed Honey and Mumford's learning styles questionnaire online. She scored highest in the activist and experimental areas. Julie agreed with these findings but is concerned that her learning styles are more focused on being active and less so on reflecting on information and hence she will not gain as much as she might from her placement. Before starting the placement Julie decided to spend 30 minutes each day reflecting after her shift and writing in a journal. She decided to write the journal on her computer, as she learned to type in the sixth form at school, even though she is not confident with technology. Two weeks into the placement Julie became aware that she had written the journal after the first three shifts, but not made an entry since. She was disappointed and considered the reasons why.

The first reason she identified was the need to care for her children. However, she realized this was an excuse and not the real reason, and with some planning she could have adapted the family's routine to incorporate her reflective time. The real reason was that she did not want to carry out the task. When reflecting further she was surprised, as while she is usually very proactive and keen regarding change and new experiences, she was concerned that learning about computers would be complex and difficult and that she would find it boring. She realized she needed to challenge her reluctance to become more computer literate, and asked a member of her student group, Andreas, whom she knew had experience working with computers, to help her in the computer lab at the university. After an hour Julie was competent in creating and formatting Word documents and has since developed a routine of reflecting and writing for half an hour after each shift.

Julie is now finding this absorbing and is seeing a great deal in practice she feels she would have otherwise missed or overlooked. In a recent assignment her reflective comments and analytical skills were identified as good strengths.

Scenario: Andreas

Andreas is 25 and in the same student group as Julie. He has no experience working in health care, having worked as an IT consultant after gaining a degree in computing. He took the same learning styles questionnaire as Julie and scored highest in the reflective and theoretical categories. Andreas was very aware of his lack of previous practice experience and concerned he would find it difficult being a student on placement. At a study day at the university two weeks into the placement he told his tutor group that he was disappointed with his progress in practice.

Andreas's placement is an assessment unit for people over 70 with cognitive impairment and severe memory problems. He explained to his group that he often felt unsure of what to do in the practice setting. Many of the service users on the unit had high levels of need, and while he watched carefully how other members of staff carried out interventions and tried to be involved as much as possible, he was not sure if he was doing it correctly.

In feeding back on his progress Andreas's mentor in practice was very positive, but Andreas was still not confident that he was really doing things correctly. The other students in his group and the tutor were supportive, explaining that at this early stage of the course the student is not expected to be highly experienced, and in contrast it is best to be aware of one's limitations of knowledge and experience in a new environment.

Andreas was reassured by this advice and later, when reflecting, remembered that he is often hard on himself and has very high expectations of his own performance. He was glad to return to the placement and surprised how much he had missed it as he had only been there for two weeks.

In his final report Andreas's practice mentor remarked that he was very popular with the staff and service users because of his willing and helpful attitude and he often correctly anticipated the care needs of service users; yet he was very discreet and always aware of respecting their dignity.

When you have read the two scenarios, consider the points below.

- When reviewing our learning needs there is often too much of a focus on our weaknesses. We are a mixture of skills and capabilities, and strengths and deficits. It is important to view our needs from a balanced perspective and in context.
- Often we work in complex ways. For example, Julie's reluctance to learn computer skills seemed to contradict her activist and experimental character but there was a rational explanation.
- To be able to learn it is important to be truthful with ourselves about our motives and to recognize when we are using defences. Not having time to complete her reflective journal because of her children masked Julie's real reason, which was that she lacked the correct motivation.
- Initiating change is difficult. In the early stages there may be little or no evidence to support continuing with the change and it can be tempting to give up if we are trying new ways of working or different behaviours in which we feel outside our 'comfort zone'. Instead it is advisable to set intermediate staggered goals and to plan change over time. This also means the change is more likely to last.
- It is necessary to be alert to our 'external radar' to detect and interpret feedback from other people for evidence as to whether we are achieving our goals or need to change our actions. Andreas's mentor and student group were supportive which he found to be useful reassurance and helped to build his confidence. The positive feedback to Julie's latest assignment suggests she is meeting her goal of developing skills in reflection.

As the Julie and Andreas scenarios demonstrate, adult learners all enter nursing with a wealth of background experience, skills, abilities and talents which often go unrecognized. The purpose of the next exercise is to encourage you to reflect on how your background has prepared you for the nursing course.

Assessing your learning style

- Write down your previous work or educational history, or read your curriculum vitae (CV). What aspects of your previous experiences, knowledge and interests prepare you for your placement?
- Which of the above learning styles, from Honey and Mumford's learning styles inventory questionnaire, do you feel apply to how you approach work situations?
- What strengths do you identify yourself as possessing?
- What areas and abilities do you anticipate you need to develop?
- What actions can you take to address these issues?
- Write an action plan with specific goals and objectives you need to achieve but which will also develop the skills you already possess. Then list appropriate actions to take and measurable outcomes which will allow you to know you have achieved your goals. What intervals will you place between achieving these steps and why?
- Discuss how you will achieve your learning objectives with your practice mentor. Include a copy of the action plan in your personal portfolio to refer to later in the course.

Practice placements

Generally your nursing training will commence with a block period of induction when you will be orientated to the university, the library and other facilities before being allocated to your first practice placement. Practice placements are specialist clinical areas where you will be based for a period of time in order to gain experience of nursing care (RCN 2002).

While the long-term focus of mental health services is on care in the community, all placement areas, whether in the inpatient or community setting, form part of a cohesive network of services for people with mental health problems (DoH 1999, 2004). By visiting a wide range of mental health services while on placement you will gain a comprehensive understanding from first-hand experience of the workings of mental health services. The independent and private sectors are also increasingly involved with the provision of mental health care and your university is likely to have study agreements with these organizations.

Your placement experience will provide you with a unique and individual insight into how mental health nursing is carried out in a range of settings, and the opportunity to begin to develop your skills and knowledge under appropriate supervision.

What to do before commencing placement

- Contact the placement area by phone or in person in advance of your start date to show courtesy to the placement and create a good impression, and so that you are aware of the working hours or shift patterns and can make any necessary arrangements in advance (RCN 2002). To gain full benefit from the experience it is expected that you will work the hours or shift patterns of the placement area. It is also worth asking about any particular conditions which may be relevant to the placement – for example, parking arrangements and access to the premises (some units have secured doors accessed by a keypad).
- Read the student handbook and the practice assessment document thoroughly (RCN 2002).
- Make yourself aware of the policy regarding confidentiality of service user information. All units will have a copy of the trust's policies and procedures.
- Ask the placement about the dress code. Some areas require the wearing of uniform, while others prefer smart casual wear. If the clinical area specifies smart casual wear, generally this does not include jeans and trainers. Discuss any policy regarding body jewellery and tattoos.
- Before commencing your placement ensure you have the appropriate uniform if required and an identification badge. The induction process at the university generally has timetabled sessions for measurements to be taken and any uniform can be collected before your placement.
- Some placements will involve travelling quite a distance which may be expensive, so plan in advance how you will afford any additional costs due to travel. If you are on the same placement with others, consider sharing lifts if you are working the same hours. If you are travelling on public transport, student travel cards offer worthwhile discounts. Remember you will almost certainly be working shifts, so acquaint yourself in advance with the times and frequency of the service to and from the placement area.
- Theoretical assignments can often be forgotten when on a busy placement for a block of time. Experienced assignment writers suggest allowing a minimum of six weeks to produce a 3000-word assignment at any level of the nursing course, and to allow additional time for background reading. It is therefore advisable to organize your workload well in advance. Ensure that you are aware of any deadlines and hand-in dates and that these are in your diary and noted on your calendar. Allocate regular study time around your placement hours.
- Time management needs to be prioritized and within practice is regarded as a basic expectation of good professional conduct (RCN 2002).

The practice mentor

While at the university you will have personal tutors to guide your development. On placement it is also a mandatory requirement of the NMC for you to have a clinical mentor from the placement area to support you in your progress as a student nurse (NMC 2006).

Mentors are nurses who:

- are on the professional registration in the same discipline of nursing as the students they are mentoring;
- have been on the professional register for at least one year;
- have continued to develop their skills and knowledge during this time;
- have successfully completed a recognized mentor training programme;
- are capable of fulfilling the requirements of the role of student mentor and assessor;
- receive regular updates on the mentor role (NMC 2006).

While practice mentors will assess student competence during the course, in September 2007 'sign off' mentors were created. These are mentors or practice educators who have undergone additional training and are responsible for 'signing off' students as proficient and safe to practice at the end of their training.

The role of the practice mentor is identified in the next panel.

The role of the practice mentor (NMC 2006)

The practice mentor is responsible for:

- organizing and coordinating the activities pertaining to learning in which the student is involved;
- supervising the student when they are engaged in learning activities in the practice setting and providing appropriate and constructive feedback on their performance;
- working with the student to identify realistic goals and monitoring their achievement;
- assessing the student's competence in skills but also their behaviour and attitudes;
- liaising with other staff including practice education facilitators and university lecturers where there is any cause for concern regarding student performance and agreeing appropriate action plans;
- providing 'sign off' mentors with evidence to support decisions made about student competence on completion of the course.

The eight areas outlined below will assist you to gain an understanding of the type of support you can expect from the mentor and the basis of the mentor-student relationship.

The student's relationship with their mentor is crucial for the placement to be successful and there are obligations and expectations for both parties. It is important to know what is expected of you while you are on placement and to take your time to learn, as the student quoted in the next panel explains.

The mentor-student relationship (NMC 2006)

- The mentor will establish an effective, trusting and mutual respectful relationship focused on learning and establishing the placement in the context of the student's overall experience.
- The mentor will facilitate learning through the use of experience and knowledge to develop learning strategies appropriate to the student's stage of learning.
- The mentor will assess the student's performance in accordance with the requirements of professional standards and promote accountability.
- The mentor will evaluate the learning experience and implement change as necessary.
- The mentor will create an environment conducive for learning and identification of learning strategies appropriate to the student which involves the multidisciplinary team, and will act as a resource.
- The mentor will work within the context of practice by establishing and maintaining professional boundaries appropriate to interprofessional care and ensuring safe and effective care through responding to developments in practice.
- The mentor will review and support students to assist them in practising evidence-based care.
- The mentor will demonstrate leadership by acting as a role model, providing appropriate feedback to the student and accessing learning opportunities within the practice setting.

A mental health student reflects on a recent placement ...

Although I am enjoying my acute inpatient placement, I began by trying to get involved in as many activities as possible including assessments, care planning, updating risk assessments, giving injections, brief solution focus therapy sessions and basic nursing care. However, now I have a feeling that I was overdoing it. I was trying to prove to myself and others that a second year student can do it all. Instead I should have been learning at my own pace as others seem to. I have a feeling that time is flying and soon I will be qualified and expected to perform at a certain level. But to do it all we need experience, experience, experience.

While the practice mentor is your main contact at the placement, it is not expected that you will work exclusively with them, but also with other members of the nursing staff of all grades and other health care disciplines, in order to gain confidence, knowledge and competence within a multidisciplinary setting. Whatever stage of training you are at, it is expected you will be appropriately supervised at all times by a registered nurse, even if they are not your supervisor, and that you will be supernumary – that is, working in addition to the employed members of staff on the unit (RCN 2002).

When commencing the placement you will receive an initial orientation on your first day regarding health and safety and evacuation pro-cedures in the event of a fire or emergency, which will be provided by a member of the team with whom you are placed. It is important to meet with your mentor as early as possible after commencing the placement to discuss the aims and goals you will achieve.

In the next section we will discuss the practice documents and learning contracts which form the framework and structure for your placement.

Learning contracts, practice documents, assessment and reflection

While on your practice placement you will be expected to complete pre-set outcomes in a *practice document*. These are mapped onto the standards of the NMC code of professional conduct. There will be increasing expectations of the level of skill, competence and autonomy at each level of progression on the course.

In your initial meeting with your mentor it is important to discuss the practice document and establish learning contracts and action plans to meet your goals for the placement. Due to the variety of different specialist settings within mental health services, and as practice documents are designed to apply to all disciplines of nursing, skills of negotiation and interpretation are required. The student together with the mentor is required to identify appropriate activities which will meet the outcome criteria, and achievement of these is clearly demonstrated within the clinical setting. The box below identifies how the same outcome criteria can be achieved in various settings.

Achieving outcomes: nutrition

In whatever environment nurses work, whether in an inpatient setting or the community, nursing skills ought to be practiced and can be learned by student nurses, although how this is achieved will vary between clinical areas.

An example is the nursing outcome of nutrition. On an inpatient mental health assessment unit where staff monitor service users' dietary intake, provide a special diet, or assist people to eat, the focus will be on a highly interventionist contribution to ensure the need for nutrition is met.

In contrast, in the community there is a greater emphasis on psychosocial interventions, and less on direct physical nursing interventions. Monitoring nutrition is nevertheless an inherent part of the nursing role, regardless of clinical setting, and this outcome can still be comprehensively addressed. Community-based staff will routinely observe how service users manage and provide for their nutritional needs although different issues may be more apparent in relation to these needs than in inpatient settings. For example, how the service user allocates their budget when purchasing food will be an active factor with regard to the pursuit of a healthy diet, whereas in inpatient settings within the NHS food is provided.

The outcome concerning monitoring a service user's nutritional needs and intake will be met in a community setting by considering the following.

- The student correctly identifying questions and making observations pertaining to the service user's patterns of eating and noting any changes.
- Cues such as references to shopping or eating and discreet, non-intrusive observations of the home will provide indications of the person's patterns of eating.
- From a health promotion perspective, action to encourage appropriate nutrition and self-care is important for the person's health. Where deficits are identified, it is important to understand the reasons for the service user not meeting their nutritional needs in order to be able to consider suitable remedies.
- Service users who experience deterioration in mood or mental health may lose the motivation to cook or self-care. Often, people do not eat well through a lack of a sense of self-worth or motivation, or loneliness as eating alone is less enjoyable than eating with others. Encouraging the service user to meet with friends for meals, if appropriate and achievable for them, represents a proactive measure.
- Economic factors may also be active if the service user is in receipt of benefits or on a limited budget; supporting the service user to optimize their budget will assist their overall health. Where the service user consumes excessive food of one type, unhealthy food or food which is harmful to health, promoting healthier choices will again benefit their overall health.
- Physical health problems such as diabetes in some cases impose dietary limitations on the person which can be neglected in some instances, where the person may experience deterioration in their mental health.
- Other services can become involved in nutritional issues, for example, occupational therapists, dieticians, day services and independent agencies.

Applying theory to practice

From your experience in practice consider a physical health need which one service user has displayed with regard to an everyday activity of living. Examples might include sleeping, communication, mobility, oral hygiene or elimination.

- Write down the different ways in which the problem affects the person's functioning in their daily life and the impact this has on their mental health.
- Identify therapeutic interventions which might assist the person with this identified need; not just in achieving the task, but in how they may be facilitated to meet this need.
- How might health care professionals from other disciplines provide useful input into the person's care?

Place your notes in your professional portfolio.

Learning contracts identify agreed activities the student will undertake to develop their understanding, meet the practice outcomes and achieve their own personal learning goals. The learning contract should proceed logically and have clear goals, actions and objectives. The more specifically individual activities are defined within the learning contract, the easier it will be to plan activities to meet them and to evaluate whether they have been achieved. While more than one learning contract can be devised, in order to allow the student to prioritize learning and to prevent excessive paperwork, it is preferable to keep them to a limited number.

Although it is the mentor's responsibility to organize and coordinate the student's learning activities, generally it is expected that students will make contact with individuals and agencies to make the arrangements when it has been agreed that the student will visit them. This is good experience and builds confidence in initiating contact with health care professionals.

A mental health student says ...
The skills I needed did not reflect the placement I was in, so I experienced considerable difficulties in completing the placement book. I now know that in the future I need to network myself out in order to complete skills that can't be achieved in the placement. That was only something I learnt from experience. As I've moved around from placement to placement, I've built up contacts and got to know staff, and they have got to know me, so I now know what clinical areas are willing to help me out if I experience difficulties like that again.

How learning outcomes will be achieved will differ depending on the clinical setting, the specific practice outcomes and the student's own learning needs. While there needs to be signed proof of the student's completion of the outcomes, unless stated in the practice document these can be achieved through discussion with the practice supervisor, although it is expected that students will be familiar with appropriate theory and policies to support their answers.

Formative and summative assessment

A fundamental part of how learning is structured while on placement is the concept of *formative* and *summative assessment*. In formative assessment the student and practice mentor meet and agree learning needs, the objectives and goals of the learning contract and the means by which these will be achieved using the practice document as a guide for the priorities (Brookhart 2001). It is possible that more than one formative assessment meeting will be necessary, and it is advisable to meet frequently with your practice mentor during the placement to review and discuss progress and ascertain whether the learning contract is still suitable and achievable. If not, then it is necessary to develop an action plan through which the practice outcomes will still be met. Summative assessment occurs at the end of the placement and involves the evaluation and review of evidence collected over time while you have been on the placement and your performance as a student mental health nurse at the relevant stage of pre-registration training (Brookhart 2001; Ecclestone 2001).

The learning outcomes are intended to provide a structure and framework across the duration of the placement and learning is intended to be incremental and gradual. Therefore, formative and summative assessments are linked and are essential to the learning process.

Where the student is not meeting the expected outcomes of the learning contract, it is necessary to identify and discuss how to improve progress and agree an action plan clearly identifying the specific measures and date(s) for review. At this stage involving the link lecturer from the university is advisable in order to support the student and mentor and to develop an action plan. All clinical areas will have a named member of the university teaching staff who works with that clinical area to support the staff and students.

Use of reflection

While on placement students are expected to develop practical skills and knowledge. The practice documentation provides evidence of meeting the required outcomes, however, crucial to the placement experience is the personal learning gained by the student.

If we never think about our work, how will we ever improve what we do, identify what we have done well, what we need to learn, why things have happened in the way they have, the risks and near misses and how to avoid them happening again? *Reflection* is the method by which experience is transformed into knowledge, and it is essential to cultivate skills in this area of learning. John Dewey is credited with first identifying the value of reflection in education, regarding it as a process of focusing carefully, thoughtfully and in detail on beliefs or knowledge and the ideas and logic on which these are based, and considering the consequences and implications which might arise (Dewey 1933).

Reflective journals

We quickly forget the fine details of events, and it is not possible to reflect on what cannot be remembered or clearly recounted (Minton 1997). To begin to reflect it is necessary to find events on which to focus, and to keep a record of your experiences in practice, in which entries are made regularly and close to the time when the events are still fresh in your mind.

Tools for reflective practice

- Keep a diary, notebook or computer log using whichever format you find most convenient and make entries at a regular and frequent intervals. A reflective diary is a private record of your experiences as a student, and a method of allowing for the reporting of thoughts, feelings and views, rather than just facts or details (Allin and Turnock 2007).
- Caution should be taken to anonymize the names and details of service users, staff or facilities you mention, because, if you misplace your journal or it is seen by anyone else, any identifying factors might constitute a breach of confidentiality (NMC 2008).
- While in a community-based setting, keep a weekly diary of your appointments and activities to help you appreciate the range of different activities in which you have been involved.
- Nursing in mental health involves working with a range of different disciplines. Make appointments to spend time with as many other health care professionals as you can, to learn about their input at first hand. Make notes of your impressions of the contrasting perspectives of these other health care professionals.
- With permission, collect copies of any written information or advice leaflets that are available, including information for service users. Pay attention to the format, content, design and layout of leaflets in relation to their intended purpose and target audience.
- Again with permission, collect copies of any admission packs, forms and assessment tools. It may be necessary to seek copyright permission or to remove headings or logos identifying the trust from the paperwork. Some clinical areas have particularly innovative or specialist assessment tools that are well worth investigating.

- You will rapidly accumulate a large amount of information which it will be necessary to organize. Use a simple system which you understand – for example, saving computer files by date order, or theme of the specialist area (e.g. Assertive outreach placement). This will allow you to access information quickly while maintaining confidentiality.

While there are no rules on keeping a reflective journal, if the document is to be a useful learning tool it is important that you find it enjoyable to produce, and that it is an *honest* account of how you feel about your practice (Allin and Turnock 2007). Reflective journals have numerous uses – for example, providing an account of significant events in your practice experience, as a method of evaluating the placement, and as a way of facilitating your critical thinking and personal and professional development.

Pieces of work from your reflective log can also be used in the professional portfolio to illustrate points of learning and achievements. To allow for personal *reflection* to occur, and for the journal to be more than simply a diary of observations on practice, it is necessary for the entries to be re-read, and consciously subjected to examination to arrive at a deeper understanding (Dewey 1933). As reflection relates to a situation or event about which we are preoccupied or perplexed, the best place to start is the first thing which comes to mind when thinking about the placement experience, or the period of duty which has just been completed. It may be difficult to understand why the incident is of interest, however, reflection often provides useful explanations as to why we are perplexed, preoccupied, confused, upset or angry and scratches away the surfaces of our emotions to access logical explanations, learning points and – most usefully – positive actions we can take to deal better with the same situation if we were to encounter it again.

A mental health student says ...

My best advice for new students is: be prepared to question everyone and everything. Never be afraid to question what you do not understand and always be prepared to question yourself.

Models of reflection

Often reflection involves personal feelings which may be decisive factors guiding the choice of the subject to begin with – for example, critical incidents, decisions we do not understand or agree with, differences of opinion or negative outcomes to care, all of which are highly emotive issues. However, these instances create memorable opportunities for learning which can leave a deep impression on the learner. It is necessary when our opinions, values, beliefs and attitudes are involved in a learning experience to apply a framework in order to manage and organize our feelings.

The model developed by Boud *et al.* (1985) is just one of a number of alternatives. Structured frameworks for reflection support the learning process, but it should not just be a theoretical activity: reflection should be incorporated into practice as a routine way of thinking and the outcomes should produce positive changes and improvements to practice. The process of reflection improves how we understand situations in clinical practice and enhances our self-awareness about the way feelings, views, beliefs and attitudes influence our practice by subjecting real-life situations to scrutiny. To really develop knowledge we are sometimes required to challenge and question the views and values we impose on events and therefore honesty and a willingness to accept other perspectives are essential.

Professional portfolios

The professional portfolio is a collection of evidence supporting personal and professional development and learning. It is not possible to state definitively what ought to be included in a portfolio other than it should summarize learning to date. As a guide on some information which ought to be included, the portfolio should be more than simply a collection of certificates and achievements but reflect the personal meaning and value of the learning to the individual and what it has contributed to their growth and understanding.

Items which might be included in the portfolio are:

- reflections on practice experience and learning;
- examples of positive practice;
- events which demonstrate the process of learning in contributing to the student's development and improved understanding with clear outcomes;
- completed assignments;
- case studies.

The portfolio should be regarded as a body of evidence summarizing your whole experience, however, entries should be selected carefully on the basis that they meaningfully contribute to your development rather than amassing an imposing catalogue of evidence. It is possible when seeking employment in the future that your portfolio will be read by your potential employer, therefore ensuring it is well organized and easy to read is important.

Some questions to consider when compiling your portfolio are:

- What have been your main achievements and learning points in practice?
- How are these demonstrated clearly in the evidence you are using?
- What are your strengths as a student nurse and how have these been demonstrated in the practice setting?

Maintaining a professional portfolio continuously will not only ensure success on the course but success in future practice, as it is an expectation of qualified nurses that they maintain a professional portfolio and engage in lifelong learning as a condition of continued registration (NMC 2008).

Integrating theory and practice

The elements of practice and theory in nursing education are the subject of differing opinion as to which ought to be more influential in preparing students to become capable practitioners. Theory can be regarded as proposed explanations for events and change with the development of knowledge (Pearson *et al.* 1996). Practice in mental health nursing is the carrying out of nursing activity in a clinical setting with people who have mental health problems.

What is theory?

- The principles of the nursing profession's ethics and values (NMC 2008).
- The findings of research and research evidence.
- The statements of policy and strategic documents.
- The views of experts, service users and independent organizations and service user groups.
- Statistics and data – for example, pertaining to prevalence of health conditions, and the results of service audits and evaluations.
- Concepts, theories and models (ideas and frameworks which can be applied to numerous specific practice-based situations).
- The rationales, knowledge and principles for carrying out interventions and procedures.

What is practice?

- The effective implementation in clinical practice of the principles, values and ethics of the nursing profession appropriate personal conduct (NMC 2008).
- Demonstrating in practice the principles and values of high quality care for patients – for example, appropriate and effective use of interpersonal communication and provision of personal nursing care, or facilitating the service user to attend to their needs; and the competent performance of clinical procedures and techniques.
- Working effectively within a health care team as a communicator, making contributions appropriate to your own position within the team to the provision of care, and working effectively within the multidisciplinary team.
- Working in accordance with principles of good practice in patient confidentiality and handling information with due discretion.
- Working to involve carers, partners and significant others in the care of patients.

While there is often perceived to be a theory-practice gap, this has been criticized as a false division (McKenna 1997). Theory and practice are not specific, separate and distinct, but loose collections of widely different sources of information, knowledge and skills. The notion of there being a theory-practice gap is also unhelpful, as students often identify with being better at either theory or practice and neglect the area in which they are less confident to the detriment of their professional development.

Theory and practice are better viewed as inextricably *linked*, and the effective use of practice-based skills involves theory and vice versa, as the scenario below demonstrates.

Scenario: Nelson

Nelson is a 33-year-old man who currently lives in a mental health unit in the community. The unit is staffed 24 hours a day by mental health nurses. Elizabeth is a third year mental health nursing student placed with the team and is two months into a three-month placement.

Nelson has a long history of severe mental health problems and has spent several years as an inpatient on various mental health units. He wishes to eventually live independently in the community and is currently staying in a self-contained flat in the unit which is specifically for service users preparing to return to independent living. The eight residents in the unit often cook meals together helped by the staff and pool their money to buy food. However, Nelson does not join in as he enjoys having his own money and spending it how he wishes, so he eats takeaways or ready meals.

Nelson can be stubborn in his opinions and defensive if challenged. He has previously been physically aggressive towards staff. Elizabeth, together with her mentor, looked up information in books, journals, online and from the local primary care trust and acquired leaflets on healthy eating and the advantages of home-cooked food, and discussed them with Nelson. She also went shopping with him and encouraged him to read the packaging on the ready meals and become aware of the nutritional content of the food he purchased.

From calculating his weekly income, Nelson and Elizabeth estimated he would save money by sharing the cooking with the other residents while also eating more healthily and developing skills for independent living. As a result Nelson joined the other residents in the cooking cooperative, with the result that he had more money to spend on other things while eating more healthily at the same time.

- In identifying evidence-based information Elizabeth was using theory on healthy eating to support her practice-based interventions.
- However, she also used practice-based skills in interacting with Nelson. It was necessary for her to communicate with him in terms which did not challenge him but supported him in making informed choices.
- Nelson's eventual choice was based not only on the benefit to his health through eating well but on the financial gain involved. Often the rationales on which people make choices depend on their personal outlook. As a health care professional it is the role of the nurse to make service users aware of the choices and alternatives available and to facilitate choice.

Integrating theory and practice is probably the most significant challenge of the nursing course, and often takes time and thoughtful reflection to achieve. The brief exercise below is intended to encourage you to begin to identify where theory is evident within your own practice.

Theory and practice

To be effective, evidence-based interventions must be appropriate to the need(s) of the service user. Reflecting on your own practice experiences, identify three interventions which you have seen or with which you were involved.

- What is the evidence supporting each intervention?
- Were they successful?
- When you have finished, place your notes in your professional portfolio.

Conclusion

We began the chapter by considering how adults learn and preparations which can be made for practice placements, before considering the role of the practice mentor in facilitating your learning in the clinical setting. The discussion then focused on tools for learning in the practice setting. We considered learning contracts, practice documents and the concepts of formative and summative assessment. In the practice setting it is necessary for the student and mentor to actively engage in negotiating and agreeing the means by which the practice outcomes and learning contract will be achieved, and how learning will occur across the full duration of the placement, rather than assessment occurring at the end of the student's allocated time in the clinical area.

We then discussed reflection, which serves as a useful tool in translating experience into knowledge. Maintaining a reflective log of practice experience is the first step in beginning to examine practice and provides material which will build your portfolio and provide a personal account of your professional achievement and development during the course. The reflective log will vary in form and content depending on personal preference.

Finally, the chapter considered how the practice-theory gap, when seen from a practice perspective, is illusory. In reality, practice placements provide an opportunity to implement and appreciate theory *and* practice at work.

References

Allin, L., and Turnock, C. (2007) Reflection on and in the workplace for work based supervisors, www.practicebasedlearning.org/resources/materials/docs/Reflection, accessed 19 December 2007.

Bloom, B.S. (1964) *Taxonomy of Educational Objectives: The Classification of Educational Goals*. London: Longman.

Boud, D., Keogh, R. and Walker, D. (1985) *Reflection: Turning Learning into Experience*. London: Kogan Page.

Brookhart, S.M. (2001) Successful students' formative and summative uses of assessment information, *Assessment in Education*, 8(2): 153–69.

Dewey, J. (1933) *How We Think*. New York: D.C. Heath.

DoH (Department of Health) (1999) *National Service Framework for Mental Health: Modern Standards and Service Models*. London: DoH.

DoH (Department of Health) (2004) *National Service*

Framework for Mental Health – Five Years On. London: DoH.

DoH (Department of Health) (2007) *Uniforms and Workwear: An Evidence Base for Developing Local Policy.* London: DoH.

Ecclestone, K. (2001) *How to Assess the Vocational Curriculum.* London: Kogan Page.

Honey, P. and Mumford, A. (1992) *Manual of Learning Styles,* revised edn. London: Peter Honey.

Knowles, M. (1984) *Andragogy in Action.* San Francisco: Jossey-Bass.

McKenna, H. (1997) *Nursing Theories and Models.* London: Routledge.

Minton, D. (1997) *Teaching Skills in Further Education and Adult Education.* Basingstoke: Macmillan.

Nicklin, P.J. and Kenworthy, N. (2000) *Teaching and Assessing in Nursing Practice,* 3rd edn. London: Baillière Tindall.

NMC (Nuring and Midwifery Council) (2006) *Standards to Support Learning and Assessment in Practice: NMC Standards for Mentors, Practice Teachers and Teachers.* London: NMC.

NMC (Nursing and Midwifery Council) (2008) *Standards of Conduct, Performance and Ethics for Nurses and Midwives.* London: NMC.

RCN (Royal College of Nursing) (2002) *Helping Students Get the Best from their Practice Placements: A Royal College of Nursing Toolkit.* London: RCN.

2

Background to mental health nurse training

Nick Wrycraft

Learning objectives

By the end of this chapter you will be able to:

- Identify the background to the current form of mental health nurse training.
- Understand how mental health nursing models inform approaches to therapeutic interactions and the planning of care in a practice setting.
- Identify the effects of the Ten Essential Shared Capabilities (DoH 2004) in shaping the perceptions of student nurses in terms of their role and practice.

Introduction

Mental health is a discipline of nursing with a distinct character which makes a specific contribution to the care of people with mental health problems. The aim of this chapter is to demonstrate how separate elements combine to shape the identity of mental health nursing. It considers the development of the discipline, nursing models in mental health, and how these values and principles are active in practice from the earliest stages of pre-registration training.

We will begin by considering how mental health nursing developed, leading to the current form of pre-registration training. It is helpful to regard nursing as working on a process of assessing need(s) and then planning care which is subsequently implemented and evaluated, allowing the cycle to then be repeated. Linking nursing to concepts and models helps us to plan and prioritize our practice and set goals and objectives together with the person experiencing the mental health problem. Therefore, we next focus on two prominent models for practice in mental health nursing. These are Hildegard Peplau's interpersonal model (1988) and Phil Barker's tidal model (Barker and Buchannan-Barker 2005).

The other crucial element of mental health nursing this chapter will consider is values-based practice. It is essential for mental health nurses to not only possess a sense and awareness of values but to implement them in practice. *The Ten Essential Shared Capabilities* (DoH 2004) were introduced with the intention of developing a mental health workforce which actively focuses on empowering people with mental health problems and advocating on their behalf. While it is necessary for mental health nurses to invest thought and actively reflect and develop values throughout their professional lives, this begins with pre-registration training, and the chapter will discuss examples of student experiences from an initiative to introduce *The Ten Essential Shared Capabilities* within a pre-registration mental health nursing training programme. The chapter concludes with a summary and reflects on the issues which have been addressed.

Several exercises and scenarios are included throughout the chapter. These will be useful for identifying areas which can be developed through further reading and reflection on practice experience, and provide action points which can be addressed on practice placements to facilitate further lifelong learning.

Before we start, here's a quote from a mental health student explaining one of the reasons they decided to become a mental health nurse.

A mental health student says …

I decided at school at 16 that I never wanted to go to university as I prefer the workplace and I was adamant that I wanted to go straight to work. I stayed on at sixth form until I was 18 to do my A levels but never enjoyed it. I had always wanted to do nursing but knew you had to go to university to train. However, when I found out that most of your time was spent on placement I was really pleased as this meant my learning experience would be in the working environment.

I feel that I learn better in practice by doing things and actually being there rather than being taught in a classroom or a lecture hall. I saw this as a big advantage as whatever we learnt at university we would eventually practice on placement throughout the three years.

The background to modern mental health nursing

For hundreds of years, until the late twentieth century, mental health care in the UK was provided in large inpatient institutions which were often isolated communities and remote from the rest of society. The early equivalent of modern mental health nurses were referred to as 'keepers' and their main role was to clean the institution, occupy the inmates and contain those who were acutely unwell or aggressive without any recognizable options for treatment (Jones 1993; Nolan 1993).

After the 1845 Asylums Act, keepers were referred to as 'attendants'. Poor working conditions, low wages, long hours and often living as well as working in the institution meant that being an attendant was not a popular choice of job, having low status and no prospects. Due to the large staffing requirements within institutions and the difficult working conditions, attracting staff was a challenge. Throughout the institutional era and and well into the 1970s there were frequent scandals and reports of abuse of inmates by attendants and, later, nursing staff. These failings were commonly attributed to a lack of adequate training and preparation of mental health nursing staff and the employment of unsuitable individuals (Nolan 1993).

The institutionalized period of mental health nursing is often portrayed as unremittingly bleak. However, standards of care across the nation were variable, with good and bad practice and it is even possible to trace comparisons with modern health care values and practice in some cases. Examples include employing people with mental health problems within the service – in many institutions former inmates who had recovered were employed and adopted a humane approach to the care of the inmates. Married couples were often jointly employed and introduced an extended family approach to working with inmates. In the eighteenth century William Battie recognized the need for staff to be carefully selected and trained and that a pleasant environment beneficially influenced mental health. At the same time the work of Joseph Tuke at the York Retreat offered an approach which treated people with mental health problems with respect and dignity and their mental health improved accordingly (Jones 1993; Nolan 1993).

Yet, frustratingly for the attendants, the development of their role was severely limited as they were employed to assist in the delivery of a medically-led approach which dominated the running of the institution but which did not yield results. Instead the actual day-to-day work of attendants was more consistent with social welfare provision as many inmates remained living indefinitely in the institutions, uncured and unwell, but removed from a society where they would be vulnerable.

The development of modern mental health nurse training

From 1845, when mental health staff first became known as 'nurses', with the term applied to female attendants until the introduction of the NHS in 1947, adult or general nursing resisted the inclusion of mental health nurses on the professional nursing register. The eventual inclusion of mental health staff was largely due to organizational restructuring with mental health services transferred from the control of local authorities to being included within the newly created NHS.

Recent developments in nurse training

As we have seen, mental health nursing emerged out of an essentially practice-based role. Traditionally, training occurred in the practice setting, and until the 1980s was based on the *apprenticeship* model where students spent most of their training in the clinical setting. This model focused on gaining practical skills and technical competence as opposed to theoretical knowledge, and, although often fondly remembered for teaching nursing in an authentic work setting, a review of nurse education in the 1980s advocated the adoption of a radical new approach (UKCC 1986).

Project 2000

Project 2000 was introduced in the 1980s to increase recruitment and professionalism in nursing and adopted a North American model pioneered by Patricia Benner (1984), which involved a much more academic approach and an emphasis on theoretical learning (UKCC 1986). While students still had placements in practice, in contrast with the apprenticeship model, they were not included as members of staff but were supernumerary, and a significant amount of time on the programme was devoted to theoretical study in the classroom.

With the enhanced academic focus of Project 2000, nurse training was transferred from local schools of nursing into universities and other higher education institutions (HEIs). Yet while Project 2000 produced skilled communicators with an awareness of research and the ability to adapt to change, feedback suggested there was a deficit of clinical skills and practical competence, and there were doubts over the competence and suitability of students for qualified practice on completion of the course. The transition of theoretical teaching into universities, with students spending more time involved in academic study, led to the accusation that there was insufficient exposure to the experience of people with mental health problems and the impact of mental illness on the

individual (Coombes, 1997; UKCC 1999; Fulbrook *et al.* 2000; Clarke and Flanagan 2003; Hughes 2004).

Problem-based learning

Reviews of Project 2000 called for an increased focus of nursing training on the acquisition of practice-based skills and knowledge (UKCC 1999). A new philosophy was adopted, known as problem-based learning (PBL) or inquiry-based learning (IBL) which has endured to the present day and seeks to bridge the gaps highlighted as a result of Project 2000. While still not returning students to the rostered workforce, the new model involves students learning proficiencies and technical competencies in 'skills laboratories' at university. Practice-based scenarios are included as part of theoretical study in order to integrate theory and practice on a 50:50 basis (Barrow *et al.* 2002; Rossin and Hyland 2003; Turner *et al.* 2003).

> ### A mental health student says...
>
> My advice to anyone starting the course would be: keep a diary, never turn up late, copy everything three times, and always have a plan 'A' and plan 'B', and if need be a plan 'C', because the course is open to change as anything would be over a three-year span.

The Nursing and Midwifery Council (NMC)

To be eligible to be registered as a nurse, all students are obliged to be successful on a course of professional training at an approved HEI, and to have completed a specific number of hours of theory and practice over the period of training. The regulation of nursing, midwives and specialist community public health nurses as a profession is carried out by the Nursing and Midwifery Council (NMC), whose main role is to protect the public through maintaining standards of practice (NMC 2006). Pre-registration nursing courses are mapped onto the competencies of the NMC, as summarized in the *Standards of Conduct, Performance and Ethics for Nurses and Midwives* (NMC 2008). Entry onto the appropriate section of the professional register obliges nurses to act in accordance with these standards of accountability, responsibility and competence in their professional practice (NMC 2008).

Mental health nursing models

In this section we will discuss various *nursing models* in order to provide a framework for how we can work in a nursing capacity with people suffering from mental health problems. Models of nursing were very popular in the late 1980s with the rise of nurse education in an academic setting and many originated in North America and were disseminated in the UK. However, the demise of Project 2000 and increased emphasis on practice-focused learning have reduced their prominence.

Models are attempts to simplify complex information by arranging it within a clear structure and making generalized statements about individual situations where there have been many instances of the same occurrence. They represent collections of theories, beliefs and knowledge which form an overall picture of nursing (Pearson *et al.* 1996; McKenna 1997). Models of nursing identify the interventions in which nurses engage, define the activity of nursing and provide underpinning beliefs about how the world works. It could be argued that as people are all different, in order to appreciate their unique individuality we should refrain from using models as they lead us to make generalized assumptions, and a central component of all our actions in mental health nursing is to focus on the individual person and their specific problem. However, the purpose of using models in pre-registration training is to learn about nursing itself and acquire guidance and structure to our developing practice. Patricia Benner (1984) reinforces this point by identifying the fact that nurses add to their knowledge base continually. While we may encounter frequent occurrences of the same problem, we will always encounter new and unique situations which the expert nurse will incorporate within their learning and personal model of nursing.

There are numerous nursing models, and one of the most prominent within UK adult nursing is Roper *et al.*'s activities of daily living model (2000). Others include Johnson's behavioural model,

Orem's model of self-care, Roy's adaptation model, Leininger's transcultural model, Neuman's systems model, King's conceptual system and theory model, Roger's model of the science of unitary beings, Newman's theory of health and Watson's model of caring (Fitzpatrick and Whall 2005).

When using any nursing model, while it is necessary to know the theory of the model, it is also important for it to be applied in clinical settings and so it is necesssary to apply your understanding of the models in your practice placement to develop your knowledge. Models of nursing are also best seen as being much more than step-by-step guides for assessing and planning care. Instead they are useful in informing our approach to nursing and forming therapeutic relationships in the many varied circumstances encountered in the practice setting.

The interpersonal model

The interpersonal model is concerned with the growth of the service user (Peplau 1988). The model is based on the idea that people have needs which can be physical – for example, food and somewhere to live – and psychological and emotional, such as feeling valued by others and engaging in rewarding social relationships (Peplau 1988; Pearson *et al.* 1996). In order for a person to experience a rewarding and enjoyable life, it is necessary that they achieve satisfaction in all these areas.

The interpersonal model assumes our environment is unstable and we are continually confronted with a variety of problems and challenges (Pearson *et al.* 1996). Peplau suggests that when a person's needs are unmet they experience stress and will either overcome this and move on in their life untroubled, or experience a problem (Pearson *et al.* 1996). The model regards the purpose of nursing as, firstly, to ensure the survival of the service user and to act as an agent of change through using interpersonal skills to achieve a therapeutic goal (Peplau 1988). Secondly, the nurse should assist the service user to understand their mental health problem(s) and work through their experiences in a creative and innovative way. In this sense mental illness is an experience within life and something from which the person can learn just as we can learn from any other event.

The model also states that the mental health nurse must be self-aware concerning their personal needs, beliefs and views in order to be able to ascertain the effect they have on service users. This is because the purpose of nursing is not to satisfy the emotional and psychological needs of the *nurse*, but to promote positive change within the life of the service user by working with their problem(s) (Pearson *et al.* 1996).

The interpersonal model consists of: orientation; identification; exploitation; and evaluation. In the practice setting these same stages are often referred to using different terms, such as assessment, planning, implementation and evaluation.

Orientation

Peplau suggests service users seek help either because they experience a 'felt need' or have expectations that health services can help in a particular way (Pearson *et al.* 1996). Information is collected and the service user and nurse together identify the nature of the problem. It is important to remember that this stage of the model is much more than 'history-taking' and represents the beginning of the nurse working therapeutically with the service user. Orientation can be very brief or prolonged depending on the need(s) of the service user (Pearson *et al.* 1996).

Identification

In identification, the relationship between the service user and nurse develops to form an agreement on the appropriate interventions to meet the service user's need(s). The nurse is identified as responsible for the care plan and the goals perceived by the nurse and service user might vary, as often there is a difference between what we want and what we need. Hence it is necessary to achieve a compromise where the service user and nurse agree on the prioritized need(s) (Pearson *et al.* 1996).

Exploitation

At this stage there is an agreement over the care plan and the interpersonal relationship functions towards achieving the mutually agreed goals of

care. However, the nurse's function can be variable, ranging from counsellor, resource or teacher to technical expert and leader (Pearson *et al.* 1996).

Evaluation

The interpersonal relationship is ended once the agreed goals have been achieved. The nurse evaluates the process to ascertain what can be learned and the new knowledge which has been gained, while the service user is no longer in need of the service.

The interpersonal model is characterized by a focus on the service user's problem(s) and the stages can be flexible in duration. In applying the model another interpretation has been used which has the acronym SOAP.

SOAP

S is the service user's subjective experience, often described in his or her own terms, or using direct quotes.

O is the objective perceptions of the nurse on how the problem affects the service user.

A is the assessment of the nurse combining the subjective (S) and objective (O) data in viewing the problem.

P is the plan resulting from the identification of the problem(s) and the combination of the subjective (S) view of the service user, the objective perception of the nurse (O) and the assessment (A).

While Peplau's model provides a useful account of how the nurse assesses the service user's need(s) through incorporating the service user's viewpoint with their own objective perception, and then assessing the collected information, the stages of implementing the care plan and evaluating its effects are absent. In some cases – for example, where the service user has ongoing contact with the health service – the reassessment of their need(s) requires consideration. In further versions of the model several other stages have been added to reflect these additional aspects of nursing, and here the acronym is SOAPIER.

SOAPIER

I is the implementation of the care plan.

E is the evaluation of the plan.

R is the reassessment of how far the problems have been resolved.

The first four stages of the SOAP acronym are demonstrated in use in the practice example below.

Scenario: Milton

Milton is 22 years old and when he was growing up his family often moved to different locations in the UK and other countries. Milton went to a number of different schools and was often teased about his accent. As a result he became very self-conscious when speaking in front of other people. He made few friends and did not do well at school, feeling this was the worst experience of his life.

Milton is studying at college and in spite of being a good student has lacked confidence and doubts whether he should continue on his course. He lives alone in a rented flat and has few friends. Over the last year he has become increasingly low in mood and begun to avoid other people. Recently he developed a chest infection and remained at home for several weeks, not answering his phone or having any contact with other people. However, as he has a good relationship with his doctor and the surgery is near to where he lives, he attended the surgery several times. After recovering Milton remained off sick from college, feeling anxious and apprehensive about returning.

On seeing him at the surgery Milton's GP became concerned at his mental state and referred him to the adult community mental health team (CMHT) with which you are placed as a student. An appointment was booked with his community psychiatric nurse (CPN) (who is your mentor) for an assessment. You attend the orientation meeting with Milton and your mentor.

Orientation

The CPN asked Milton to describe the problem which led him to attend the appointment. Milton's subjective perception of the problem was that he feels 'feels awkward around other people ... like they are staring at me and thinking the way I talk is funny'. Milton explained he felt vulnerable going out, that people were making judgements about the way he looked and spoke, and felt he should not be at college. Milton seemed very low in mood, and avoided eye contact. When asked if he had thought about ending his life, Milton replied he wished he were dead but had no active plans to carry out this wish.

When discussing his past Milton stated he had always felt criticized by others when he was at school and as though he were not good enough even though he had achieved good qualifications.

The CPN asked what help Milton wanted and he replied that he wanted to be able to feel more confident and not so self-conscious and ashamed about himself. The CPN suggested their objective perception of the problem was that being teased at school led Milton to feel low self-esteem and to experience feelings of low mood. Milton agreed to meet with the CPN and you again to discuss a care plan.

Identification

At the next meeting the plan of care was discussed. The CPN asked Milton what his goals were. Milton wanted to be able to function in a social situation without experiencing feelings of low self-esteem and fear; to get a good job and have a wider social circle and maybe even a girlfriend. The CPN suggested a realistic goal for the therapeutic relationship would be to take smaller steps first, and for Milton to work on managing to feel comfortable in situations with other people, and then for his other goals to be addressed.

Exploitation

It was agreed Milton would attend meetings each week with the CPN and you for the next six weeks.

At the sessions a number of strategies were used. Initially the CPN worked with Milton to identify the process by which he felt low self-esteem in social situations, and how these feelings escalated his anxiety and influenced the thoughts he experienced. Role play was also involved, and Milton was required to explore the perspective of other people with whom he came into contact.

In later sessions Milton was encouraged to look at strategies for diverting his feelings and negative thoughts in challenging situations and then at alternative methods of addressing these issues.

It was agreed that Milton would practise exercises outside the sessions and feed back on his progress. As he has few social contacts Milton carried out these exercises when he was at college, and found them useful in making him feel more comfortable in that environment.

Evaluation

At the end of the six weeks Milton had made great progress and invested considerable effort on the work between sessions. Milton felt comfortable among other students at college and did not think people were laughing at him. He described feeling generally better, less anxious and more confident in day-to day-life. While he was content to no longer attend weekly sessions a further appointment four weeks later was planned.

At that appointment Milton was continuing to make positive progress and had made friends with other students on his course.

The tidal model

Probably the most prominent model in modern mental health nursing is Phil Barker's tidal model which functions on the premise that people are defined by their experience. The tidal model was developed within a practice-based setting and has enjoyed enduring success and popularity (Barker and Buchannan-Barker 2008). The model connects human experience with the metaphor of water and tides, both of which are changeable and fluid. While our experiences appear to have boundaries which impose finite limits on us, as we progress towards the 'horizon', our own perception of our limitations and boundaries shifts. The comparison with the horizon invokes on the one hand the unlimited nature of personal experience, yet simultaneously the notion of our self-imposed illusory boundaries (Barker and Buchannan-Barker 2005).

The tidal model proceeds from four core assumptions, shown on the next page.

Assumptions of the tidal model (Barker and Buchannan-Barker 2005)

1 Mental health nursing relates to the person's future development, as opposed to the origins of distress, and interpersonally involves the nurse and service user. Barker and Buchannan-Barker emphasize the purpose of nursing as focusing on working with the person's immediate needs in the present, as opposed to seeking to identify the origins of the problem. However, this does not dismiss the importance of the person's past and in fact it is acknowledged that this has a significant influence; however, the model prioritizes the person before us in their present condition.

2 Only the person undergoing mental distress accurately experiences the problem. Mental illness is often assessed through the person's observable behaviour and the assumptions of health care professionals about what it means, yet this does not necessarily yield a true picture of the nature and extent of what the person is experiencing.

3 The correct function of nursing is for the practitioner to help the person rediscover their life through reconciling their past and present and realizing future opportunities through working collaboratively in an interpersonal relationship.

4 Mental illness is experienced as a disturbance of living and the activity and focus of the mental health nurse, probably uniquely among other branches of nursing, are on the person's relationship with what is defined as mental health and illness.

There are six principles of implementation of the model, outlined below.

Furthermore, Barker and Buchannan-Barker (2005) suggest that there are four questions which need to be asked when using the tidal model, as shown below.

Implementation of the tidal model (Barker and Buchannan-Barker 2005)

1 Curiosity: the mental health nurse aims to find out about what the person, thinks, feels and knows about themselves.

2 Resourcefulness: the mental health nurse aims to identify the person's positive coping mechanisms.

3 Empowering the person: by working on the need the person prioritizes at that time and working with them in collaboration.

4 Viewing the crisis as an opportunity: to allow the person to radically redirect their life, goals and priorities.

5 Setting small-scale, achievable goals.

6 Identifying the simplest actions to generate change for the person.

Questions when applying the tidal model

1 Why is the problem important to the person at this point in time?

2 What interventions or solutions have worked in the past for the person, or might work now?

3 How does the person explain or understand the problem?

4 What is the least restrictive intervention which can be offered? Interestingly Barker and Buchannan-Barker suggest this is likely to be the option involving the *least* intervention from nurses and the *most* action or exercise of choice on the part of the service user.

Due to its focusing on the present rather than the past, the tidal model is suited to working with people in crisis. Below is a practice-based example illustrating the application of the model.

Scenario: Aaliyah

Aaliyah is 19 years old and her family moved to the UK when she was very young. She described feeling as though she existed between two cultures but did not belong to either. When she was 14 Aaliyah ran away from home and has not had any contact with her family since.

After leaving home Aaliyah describes becoming involved with illicit drugs which she began to use in large quantities. She has had several relationships with boyfriends who treated her badly. Aaliyah has been self-harming on a regular basis. Recently, after a violent argument with her current boyfriend, she set fire to their flat and injured herself repeatedly with a sharp blade. The emergency services found her in a distressed and confused state. She was taken to a mental health unit and agreed to be admitted informally.

You are a student on placement at the unit and your supervisor is Aaliyah's keyworker. During the early stages of her admission Aaliyah's mood was very low. While her recollection of recent events was vague she recounted escalating drug use and self-harm, as well as feeling increasingly desperate and unhappy, culminating in the argument with her boyfriend and the fire. She felt that her life until now had involved so many negative events that she could not envisage an improvement and was scared and reluctant to think about the future. While she described feeling ambivalent about her life, she had no conscious plans for suicide but said she did not care if she lived or died. During the early stages of her admission Aaliyah was placed on one-to-one close observations.

Aaliyah remained on the unit for several weeks, during which you regularly worked with her. The tidal model focuses on the person's future development. In applying the stages of the model to Aaliyah's situation the following observations were noted:

Curiosity
From working with her on the ward it is evident from her behaviour that Aaliyah feels a low sense of self-worth and self-esteem, suggesting that her feelings dominate her self-perception. Often she expresses her views and opinions very effectively, especially when supporting others, and it appears these are skills of which she is unaware.

Resourcefulness
Aaliyah enjoys solving problems and is highly adaptable to different social environments. She enjoys the company of other people and new challenges and experiences.

Empowering the person
The inpatient unit provided a safe and secure environment where Aaliyah could work through the crisis phase of her experience. On the unit the staff spent individual time with her, discussing how she felt and her future goals and aspirations.

Viewing the crisis as an opportunity
The crisis caused a disruption to the established pattern of Aaliyah's life and provided her with the opportunity to review her goals and priorities and identify her choices in life.

Setting small-scale, achievable goals

In the inpatient setting the goal of care was to stabilize Aaliyah's mental health and to restore a sense of equilibrium to allow her to see a potential positive future.

Identifying the simplest actions to generate change for the person

On the unit it was initally agreed for Aaliyah to receive 45 minutes of one-to-one time with her allocated mental health nurse each shift, and for her to become involved in the group activities on the unit. After the first week Aaliyah appeared to be much improved and began to consider her goals and priorities on leaving the unit.

Aaliyah remained on the unit for three weeks. Following her discharge she left to stay with a friend but continued to attend a day hospital for one-to-one sessions each week and an open group with other service users. A goal identified by the staff for Aaliyah in her care plan at the day service was to encourage her to become aware of her skills of self-expression. After several months on a waiting list Aaliyah was allocated a housing association flat situated in a different locality than she had lived in previously, in accordance with her wishes to avoid coming into routine contact with her former friends and the possible temptation of her previous lifestyle.

While it has been presented in clear and specific stages so that you can see the main points, the tidal model is not intended to be a highly defined structure, as to implement it in the same way every time contradicts the notion of each person's narrative or story being unique. Instead, the model ought to be implemented flexibly to incorporate the different experiences of each service user (Barker and Buchannan-Barker 2005).

Student nurses often find this model elusive and difficult to apply in practice. One reason is because it is presented in very personal and emotive language, referring to feelings and experiences. Therefore, once you have read about the model, it is best applied in the practice setting to help you develop personal knowledge and understanding of how it works.

The following two exercises are designed to assist you in developing knowledge of the interpersonal and tidal models, to consider your opinions and to build them into your developing perspective and approach to practice.

Comparing and contrasting the interpersonal and tidal models

- Read through the descriptions of the two models again.
- Now on a piece of paper write 'the interpersonal model' as one column and 'the tidal model' as another.
- Taking them one at a time, write down the positive features of each model.
- After you have done this, read what you have identified as the positive features.
- Which model do you find more useful and why? The answer does not have to be based on the most positive points. It may be those you identify for one or other model are fewer, but of greater significance.
- When you have finished, place your notes in your professional portfolio and make a note in your diary, or on your calendar, to repeat this exercise after one year on the course.
- After a year, repeat the exercise but do not refer to your original notes.
- When you have completed the exercise, compare the notes you have just made with those you originally made.

- Have you said anything new or different than when you carried out the exercise before? If so, how do you account for what you have said?
- What do you believe you have learned about practice during the intervening time?

When you have finished, place your notes in your professional portfolio.

Applying the interpersonal and tidal models

Often in practice settings different frameworks are used depending on the documentation applicable to the area. From your placement experience select the case of one service user newly referred to the service with which you are placed, and in whose assessment and planning of care you have been involved. Now answer and reflect on the following points.

Apply the stages of the interpersonal and tidal models to the assessment of need and planning of care.

Do the models identify any other areas of need which were not considered in the actual assessment and planning of care?

- Comparing the three versions of the assessment and planning of care provided by the two models and the actual case, are they all focused on the service user's needs? In the actual assessment were any assessment tools used, and if so why?
- Reflect on the skills you observed the qualified nurse using in developing a therapeutic relationship with the service user. Examples might include how they engaged with the service user, the technique(s) used to identify the problem(s), how they investigated the issues, and the approach used to consider the impact of the problem(s), exploring the possible solutions and options.
- Comparing your application of the stages of the model to the actual case, were the assessment and planning of care focused on the need(s) of the service user?
- When participating in the assessment of the care needs of service users, what techniques did the nurses use to develop therapeutic relationships?

When you have finished, place your notes in your professional portfolio. Now apply this exercise to the assessment and planning of care of other service users. In future placements, your knowledge and understanding of nursing models can also be developed by:

- Identifying useful tools and methods of assessing the needs of service users in the practice setting.
- Exploring and applying other nursing models in the practice setting.
- Discussing assessment and care planning with practice mentors.

The Ten Essential Shared Capabilities

Finally in this chapter we will discuss *The Ten Essential Shared Capabilities* (10 ESC) (DoH 2004) and their impact on our understanding of the practice of mental health nursing. While the specific implementation of the 10 ESC is discussed in more depth later in this book, here we consider how students found that learning about the 10 ESC has enhanced their emerging development as future mental health nurses.

Background

The 10 ESC were developed from a study of the mental health workforce, people receiving mental health services and carers, which revealed deficits in the way that mental health professionals provided care to people with mental health problems. The 10 ESC are principles which the study identified would enhance the practice of mental health professionals. Through reflecting on these we can develop our understanding of how we can incorporate them into our practice and work to place the person with a mental health problem at the centre of that practice.

Since their introduction the 10 ESC have repeatedly been emphasized in government documents as a priority for the future development of the mental health workforce. They are listed below.

The 10 ESC

- Working in partnership
- Respecting diversity
- Practicing ethically
- Challenging inequality
- Promoting recovery
- Identifying people's needs and strengths
- Providing service user-centred care
- Making a difference
- Promoting safety and positive risk
- Personal development and learning

Central to carrying out the 10 ESC in practice is ensuring you have incorporated their real meaning into your personal and professional values. Yet there is evidence to suggest that these principles have been slow to filter through into practice. Repeatedly students have identified that there is limited awareness of the 10 ESC in practice areas among qualified staff and mentors. Among the reasons suggested for this was: 'The lack of information that current mental health professionals have of the 10 ESC; the pressures of having other priorities such as practice documents and reports due'.

However, it is frequently stated that the 10 ESC are an *expectation* of good clinical practice, in that, because trainee nurses are finding them helpful, they can be expected to have a beneficial influence as new staff join the profession. In reflecting on learning about the 10 ESC in pre-registration training, one student mental health nurse remarked: 'They are values that we apply every day but the 10 ESC give a platform to refer to. I discovered that the 10 ESC are within the CPA policy and I have been able to use this to apply the values to practice.' Another student remarked: 'I believe as a student nurse I contribute to making a dif-

ference by going the extra length to treat patients with dignity, especially attending to personal care. Taking a genuine interest helped me to build trust with the patients.' The values of the 10 ESC are therefore not only evident in the student's beliefs but implemented in actions and interventions with service users which are appropriate to their needs.

The linkage of theory and practice in this manner applies to both physical and psychological interventions. Another student stated that after training in the 10 ESC: 'I now make it my responsibility to talk to clients about their strengths. I feel ... people's strengths are very much overlooked.'

Central to the 10 ESC making a genuine impact on improving practice are positive changes to that practice and the way in which students understand their role. Often these changes are only slight or subtle, yet they have a significant effect on the service users who receive the care. In the next panel are a number of examples of instances where student mental health nurses reported that an awareness of the 10 ESC made a positive impact on a practice situation.

Improvements in practice

- 'I don't see many carers or relatives in my current placement, however, when I do I always talk to them about the individual concerned. I think that involvement of carers and relatives will be of greater use in the community.'
- 'A service user was reluctant to come to the unit for an outpatient appointment because of stigma. So a domiciliary visit was arranged.'
- 'Respecting diversity in my practice area was an issue [for] a client, who because of his religion does not eat meat or engage in certain things ... I kind of followed in line ... and accommodated it.'

Therefore the 10 ESC ought to be rooted within practice.

Grounding the 10 ESC in practice means that

students are able to identify their practice skills with regards to the 10 ESC, and also their learning needs. As one student said:

'I have developed an understanding of the role of the service user/carer input into an individual's care. This has allowed me to further develop the relationship so that I am more effective as a professional.' Yet practicing values-based care is not only learned: it needs to be continually reviewed and relearned in the face of continual challenges. As another student recognized: "[There is a] need to work alongside service users and honestly to continue to question the care I provide and my

motives, recheck self-awareness and the ethos of the service I work in ... '

Finally, the 10 ESC are more than a guide for practice. They need to be reflected upon and absorbed within the student's personal and professional values in order to obtain real personal motivation, and so that the student's philosophy of nursing practice reflects their view about the way the world works.

In the next box are several statements from students summarizing their learning following a workshop-based programme in their mental health nurse training on the 10 ESC.

Personal values

- 'Everyone is just the same. We have to treat each other equally without looking at gender, race or creed. Therefore equality has to be maintained and it will be nicer if everyone puts themselves into someone else's shoes, thus you will see how it feels.'
- 'The most important thing I have learned is that mental illness can affect any individual and with good, fair and caring interventions recovery can be achieved. How the mental health nurse approaches and liaises with the client is a priority to their care.'
- 'The most important thing to me in the 10 ESC is the promotion of recovery. People go through the journey and back to their old life, [it] gives me joy knowing that I contributed to that.'
- 'I feel that even if society changes rules and legislation changes, what I have learned by doing this pack/workshop will always be ingrained in my ways of working and doing things. Added to this would be the core values of respect to another human being [who] like me has the same right to be in the world I live in, despite and in spite of their colour, creed, disability [or] religion.'

The 10 ESC revised

As a reminder, the 10 ESC are:

- Working in partnership
- Respecting diversity
- Practising ethically
- Challenging inequality
- Promoting recovery
- Identifying people's needs and strengths
- Providing service user-centred care
- Making a difference
- Promoting safety and positive risk
- Personal development and learning

Read the above quotes from students and the reiterated list of the 10 ESC.

- Now write a brief statement identifying what you personally value and prioritize in terms of your understanding of nursing.

- Next consider what your skills in the 10 ESC are and write down how you will use and develop these in practice.

- When you have finished, place your notes in your professional portfolio and put a note in your diary or on your calendar to review them in six months.

- When you review your statements, consider your practice experience in the intervening time.

- Have things happened to cause you to change or review your personal understanding of nursing? If so, what? Has the change been positive and confirmed or enhanced your commitment, or negative, leading you to question your understanding of the importance of the role of values in nursing practice? Alternatively, there may be no difference and your opinions and values are unaltered.

- Next consider whether you have practiced and developed the skills you prioritized. What have you learned about these? Can you develop these skills further?

- Now write down further goals for developing your practice – this may involve acquiring or gaining proficiency in new skills.

When you have finished, place your notes in your professional portfolio.

Conclusion

This chapter began with a brief discussion of the development of the role of the mental health nurse and the emergence of modern nurse training. We then considered the interpersonal and tidal mental health nursing models of Peplau and Barker. While both models provide useful structures within which to assess the needs of, and plan care for, service users, they are not intended to represent rigid frameworks. Instead these models allow the nurse to focus on the service user's needs and offer guiding principles which can be applied in assessing, planning, implementing and evaluating care. The value of these models is to provide a guiding idea of nursing, which can be applied in practice placements to develop your own experience-based knowledge of mental health nursing.

We ended the chapter by considering the 10 ESC, as these embody principles which service users value. The 10 ESC provide a framework for integrating personal commitment and self-awareness in practice which is useful for students, as developing these skills in training will provide you with a basis from which you can continue to learn throughout your career.

References

Barker, P. and Buchannan-Barker, P. (2005) *The Tidal Model: A Guide for Mental Health Professionals*. Hove: Brunner-Routledge.

Barker, P. and Buchannan-Barker, P. (2008) Reclaiming nursing: making it personal, *Mental Health Practice*, 11(9): 12–16.

Benner, P. (1984) *From Novice to Expert: Excellence and Power in Clinical Nursing*. Menlo Park, CA: Addison-Wesley.

Clarke, L. and Flanagan, T. (2003) *Institutional Breakdown: Exploring Mental Health Nursing Practice in Acute Settings*. Salisbury: APS Publishing.

Coombes, R. (1997) Off at the deep end, *Nursing Times*, 93(40): 16–17.

DoH (Department of Health) (2004) *The Ten Essential Shared Capabilities: A Framework for the Whole of the Mental Health Workforce*. London: DoH.

Fitzpatrick, J.J. and Whall, A.L. (2005) *Conceptual Models of Nursing: Analysis and Application*, 4th edn. Upper Saddle River, NJ: Pearson Education, Inc.

Fulbrook, P., Rolfe, G., Albarran, J. and Boxall, F. (2000) Fit for practice: Project 2000 student nurses' views on how well the curriculum prepares them for clinical practice, *Nurse Education Today*, 20: 350–7.

Hughes, S.J. (2004) The mentoring role of the personal tutor in the 'Fitness for Practice' curriculum: an all Wales approach, *Nurse Education in Practice*, 3: 1–8.

Jones, K. (1993) *Asylums and After: A Revised History of the Mental Health Services from the Early 18th Century to the 1990s*. London: The Athlone Press.

McKenna, H. (1997) *Nursing Theories and Models*. London: Routledge.

NMC (Nursing and Midwifery Council) (2006) *Standards to Support Learning and Assessment in Practice: NMC Standards for Mentors, Practice Teachers and Teachers*. London: NMC.

NMC (Nursing and Midwifery Council) (2008) *Standards of Conduct, Performance and Ethics for Nurses and Midwives*. London: NMC.

Nolan, P.A. (1993) *A History of Mental Health Nursing*. London: Chapman & Hall.

Pearson, A., Vaughan, B. and Fitzgerald, M. (1996) *Nursing Models for Practice*, 2nd edn. Oxford: Butterworth-Heinemann.

Peplau, H. (1988) *Interpersonal Relations in Nursing*. Basingstoke: Macmillan.

Roper, N., Logan, W. and Tierney, A. (2000) *The Roper-Logan-Tierney Model of Nursing: Based on Activities of Living*. Edinburgh: Churchill Livingstone.

UKCC (United Kingdom Central Council for Nurses, Midwifery and Health Visiting) (1986) *Project 2000: A New Preparation for Practice*. London: UKCC.

UKCC (United Kingdom Central Council for Nurses, Midwifery and Health Visiting) (1999) *Fitness for Practice*. London: UKCC.

Mental health and recognition of mental illness

Nick Wrycraft

Learning objectives

By the end of this chapter you will have:

- Gained an understanding of what is meant by mental health/ill health.
- Been introduced to an understanding of the range and different types of mental health conditions.
- Developed an awareness of some of the factors which can predispose individuals to experience mental health problems.

Introduction

In this chapter we will discuss mental health and ill health, and gain an understanding of the range of mental health problems which people experience and the factors which can contribute to this. Mental health is a complex phenomenon and we begin by discussing the concepts of mental health and ill health and how legislation defines mental illness. Many different disorders are embraced within mental illness and we will look at a number of mental health conditions and identify their characteristics.

Finally, we will consider some social factors which can predispose people to experience mental illness within three broad categories: social and economic, gender and ethnicity.

Scenarios and examples of mental health problems will be presented during the chapter to illustrate the clinical and professional complexities involved. Answers are provided to the scenarios of Dave, Sophie, Asifa and George at the end of the book. Several exercises will help you identify areas for your professional development through further reading and reflection on practice experience, and action points which can be addressed on practice placements.

What is mental illness?

At any one time mental ill health can affect one in six people of working age (DoH 1998; NIMHE 2004) and accounts for one-third of all illness in the UK (DoH 2007). It is estimated that nearly half of all women and a quarter of all men will experience depression, which is the most frequently occurring mental health problem, before they reach 70 years of age (DoH 1998; NICE 2002). Yet many people with a mental health problem continue to carry on their daily lives in the community in exactly the same way as other people who are perfectly healthy and well. Therefore we need to establish what mental illness really is.

To a large extent how mental health and ill health are understood depends on the reason why we are making the distinction, and in nursing there are two reasons which are very important. First, identifying mental illness is necessary so that the person can be offered appropriate specialist help. Second, we are obliged to define mental health and ill health in relation to the law, as some people with acute mental health needs lack insight into their condition and require assessment for compulsory treatment in accordance with mental health legislation.

There are many different understandings of mental health. Here are just two:

> Mental health is about the way human beings adjust to the world, and are effective, happy, efficient, content, and maintain an even temper, an alert intelligence, socially considerate behaviour and a happy disposition.

> (Eaton 1951: 88)

[Mental health is] the capacity to live life to the full in ways that enable us to realise our own natural potentialities, and that unite us with rather than divide us from all the other human beings who make up our world.

(Guntrip 1964: 25)

but which marks the end of the person's coping resources. However, mental illness is a highly individual experience and equally a person who has not been exposed to difficult life events may become mentally ill.

The continuum usefully differentiates between

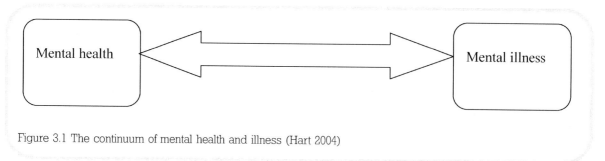

Figure 3.1 The continuum of mental health and illness (Hart 2004)

However, both these definitions speak about what mental *health* is and for the purposes of our interest as mental health professionals we want to identify what mental *illness* is. A useful concept which links mental health and ill health is the continuum shown in Figure 3.1, which has complete mental health and well-being at one end and mental illness at the other.

There are numerous different points along the continuum with various degrees of mental health and illness and our position on it can change as time passes (Hart 2004). At certain key points people are more prone to mental illness. Significant life events such as moving home, redundancy, divorce and bereavement can all contribute to a person developing a mental health problem (Holmes and Rahe 1967).

Yet it should not be assumed mental ill health is an *inevitable* consequence of difficult life events as two individuals might have identical circumstances yet one person develops a mental health problem while the other does not. Often an accumulation or series of distressing factors culminate in the person experiencing a crisis which may be triggered by an apparently quite innocuous event

mental health and mental illness, identifying them as separate. However, complete mental health would appear to be an unobtainable utopian state, as in order to appreciate that we have mental health it is necessary to be able to understand what it is to experience mental ill health. This reinforces the notion of the continuum and our ability to move along it as we experience varying stages of mental health and ill health.

Everyone experiences symptoms of mental ill health at some time in their life. In many circumstances, while these feelings are uncomfortable, they are time limited or in response to specific events. For example, it is perfectly normal to be anxious about a driving test or exam. Due to the fight or flight instinct, heightened alertness occurs in response to a perceived threat of danger and serves a useful role in self-preservation and efficient performance of some tasks through increased attention or awareness (Wilson 2001). While these feelings and experiences are not pleasant, they can be viewed as an opportunity to learn and experience personal growth. By successfully negotiating the problem, the person arrives at a new understanding.

Coping with anxiety

Consider a time in practice when you have felt anxious, for example, on the first day of the course, meeting your new study group, or when being assessed carrying out a technical skill under supervision by a qualified nurse. Write down your answers to the following.

● What physical changes did you notice in yourself?
● What helped you to feel less anxious?
● Did you adopt any strategies to help you cope?
● What learning points can you translate to your practice on coping with feelings of anxiety?

When you have finished, place your notes in your professional portfolio.

Mental illness can be said to occur where the response to a stressor is prolonged, or is triggered by inappropriate events, or where the person's quality of life is impeded and they experience significant distress over a sustained period of time.

It should also be remembered that mental illness is prone to misinterpretation as frequently people who are experiencing a mental health problem display erratic or unusual behaviour, have an inaccurate perception of reality or express views which differ from the majority of the rest of society, hence they can be confused with people who are eccentric, or whose lifestyle and views differ from those of other people (Hart 2004).

The Mental Health Act

Within the specialist mental health services our definition of mental illness is determined by legislation. Until very recently the Mental Health Act 1983 provided four criteria for determining mental illness (DoH/Welsh Office 1999), which were:

● incomplete development of the mind;
● psychopathic disorder;
● disturbance which prevents normal development;
● a mental disturbance which interferes with normal behaviour and daily life.

The Mental Health Bill of 2006 (DoH 2006) revised the legislation to use just *one* definition of mental health ('any disorder or disability of mind') which instead focuses on the problem(s) the service user is experiencing, rather than diagnosis within the above criteria. It is still too early to assess the impact of the new legislation, however, mental health nursing and the law are discussed in greater depth in Chapter 5.

Mental health conditions

In this section the range of different mental illnesses will be discussed and scenarios provided of individuals experiencing these problems.

Classifying mental illness

Within medical care there are two systems for classifying mental illness: the International Classification of Diseases (ICD) produced by the World Health Organization (WHO), and the *Diagnostic and Statistical Manual* (DSM) of the American Psychiatric Association (APA). The ICD provides standardized descriptions to define mental health problems and includes directive information to allow for differentiation between illnesses and for diagnosis (Katona and Robertson 2000). In contrast, the DSM states which symptoms are required, often specifying the number and identifying the necessary length of time for which a symptom has to be present for a diagnosis to be made. The ICD and DSM criteria are generally the same in their definition of mental illnesses (Katona and Robertson 2000). While you may still encounter these systems being used by doctors when assessing service users in a multidisciplinary or inpatient setting, the increasing influence of psychosocial approaches within mental health nursing and a wish to avoid stigma and labelling of mental illness have led to the avoidance of diagnosing service users within nursing.

Mental illness is an umbrella term, as it covers a range of disorders with varied causes. Opinions vary as to whether different mental health conditions have biological, psychological or sociological causes, and in some cases more than one of these factors may be active. However, traditionally mental health problems have been defined as either *functional* or *organic*.

- *Functional mental health problems* can be divided into psychotic disorders, which include schizophrenia, and mood disorders and other affective disorders, for example, depression, anxiety, obsessive-compulsive disorder (OCD), phobias, anorexia nervosa and bulimia nervosa. Other types of functional mental health problem include personality disorders, where a person's attitudes and behaviour lead them to make chaotic life choices, for example, in relationships, employment, housing and other areas of their life.
- *Organic mental health problems* are caused by the effects of physical illnesses on the functioning of the brain. They include dementia-type illnesses, infectious causes and alcohol and substance misuse.

There are a wide range of different types of mental health problem, and the next panel presents an overview. The types of problems listed will be briefly discussed, but for a comprehensive understanding the reader is advised to consult more specific texts.

Types of mental health problem

- Depression and anxiety.
- Bipolar mood disorders.
- Psychotic disorders and schizophrenia.
- Personality disorders.
- Psychoactive substance misuse.
- Self-harm.
- Eating disorders.
- Dementia.

Characteristics of depression

Depression can be regarded as evident in *four* areas of a person's functioning.

- Symptoms of pervasive *low mood*, and a loss of interest in activities the person previously pursued. The person may experience preoccupation and a reduced ability to think, concentrate and make decisions. They will also feel worthless and ashamed or a sense of blame or guilt (Lagerquist 1997) .
- *Physical symptoms* may be evident where the person may experience loss of sexual appetite (libido), eats much more or much less, leading to weight gain or loss, experiences sleeplessness (insomnia), or sleeps excessively (hypersomnia) and experiences changes in energy, for example, feeling unusually lethargic or lacking in energy (Katona and Robertson 2000).
- *Cognitive changes* may mean that the person has difficulty concentrating, is unable to remember information, or feels indecisive and experiences uncommonly negative thoughts of self-harm and/or suicide (Lagerquist 1997).
- Finally there may be *behavioural factors*, for example, loss of interest in personal appearance and avoiding people in social settings (Lagerquist 1997; Brosan and Hogan 2007). The person may appear to lack animation and speak in a monotonous voice. Conversations may be repetitive and the person may be reluctant to engage eye contact or expand on answers to questions (Lagerquist 1997).

Depression

Depression and anxiety are the most commonly occurring mental health conditions. Generally people experience a mixture of depression and anxiety, however, to make it easier for you to understand the characteristics of both illnesses, here they are discussed separately.

Often depression can be triggered by an ongoing life-limiting physical condition, or where the person also has a physical health problem (comorbidity) – for example, diabetes, chronic obstructive pulmonary disease (COPD) or cardiac problems (Kisley and Goldberg 1996). The effect on the person's wider social network, family and life situation also ought to be considered, as people do not exist in a vacuum and their behaviour both affects and is affected by significant others.

Scenario: Dave

Dave is 52 and experienced a heart attack approximately 18 months ago. He described himself before the heart attack as a 'happy go lucky' and sociable person who never worried about anything. Before the heart attack Dave worked as a builder and was often away from home on jobs for long periods of time. He admits that he often did not eat well and was overweight.

After having the heart attack Dave changed his lifestyle, taking regular exercise and eating healthily but has begun to feel low in mood and had difficulty sleeping, waking up early in the morning and generally losing interest in life. He has not worked since the heart attack, has abandoned many former interests, has lost contact with friends and lacks motivation.

Due to losing interest in eating Dave has lost a lot of weight and his wife is worried about his physical health. Dave feels he has lost confidence and is reluctant to leave home. Recently he has been asked to look after his 3-year-old grandson while his daughter-in-law works. Dave wants to do this, but worries he will have another heart attack while caring for the child. On several occasions recently he has had chest pain and attended the accident and emergency (A&E) department at the local hospital, but in spite of extensive investigations no physical problems were found. Dave experienced this pain again during a weekend when his GP was unavailable so his wife drove him to A&E.

Applying theory to practice

Under the supervision of a qualified member of staff you are assigned to assess Dave's condition. Write down your thoughts in response to the following questions.

- What effect do you think his state of mind might be having on his physical condition?
- What verbal and non-verbal communication might you notice which would suggest Dave is depressed?

When you have finished this exercise, place the notes you have made in your professional portfolio.

Anxiety

Anxiety is a state where a person is preoccupied and displays heightened or exaggerated concern and attention to specific issues. Certain levels of anxiety are part of normal life, and even necessary in order for us to recognize risk and to enhance concentration in important circumstances – for example, in an exam or on a driving test. Yet where such anxiety is prolonged and exerts a detrimental effect on the person's functioning and quality of life, they may experience a mental health problem.

There are physical and psychological characteristics associated with this problem. Common physical characteristics are summarized in the next panel.

Physical characteristics of anxiety

- Increased heart rate.
- Increased rate of respiration.
- Increased rate of passing urine (micturition) and diarrhoea; or constipation.
- Dry mouth.
- Poor appetite, feelings of nausea, tightness in the stomach or 'butterflies'.
- Increased discharge in menstruation.
- Increase or reduction in body temperature.
- Increase or reduction in blood pressure.
- Dilated pupils.

(Lagerquist 1997)

Among the psychological characteristics of anxiety are that the person will feel restless and tense and may appear to be agitated, or easily become irritable. Often the person experiences feelings of fear or terror over a sustained period of time and is indecisive and preoccupied, with 'tunnel vision' causing them to focus intently on specific issues, frequently minor, in detail to the exclusion of all else, and have an exaggerated view of the importance of certain events. The person may not be aware of the wider environment, is oblivious to what other people say to them and unable to concentrate or remember new information or perform tasks which they can do with ease when well (Lagerquist 1997).

Anxiety can present at varying levels from mild to severe, and frequently occurs alongside other mental health problems. At the more extreme end are *panic attacks*, which can be said to occur where physical symptoms are experienced due to the body being highly responsive. Symptoms include palpitations, chills, hyperventilation, dizziness, chest pain, choking, nausea and stomach churning.

It has been suggested that panic attacks have a physiological basis and are a fear response triggered in reaction to a perceived but unidentified threat (Hart 2004). In addition to the disabling physical effects, which will increase the person's agitation, they will experience racing thoughts, a feeling that everything is happening quickly, an inability to focus or concentrate and difficulty articulating their thoughts. They may feel they are losing control of their thoughts and 'going crazy' (Katona and Robertson 2000). Other forms of anxiety include phobias, of which there are several types.

Types of phobia

- Agoraphobia is anxiety pertaining to places or situations from which it may be difficult to escape or receive help if the person were to experience a panic attack.
- Specific phobias are anxiety caused by a particular object or phenomenon, common examples being flying or spiders.
- Social phobias are anxiety and persistent fear where the individual is in proximity to other people with whom they are unfamiliar.

(Katona and Robertson 2000)

Obsessive compulsive disorder or OCD comprises of obsessive thoughts and compulsive actions. The obsessive thoughts develop from a wish to stay safe. While this is a logical concern, in OCD the person becomes preoccupied with a specific issue and has negative feelings in which they have an exaggerated sense of responsibility. These thoughts lead to compulsions, which are actions resulting from, and in response to, urges to perform stereotypical behaviours intended to avoid feared outcomes and reduce the anxiety and distress the person is experiencing (Brosan 2007).

For example, Sally is a mother with a young baby. Her obsession has developed from a preoccupation with fear about her child becoming ill from an infection acquired in the home. She experiences increasing anxiety and feelings of guilt, and her compulsions are that unless she cleans the home to an exceptional standard, her child will fall ill and die, and it will be *her* fault. Sally establishes a rigorous cleaning ritual, yet is still concerned whether this is sufficient to keep her child safe.

The cycle of OCD is often progressive, and in spite of repeatedly performing compulsions, instead of the negative thoughts, fears and obsessions dissipating, they remain unchanged, or become even more insistent, leading to the person performing more extreme, elaborate or frequent compulsive acts or rituals. Often the person is aware they are experiencing obsessive thoughts, and do not want to perform the compulsive acts or rituals, but experience the obsessive feelings to such a powerful extent they are unable to resist (Hart 2004).

In Sally's case her compulsions increased in severity. She began to cancel social engagements to avoid leaving the home and entering an environment where her baby might acquire an infection. She became increasingly isolated, preoccupied with her obsessive thoughts and exhausted from continually cleaning, yet unable to break her routine out of fear of the consequences. Sally and her partner were invited to a family occasion which she felt she could not attend due to her problem. Sally visited her family doctor and was referred to counselling and is now working with a therapist and making a gradual improvement.

Bipolar mood disorders

Bipolar disorder affects mood, thinking and behaviour and is characterized by mood swings. When in a high phase the person can display grandiose behaviour and express delusions, but when low they become deeply depressed. Often changes to the person's mental health are clearly noticeable, as their behaviour contrasts significantly with when they are mentally well.

The symptoms outlined below refer to a person in the elevated phase and can be reversed when the person is in a low mood. Due to the impulsive and emotion-driven nature of the condition people with bipolar mood disorder present a high risk of suicide.

Symptoms of bipolar disorder

- Mood
  - Elevated and expansive or euphoric
  - Irritable and impatient
  - Rapidly changing
- Thought
  - Flight of ideas
  - Grandiose delusions
  - Jealous or persecutory views
- Speech
  - Rapid delivery
  - Loud in volume and expansive
  - Singing or rhyming words together
- Behaviour
  - Emotionally inappropriate and disinhibited
  - Uncharacteristic actions, for example, overspending
  - Unusual or colourful choices of clothing
- Bodily functions
  - Insomnia
  - Increased activity levels
  - Increased appetite
  - Increased libido
- Perceptions
  - Illusory ideas
  - Misunderstanding of other people's communication
  - Jumping to conclusions
  - Lack of insight and congruence with reality

(Hart 2004)

Psychotic disorders and schizophrenia

Psychosis leads the person to lose touch with reality and attribute personalized or unusual meanings to events or phenomena. Psychosis is frequently a response to traumatic events or problems at a particular time in life (e.g. starting university and living away from home, divorce, bereavement, redundancy or as a result of the use of illicit substances). Psychosis is an acute mental illness, however people can experience an episode of psychosis and fully recover.

Schizophrenia is often mistakenly thought to be 'split personality'. Instead it is a *fragmentation* of the person's perception and grasp of objective reality, which affects their mood, thinking and behaviour, and makes it difficult for them to be able to separate their own thoughts and perceptions from what occurs outside of them.

Symptoms of schizophrenia

- *Delusions*, which are fixed beliefs and are commonly held quite firmly.
- *Hallucinations* in the form of perceptions caused by no apparent external stimuli, for example, hearing voices, but these can also occur through the other senses.
- *Disorganized thinking and speech* where the person makes statements and/or carries out actions which are inappropriate, or for no apparent reason (Katona and Robertson 2000).

While the cause of schizophrenia is not definitely known, it is felt some physical factors are active (Wilson 2001). The onset of the illness is usually between the ages of 15 and 27, and as this is often a time of great upheaval and change in people's lives and development there has been much speculation that biological, psychosocial and environmental factors may all contribute to people developing a schizophrenic illness (Lagerquist 1997).

Schizophrenia is an illness you will encounter frequently within specialist mental health services, and there are several distinctly different forms, which are outlined below.

Subtypes of schizophrenia

- *Catatonic*: often people will display a fixed posture and may remain silent (mute) for long periods of time and not engage with their environment, be non-responsive and in some cases neglect their self-care and hygiene needs over a period of time. The person may also be prone to aggressive outbursts or frantic activity.
- *Disorganized*: using inappropriate mannerisms and inappropriate responses or incoherent language in conversation; tending to be withdrawn and preoccupied.
- *Paranoid*: disturbed thought content with a persecutory or hostile nature which can also be grandiose and often on a recurrent theme, for example, elaborate beliefs pertaining to the army, organized crime, conspiracy theories or religion.
- *Undifferentiated*: mixed symptoms of schizophrenic-type illness.

(Lagerquist 1997)

Schizophrenia is acutely distressing for the person, their family and significant others, yet the subject of much fear and stigma from the general population which limits the opportunity for social inclusion and the meaningful participation of people with a psychotic or schizophrenia-related illness.

Personality disorders

Personality disorders are a controversial area of mental health, and for many years there was debate over whether they were mental health problems at all. However, increasing awareness of the effects of personality disorders has led to their recognition as mental illness by statutory mental health services. Often personality disorders are characterized by consistent character traits and patterns of negative behaviour.

Personality disorders are established patterns of maladaptive thinking, feeling and behaving which differ significantly from the expectations of the person's culture and produce detrimental outcomes (Lagerquist 1997). Characteristics include repeated chaotic interpersonal relationships and behaviour. The person's inner conflicts are expressed through the way in which they relate to others (Lagerquist 1997). Personality disorders are often first evident in childhood and continue into adulthood, and there is no identifiable cause (Katona and Robertson 2000).

There are numerous classifications of different types of personality disorder. However, these can be divided into three areas, or clusters, as outlined below.

Classifications of personality disorders

- **Cluster A**
  - *Paranoid:* characterized by being aloof towards others and lacking trust, even in interpersonal relationships; being unwilling to confide in others, and oversensitivity to criticism; interpreting negative meanings in other people's comments.
  - *Schizoid:* the person actively avoids social contact with others and has a limited range of emotional engagement in all areas of social activity.

- **Cluster B**
  - *Borderline* (also called impulsive): the person has chaotic, unstable and turbulent interpersonal relationships and is prone to self-damaging and risk-taking behaviour together with suicidal or self-harming behaviour and paranoia.
  - *Histrionic* (also called narcissistic): the person seeks attention from others, can be manipulative and fails to form appropriate or helpful relationships. Often the person has a changeable mood and displays immaturity in their attitude.
  - *Dissocial* (also called psychopathic and sociopathic): characteristic of this form of personality disorder is a lack of awareness of the rights of others and an inability to maintain relationships. Frequently people with this form of personality disorder are impulsive and aggressive, and prone to dangerous risk-taking, with a lack of tolerance of others and a lack of conscience, meaning there is an inability to learn from experience.

- **Cluster C**
  - *Avoidant (anxious):* the person feels inadequate and is reluctant to become involved in social settings and seeks to maintain physical security.
  - *Dependent (asthenic):* the person depends on others to an excessive extent in interpersonal relationships, is 'clingy', avoids disagreement out of concern at losing support and is reluctant to make decisions without significant reassurance.

(Katona and Robertson 2000)

There are other types of personality disorder which the learner might wish to read about in more detail in other sources of literature.

Substance misuse

There are a wide range of substances which can be misused. These include nicotine, caffeine, alcohol, amphetamines and associated compounds, cannabis, cocaine, opioids, hallucinogens, inhalants, sedatives, hypnotics and anxiolytics. The effects vary depending on the choice, amount taken, frequency of use, individual susceptibility to the effects, and the combination of substances used. Frequently people experience low mood, personality changes, and become more impulsive when under the influence of substances, or have impaired judgement. Often people experience substance misuse problems alongside other mental health problems.

Characteristics of substance misuse

- A preoccupation with and persistent desire for the substance.
- Activities to acquire continual supplies of the substance.
- Absence of control in taking the chosen substance.
- Tolerance to the chosen substance, leading to an increased intake being required to achieve the same effect.
- Psychological and/or physical dependence leading to difficulties with withdrawal, reduction or abstention.
- Reduction in participation in other activities.

(Hart 2004)

Self-harm

Self-harm is often regarded as the same as attempted suicide. While it appears that the two can be distinguished on the basis of the intent of the person, as in the first case the person intends to injure him or herself, while in the second they aim to end their life, in practice it is not so easy to clearly place a person's motive in one or other category. Furthermore, self-harm often has the potential for lethal consequences, whether the person intends this to be the case or not.

Self-harming behaviour also includes actions such as tattooing, piercing, plastic surgery or other cultural acts – for example, tribal scars which are clearly not carried out as attempts to cause long-term harm (Noonan 2005). Instead, as with mental health and illness it may be more useful to view self-harm and suicide as situated at the opposite ends of a continuum, with levels of severity of self-harm and those actions which are severely damaging to the person closer to attempted suicide (Noonan 2005) (see Figure 3.2).

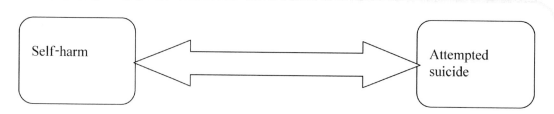

Figure 3.2 The continuum of self-harm and attempted suicide

Self-harm can take many different forms and methods, ranging from cutting and burning the skin to deliberate overdose and substance misuse. People frequently self-harm to relieve pent up feelings of emotion or anger or to express pain and feelings of self-loathing or worthlessness. Teenagers and young adults experience feelings of alienation or rejection which can cause self-harm to be an accepted activity which among their peer group can be regarded alongside other aspects of lifestyle choice, including clothing, music and substance misuse.

Often self-harm is repeatedly focused on certain specific parts of the body. Frequent areas which are the focus of self-harm are the wrists, upper thighs, inner arms and upper chest, although self-harm can also include skin picking and the deliberate breaking of bones. The most commonly used implement of self-harm is knives or blades, yet it can occur in subtle and varied forms. People who self-harm tend to be ashamed of their behaviour and conceal their injuries and the means by which they carry out this activity, and so the chosen methods vary and can be very discreet.

Scenario: Sophie

Sophie is 14 years old. Her school is located near to the hospital. At 2 p.m. she is visiting her father John who is in hospital for observation after falling from a ladder and possibly incurring some internal injuries. She is dressed in a dishevelled manner and seems preoccupied and low in mood. When you ask if she is okay, Sophie avoids eye contact, replies in an offhand way and appears to become defensive, explaining that due to a teacher being taken ill she has been granted a 'non-pupil afternoon' and this often happens. As you leave the bedside you notice the left-hand sleeve of her shirt is rolled up and the inside of her forearm has raised horizontal pale welts from what you think is scarring. The other sleeve is pulled down and what appear to be bloodstains have soaked through the material.

Questioning clinical practice

- Think about and then write down how you would attempt to engage with Sophie, describing the techniques you would use.
- Is it in accordance with the NMC code of professional guidance (2008) (discussed in Chapter 1) to ask further questions about Sophie's well-being, or is that exceeding the acceptable role of the nurse?

Place your notes in your professional portfolio.

Eating disorders

Eating disorders incorporate a range of problems. In some cases the person does not eat because they mistakenly believe they are overweight and introduce a rigorous regime of dietary control and deprivation of food (*anorexia nervosa*). Alternatively the person binge eats large amounts of food and then purges through vomiting or using laxatives (*bulimia nervosa*). It is also important to consider persistent overeating which leads to weight gain and obesity. Frequently obesity coexists alongside other mental health problems yet can predispose the person to other health problems. It is increasingly being highlighted as an area of concern for general health within the population. However, in this section we will next focus in more detail on anorexia nervosa and bulimia nervosa.

Anorexia nervosa is a disorder in which the person does not believe they are of normal weight and size and has a distorted perception of their body and powerful aversion to food. The person reduces their intake of food and severely limits their diet, yet still often has a preoccupation with food, often hoarding certain products and becoming acquainted with the nutritional values of foods to avoid high calorie items. The person may

also be hyperactive and engage in exercise or other activity associated with weight loss, or which will use up calories (Lagerquist 1997).

The physical effects of anorexia, in addition to obvious significant weight loss, include delayed physical development in the case of younger people, loss of energy and vitality, amenorrhea (the absence of three or more menstrual cycles) in women, low sex drive, a low heart rate (bradychardia), dryness of the skin and hair and the presence of 'lanugo' or an excess of fine hair on the body and face. The person may experience constipation, and at the advanced stages impaired functioning of the organs (Lagerquist 1997).

It has been noted that there is a high incidence of anorexia nervosa among people with obsessive or perfectionist personalities and also where other family members also have eating disorders. It is also evident in some instances where the person wishes to avoid the onset of sexual maturity (Katona and Robertson 2000).

While some people with anorexia nervosa also often carry out bulimic behaviour, not all people with anorexia also have bulimia. Characteristic of bulimia nervosa is the consumption of large amounts of food at one time, and a loss of control followed by vomiting or purging by using laxatives and diuretics (Katona and Robertson 2000). In common with anorexia nervosa the person is concerned with retaining a low body weight and shape. Physical damage to the oesophagus may occur as a result of repeated forced vomiting, while there may be damage to the teeth occurring as a result of vomiting food containing acid from the stomach. The person's weight will also often fluctuate (Katona and Robertson 2000).

Identifying an eating disorder can be difficult. Often people feel ashamed and a sense of guilt, and will be secretive about their behaviour. Also the media has a preoccupation with unrealistic weight and body shape regarding women (and increasingly men) which can exert a pervasive but subtle influence by reinforcing unhelpful beliefs in people with a predisposition to an eating disorder.

Scenario: Asifa

Asifa is 25 years old and a student nurse in your intake. She moved from her home some distance away to live in university accommodation when she began training and at the same time ended a long-term relationship with her boyfriend.

While on placement Asifa does not eat, providing the reason that shifts interrupt the usual pattern of meals. She also does not keep food in the kitchen she shares in a communal flat with other students, as she lives on a bursary and enjoys spending her money on clothes and travel.

During the 18 months of the course to date Asifa has lost a significant amount of weight and often looks pale and tired. On more than one occasion you have heard other people remark to Asifa that she appears to be underweight.

Asifa responds to these comments as compliments, stating that it is fashionable to be thin, and that when growing up her mother always criticized her for being overweight, but now she is able to live up to the ideal of being slim. Recently on a particularly busy shift Asifa appeared to faint and lose consciousness briefly but when recovering would not seek help. She increasingly appears to have difficulty concentrating and focusing on her work, and her recent marks in assignments are lower than previously on the course.

Questioning clinical practice

Think carefully about the dilemmas posed by the scenario, and then write down your responses to the questions below.

- Are you obliged to notify the university of your concerns about Asifa? If so, how would you describe what these concerns are and the rationale(s) to support your observations?
- Within the scope of the NMC guidance on professional conduct (2008), are qualified members of nursing staff obliged to report similar instances regarding colleagues?

Once you have answered these points, read through the guidance on professional conduct and see if your thoughts, feelings and views match the professional guidelines prescribed by the NMC. Place your notes in your professional portfolio.

Dementia

Dementia is not a single disease but group of different illnesses which all cause degenerative changes in brain tissue and a progressive decline in cognitive functioning. Typical changes which occur in dementia are loss of memory, confusion and change in personality, mood and behaviour (Hart 2004). Examples of dementia-type illnesses are Alzheimer's disease, Lewy body, vascular disease and Pick's disease. Cerebral haematomas or space-occupying lesions in the cerebral cortex can also produce similar symptoms to dementia. While commonly it is regarded as a disease of older age, it is not inevitable that as people age they experience dementia. Dementia can occur in younger people as a result of conditions such as Korsakoff syndrome and Creutzfeldt-Jacob disease (CJD).

Scenario: George

George is 78 years old and was bereaved of his wife Joan 18 months ago. George's daughter Sarah became concerned as shortly after this event she went away with him on holiday and found that he could not remember where his room was and became very easily confused and disorientated. When he returned home George often did not know where he was, and recently on some occasions has not known who Sarah is. When she asked him about this, George said it was all a part of the ageing process. Lately George has been forgetting to wash, eat and generally neglecting his needs. Late on one Sunday evening Sarah was phoned by a neighbour of George's who found him wandering outside his house and only partly clothed. Not knowing where else to go Sarah has brought George to the A&E department; he is very confused and not able to provide any information, while she is very tearful and when registering his details with the receptionist explains that she can no longer care for her father and needs urgent help.

Applying theory to practice

● What techniques would you use in a conversation with Sarah to provide support and reassurance while also gaining information to be able to effectively assess George? Write down how you would approach this situation and then consider why you chose these methods.

Place your notes in your professional portfolio.

While we have considered a range of specific mental health conditions, people do not experience mental health problems in isolation from their environment. Instead the circumstances in which people live exert an important influence over whether they develop mental health problems. In mental health nursing it is essential, if we are to gain an accurate understanding of how the illness affects the person, to gain a good picture of the background and environment within which the person lives and functions. In the final section of the chapter we will consider a very brief overview of some environmental factors which affect people's mental health.

A socioeconomic perspective on mental health

Associations between social and economic deprivation and physical and mental health have long been established (Townsend *et al.* 1992; SCMH 1998). Factors including poor housing and physical environment, and whether a person has a long-term physical health problem also increase the likelihood of mental ill health (Ford 2005). Living in poor housing, on a low income or state benefit, having caring responsibilities, and with a limited network of social support all predispose a person to experiencing a mental health difficulties. However, these factors are *risk factors* rather than *predictors*; many people still manage in these circumstances and are unaffected.

It has been identified that work and meaningful occupation are linked to better mental health, and people experience improved self-esteem and sense of identity, and feel they are contributing usefully to society when in work or pursuing an occupation (DoH 1998, 1999; NSIP 2006). However, the severely mentally ill have the lowest employment rates of any of the main groups of disabled people (NSIP 2006). Within wider society, stigma and negative perceptions of mental illness often lead to a lack of opportunities for employment and other opportunities for people who have experienced mental health problems (DoH 1998, 1999; NSIP 2006).

To combat the negative effects of stigma and support people with mental health problems returning to work the government has invested significant effort in assisting people with mental health problems to gain or return to work and promote social inclusion (DoH 2004a, 2004b, 2004c; DWP 2004; Social Exclusion Unit 2004; DoH/DWP/HSE 2005; Till 2007). In some cases part-time or voluntary work may be suitable depending on the individual's needs and situation (Allen 2008). The example below illustrates the positive benefits of supporting people in returning to work after experiencing a mental health problem.

Returning to work

The following is an extract of a personal account from the document: *Vocational Services for People with Severe Mental Health Problems: Commissioning Guidance* (NSIP 2006: 9).

I am middle aged and have been working in a large organisation as a junior manager for 25 years. Nine years ago I suffered a nervous breakdown and was diagnosed with schizophrenia. I was in hospital for several months. I received excellent psychiatric help and returned to work at the same organisation after a year. I have since received excellent support from the organisation ...

Offering a different perspective on mental health in the workplace, people often persevere with problems and lead apparently normal lives while undergoing mental distress. Yet at the same time we are involved with increasingly demanding working lives, which are both stressful and demanding of our time and emotional resources which can worsen mental health and well being (Parsons 1999). The government has recently supported initiatives to reduce the stress experienced by staff in the workplace, including readily available counselling, subsidized memberships to gyms and initiatives to promote mental well-being (Brown 2007).

Gender

It has been noted that fewer women are in receipt of specialist mental health services than men (Repper and Perkins 1995; Owen and Milburn 2001). Among explanations to account for this are different expectations of the roles of men and women from health care practitioners (Perkins and Rowland 1991; Ussher 1991). A number of practical factors might act as disincentives to women to seek help. These include:

- women are often the primary carer for their children and may not be able to arrange childcare to be able to attend appointments;
- women may feel a sense of blame or recrimination because experiencing a mental health problem conflicts with the role expectations of a woman in society;
- mothers may fear losing custody of their children, or being subject to investigation from social services if they admit to having a mental health problem;
- a frequent symptom of mental illness is a loss of self-esteem and sense of self-worth, hence, as a parent the woman may place her own needs behind those of her children and partner;
- often women will experience abuse within domestic relationships which is traumatic and distressing, and do not seek help due to self-blame and guilt.

In contrast, if we focus on men it could be suggested that when mentally unwell they present as more dangerous and a risk to themselves and others, which accounts for the higher representation of men in inpatient areas. This would appear to be supported by the facts, as while the rate of people committing suicide has fallen, overall the majority are still male, and there is a preference among men who commit suicide for the use of violent methods (University of Manchester 2006).

Ethnicity

The increasingly rich ethnic and cultural mix of the population of the UK provides challenges for the mental health services. People coming to the UK from other countries have in many cases experienced traumatic or turbulent events such as war, rape, bereavement and loss of family members or their home, all of which can predispose people to mental illness. Issues such as differences in language, culture and customs can also account for a failure to identify mental illness or mental illness to be suspected where it is not.

An example of the experience of one group is the African-Caribbean population where there are more compulsory admissions, more diagnoses of schizophrenia and more instances of medication administered by force than in other social groups (Harrison *et al.* 1989; Lloyd and Moodley 1992; Thornicroft *et al.* 1999). Among explanations for this phenomenon are that African-Caribbean households experience worse circumstances in most socioeconomic indicators and far higher unemployment among young males than their white counterparts (SCMH 2002).

People do not exist in vacuums but are influenced by a number of factors. In order for mental health nurses to understand how a mental health problem affects the person we need to appreciate their environment and the effects of socioeconomic circumstances, gender and ethnicity on mental health. In Chapter 6 we go further and not only consider how we perceive mental illness but how we can promote positive mental health.

Conclusion

The chapter addressed several core areas of knowledge essential for student nurses. We began by discussing a definition of mental health and ill health, before considering the different types of mental health conditions, and then concluding with an outline of some factors which can predispose a person to experiencing mental illness.

It is important that readers reflect on the meaning of the terms 'mental health' and 'ill health' and consider how their personal understanding influences their work with service users. Yet it is also necessary to be aware of how professional practice is guided by the code of professional practice which regulates nursing (NMC 2008) and the specific terms of legislation which define mental illness.

In order to practice effectively and be able to recognize and differentiate between illnesses it is also necessary for students to become aware of the characteristics of different mental health problems. However, our experience of mental health and propensity to experience mental illness are frequently subject to influences within our environment, and it is important for mental health workers to be aware of how these factors are active.

Readers are encouraged to consider and reflect on the issues discussed in this chapter, return to them throughout their training and seek to apply them widely in their practice settings to enhance their knowledge and understand how and why people experience mental illness.

References

Allen, D. (2008) Volunteering works, *Mental Health Practice*, 11(9): 6–7.

Brosan, L. (2007) *An Introduction to Coping with Obsessive Compulsive Disorder.* London: Robinson.

Brosan, L. and Hogan, B. (2007) *An Introduction to Coping with Depression.* London: Robinson.

Brown, C. (2007) Employers to urge staff to lead healthier lives, *The Independent*, 28 December: 20.

DoH (Department of Health) (1998) *Modernising Mental Health Services: Safe, Sound and Supportive*, Mental Health Service Circular, HSC 1998/233: LAC (98)25. London: DoH.

DoH (Department of Health) (1999) *National Service Framework for Mental Health: Modern Standards and Service Models.* London: DoH.

DoH (Department of Health) (2004a) *The Ten Essential Shared Capabilities: A Framework for the Whole of the Mental Health Workforce.* London: DoH.

DoH (Department of Health) (2004b) *National Service Framework for Mental Health – Five Years On.* London: DoH.

DoH (Department of Health) (2004c) *Choosing Health: Making Healthier Choices Easier.* London: DoH.

DoH (Department of Health) (2006) *Mental Health Bill, 2006: Summary Guide.* London: DoH.

DoH (Department of Health) (2007) *Breaking Down Barriers: Clinical Case for Change. Report by Louis Appleby, National Director for Mental Health.* London: DoH.

DoH/DWP/HSE (2005) *Health, Work and Well-being: A Strategy for the Health and Well-being of Working Age People.* London: DoH.

DoH/Welsh Office (1999) *Code of Practice: Mental Health Act, 1983.* London: HMSO.

DWP (Department for Work and Pensions) (2004) *Framework for Vocational Rehabilitation.* London: DWP.

Eaton, J.W. (1951) The assessment of mental health, *American Journal of Psychiatry*, 108: 81–90.

Ford, R. (2005) The policy and service context for mental health nursing, in I. I. Norman and I. Ryrie (eds) *The Art and Science of Mental Health Nursing: A Textbook of Principles and Practice*, pp. 99–127. Maidenhead: Open University Press.

Guntrip, H. (1964) *Healing the Sick Mind.* London: Allen & Unwin.

Harrison, G., Owens, D., Holton, A., Nelson, D. and Boot, D. (1989) A prospective study of severe mental disorder in Afro-Caribbean patients, *Psychological Medicine*, 19: 683–96.

Hart, D.A. (2004) Common mental health problems, in S.D. Kirby, D.A. Hart, D. Cross and G. Mitchell (eds) *Mental Health Nursing: Competencies for Practice*, pp. 79–94. Basingstoke: Macmillan.

Holmes, T. and Rahe, R. (1967) The social readjustment rating scale, *Journal of Psychosomatic Research*, 11: 213–18.

Katona, C. and Robertson, M. (2000) *Psychiatry at a Glance*, 2nd edn. Oxford: Blackwell Science.

Kisley, S. and Goldberg, D. (1996) Physical and psychiatric comorbidity in general practice, *British Journal of Psychiatry*, 169: 236–42.

Lagerquist, S.L. (1997) *Psychiatric Mental Health: Care at a Glance.* New York: Lippincott.

Lloyd, P. and Moodley, P. (1992) Psychotropic medication and ethnicity: an inpatient survey, *Social Psychiatry and Psychiatric Epidemiology*, 27: 95–101.

NICE (National Institute for Health and Clinical Excellence) (2002) *Computerised Cognitive Behaviour Therapy for Depression and Anxiety.* London: NHS R&D HTA Programme, NICE.

NIMHE (National Institute for Mental Health in England) (2004) *Enhanced Services Specification for Depression Under the New GP Contract.* York: The National Primary Care Research and Development Centre and the University of York in partnership with the North West development centre of NIMHE.

NMC (Nursing and Midwifery Council) (2008) *Standards of Conduct, Performance and Ethics for Nurses and Midwives.* London: NMC.

Noonan, I. (2005) Therapeutic management of attempted suicide and self harm, in I. Norman and I. Ryrie (eds) *The Art and Science of Mental Health Nursing: A Textbook of Principles and Practice*, pp. 747–69. Maidenhead: Open University Press.

NSIP (National Social Inclusion Programme) (2006) *Vocational Services for People with Severe and Enduring Mental Health Problems: Commissioning Guidance.* London: NSIP.

Owen, S. and Milburn, C. (2001) Implementing research findings into practice: improving and developing services for women with severe and enduring mental health problems, *Journal of Psychiatric and Mental Health Nursing*, 8: 221–31.

Parsons, S. (1999) Working with depression, *Mental Health Practice*, 3(4): 32–6.

Perkins, R. and Rowland, L. (1991) Sex differences in service usage in long-term psychiatric care: are women adequately served? *British Journal of Psychiatry*, supplement 10, 158: 75–9.

Repper, J. and Perkins, R. (2002) *Social Inclusion and Recovery: A Model for Mental Health Practice.* Oxford: Baillière Tindall.

SCMH (Sainsbury Centre for Mental Health) (1998) *Keys to Engagement: Review of Care for People with Severe Mental Illness who are Difficult to Engage.* London: SCMH.

SCMH (Sainsbury Centre for Mental Health) (2002) *Breaking the Circles of Fear: A Review of the Relationship Between Mental Health Services and African and African Caribbean Communities.* London: SCMH.

Social Exclusion Unit (2004) *Mental Health and Social Exclusion.* London: ODPM.

Thornicroft, G., Davies, S. and Leese, M. (1999) Health services research and forensic psychiatry: a black and white case, *International Review of Psychiatry*, 11: 250–7.

Till, U. (2007) The values of recovery within mental health nursing, *Mental Health Practice*, 11(3): 32–6.

Townsend, P., Davidson, N. and Whitehead, M. (1992) *Inequalities in Health.* London: Penguin.

University of Manchester (2006) *Five Year Report of the National Confidential Inquiry into Suicide and Homicide by People with Mental Illness: Avoidable Deaths.* Manchester: University of Manchester.

Ussher, J. (1991) *Women's Madness: Misogyny or Mental Illness?* Hertford: Harvester Wheatsheaf.

Wilson, E.O. (2001) *On Human Nature.* London: Penguin.

Risk assessment: practicing accountably and responsibly

Nick Wrycraft

Learning objectives

By the end of this chapter you will have gained:

- An understanding of the concept of risk applied to mental health and illness.
- An appreciation of the relationship of risk, responsibility and mental health.
- Knowledge of risk management in mental health nursing.
- An appreciation of practice-based risk assessment.
- An appreciation of the value of positive risk.

Introduction

Risk assessment is one of the most important areas of the work of mental health nurses. Due to the highly varied situations encountered in practice and the many different forms that 'risk' assumes, it is not possible to provide clear guidelines. Instead this chapter encourages you to integrate the skills we possess as people and that we use in our daily lives with a nursing-focused framework of assessment. Through using this approach we can justify observations and interventions and develop appropriate risk management strategies when working with people with mental health problems.

The role of the mental health nurse involves identifying where risk is present for people experiencing mental health problems and so we begin by considering the issues of risk, responsibility and mental health. However, at the same time mental health services are increasingly concerned to optimize the autonomy of service users. Balancing these competing considerations is a complex yet important challenge. We then consider the recent emergence of risk assessment as a priority within NHS organizations.

The chapter will then shift focus to the practice setting and discuss risk assessment in mental health services, and outline a suitable framework to guide the appraisal of risk before considering risk management interventions. Finally, we explore risk assessment in practice, focusing on issues including communication, confidentiality and positive risk-taking before ending with an overview of the chapter.

The discussion will involve practice-based scenarios from inpatient settings. This is for two reasons: risk assessment is frequently prevalent among the reasons for admitting people to inpatient care, and scenarios from the inpatient setting offer a 'close up' and detailed focus on people with mental health problems which is only possible in such a setting. However, it is expected that the principles of risk assessment and management which are discussed can be transferred to any practice setting. Answers to the scenarios are provided at the end of the book. Exercises will assist you to identify areas of learning which can be developed through further reading, reflection on practice experience and the identification of action points to facilitate learning.

An understanding of risk

Whether we are aware of it or not, we are expert risk assessors and are constantly engaged in a highly sophisticated risk assessment process. In everyday decisions we assess and mange risk all the time. For example, simply leaving our home and crossing the road involves a complex array of decisions and actions to ensure our safety.

As student nurses, before applying risk assessment skills to a practice setting, it is helpful to consider how we perceive risk in our own lives.

Our personal response to risk

The intention of this exercise is to encourage you to consider how you have reacted in a situation where risk was present, rather than responding to a high level of danger. Think of a time when you were either frightened, or in a dangerous but non-life-threatening situation. Write down the circumstances of the situation.

- What were you thinking?
- How did you feel?
- How did you react?
- What was the outcome of the situation?
- How do you feel about it now?
- Is there anything you would have done differently?

Often in these situations time seems to pass very quickly or to slow down. In some cases people also act in a certain way which helped the situation but they do not know why.

Reflect on the above and consider whether your 'fight or flight' instinct was active in the example you have chosen and if so, how was it evident? What have you learned about how you respond in risky situations? Now place your notes in your professional portfolio.

The relationship of risk, responsibility and mental health

In our lives we are responsible for our behaviour and conduct. Where our behaviour transgresses the rules of society there are laws determined by the government to protect those around us. These are enforced by the police and the courts.

Even in the case of impetuous or spontaneous acts, while there may be some consideration of mitigating factors, the individual bears responsibility for their actions. However, this system rests on the premise that as individuals we are responsible for our actions. The legislation regarding mental health has evolved over time to reflect a balance of the consideration of both health and justice. In English and Welsh law, if a person's judgement is impaired as a result of mental illness it is required for there to be adequate and suitable provision made for the treatment and care of the person and to preserve the safety and protection of the general public (DoH/Welsh Office 1999; DoH 2006).

Within the law the knowing refusal to accept treatment is valid even where the person has a mental health problem, if their refusal is based on an understanding unimpaired by mental illness. Therefore a person who is mentally ill can still refuse mental health treatment. In instances where mental illness impedes the person's capacity to consent and the person needs urgent mental health treatment, there is legal provision under the Mental Health Act 2007.

The current balance of the law protecting the public and providing care and treatment as necessary for mentally ill offenders has generally been regarded as fair and equal, both respecting and preserving the rights and responsibilities of the individual and the general public. This would appear to have been substantiated by the findings of the recent eight-year multi-stakeholder review of the Mental Health Act 1983, which only chose to make amendments to the legislation rather than wholesale revisions. The changes that were made, such as widening the definition of mental illness, extended the spirit of the legislation by ensuring mental health care will become accessible to more people than previously (DoH 2006).

A mental health student says ...

My first ever placement was a low secure acute inpatient setting. I was incredibly nervous starting the course with my first ever placement being in an area caring for individuals who were acutely unwell. Initially the ward was very daunting and almost intimidating. However, after one shift I was at ease.

My mentor was brilliant as she always ensured that I had a debriefing after any specific incidents. My ward manager played a huge part in me being accepted on the ward. He made me feel part of the team from day one, which boosted my confidence and resulted in me presenting as more professional to the clients.

In terms of assessing propensity towards risk-related behaviour, it is necessary to understand the way in which the world may appear to the person and how mental health problems can lead to the display of certain behaviours. Through gaining close insight it is possible to begin to appreciate how the problem affects the person, the risks to which they are prone and how the nurse can best support them, while minimizing risk at the same time.

Mental illness and risk

People with mental health problems experience particular kinds of risk directly due to their illness. A person's awareness of potential sources of danger around them can be heightened or reduced. Spend a few minutes considering the two scenarios below. On a piece of paper under the headings of Scenario 1 and Scenario 2, write down your answers to each of the two questions for both of the examples.

Scenario 1

If you have ever watched a film about a conspiracy theory, try to imagine this has suddenly become a reality and there is a secret plot to silence you speaking out. Being apprehended by the police and taken to a mental health unit is likely to add to the evidence supporting your delusional beliefs. If you feel there is a risk to your well-being and these people mean to do you harm, you are likely to not believe their reassurance, and believe they are lying to you. People may be trying to placate you, or not listening to what you are trying to tell them, or appreciating the importance of the conspiracy.

Now, switching character from the person experiencing the problem to the perspective of the nursing staff, consider the following.

- What might be the risks to the person in this situation?
- What response from the nursing staff can help or empower the person in this situation?

Scenario 2

If a person is experiencing advanced stages of cognitive impairment their ability to manage a safe environment also becomes impaired. Imagine you cannot judge distances or react to physical risks. You are sitting at a table with a hot meal in front of you. You feel hungry but cannot understand how to use the cutlery beside the plate.

Now, switching to the perspective of the nurse again, consider the following.

- What are the risks for the person when eating?
- How can the nurse provide support which empowers the person, respects their dignity yet will also represent a psychosocial interaction?

Now place your notes in your professional portfolio.

Both people in the scenarios above would be regarded as experiencing an acute mental health problem, and it is likely they will require significant support from the mental health services to improve their well-being.

The importance of risk assessment in mental health services

Following a number of high profile tragedies concerning people with mental health problems and the inquiries which followed, there has been a concerted effort in recent years to improve the effectiveness of mental health services in identifying and reducing risk (DoH 1999).

As a result the CPA (Care Programme Approach) was developed from a wish to increase communication of information between different disciplines; to encourage more organized care with identified lines of responsibility; and to ensure a named individual practitioner acts as the CPA coordinator (Morgan and Wetherell 2005; Salter and Turner 2008). Furthermore the *National Service Framework for Mental Health* identified reducing the number of suicides as a central priority of services (DoH 1999). As a result of these initiatives significant improvements have occurred, and there has been a noticeable and continuing reduction in the number of suicides (University of Manchester 2006).

Supporters point out that the CPA has become established as an effective system providing a useful framework and process of documentation throughout the mental health services. It has also successfully promoted the effective coordination and planning of services, while offering people with mental health problems and their carers and families the expectation of a specific standard of service for their needs. However, critics argue that the scrupulous completion of paperwork does not represent the delivery of effective care or any reduction of the actual level of risk which may be present (Salter and Turner 2008). Experienced mental health nurses often express the opinion that the increased emphasis on recording risk achieves government targets and records their activities, yet wastes their extensive skills in working with individuals who have mental health problems.

While it is a crucially important aspect of mental health nursing, risk assessment generates uncertainty and anxiety not only within individuals but also organizations. Even with the completion of extensive documentation, when there are untoward events it is argued that apportioning blame is a characteristic of modern cultures within the public services (Morgan and Wetherell 2005). In this environment there is the potential for mental health nurses to feel vulnerable and at the mercy of competing pressures between their professional obligations towards service users on the one hand, and the expectations incumbent upon them as employees to record risk on the other. While poor performance ought never to be excused, instead it is better to promote reasonable accountability and rational assessment of risk, and this is within the spirit of the CPA and in accordance with the standards and professional values of nursing (NMC 2008).

While as nurses we seek to promote the safety of people with mental health problems, some present a high and continuous level of risk which is often how they come into contact with mental health services in the first place. The answer is not to abandon risk assessment and management as it is clear that focusing on this as a priority has yielded results. Instead it is necessary that we carefully consider how we can reasonably and accountably use our skills to assess and manage risk within our role as mental health nurses. Therefore the most effective risk assessment is as part of an overall care assessment and should not be viewed as separate from other aspects of care but part of the overall process, and integral to the nursing role.

How risk assessment contributes to mental health nursing

While trusts will have specific policies and procedures and uniform systems of paperwork guiding the management and recording of risk, the exact form of risk assessment will vary depending on the specific nature of the clinical environment. For example, day hospital risk assessments will differ from community mental health teams and inpatient settings based on the different forms of interaction. Also, some specific areas of risk will be relevant to specific individuals depending on their mental and physical health status.

Risk in mental health can be grouped into a number of specific categories, as shown in the next panel.

Categories of risk

- Suicide.
- Violence and or aggression.
- Self-harm.
- Neglect.

Each of these categories is considered in greater depth in the next panel to identify which factors may lead a person to be considered to be of higher risk in each area. The list is not intended to be definitive, as there may be additional factors; or it may be felt that the presence of some of these factors do not predispose the person to be at risk. Accurate risk assessment ought to focus on the individual being assessed and be flexible in order to accurately identify relevant risk factors, and the extent and way in which they are active in the person's life.

Risk assessment

Suicide

- Expresses helplessness/hopelessness.
- Expresses the belief they cannot control their life.
- Lives alone with no significant others (is bereaved of a spouse, or partner) and has a limited social network.
- Has recently experienced significant life events (e.g. loss of a close relative, redundancy or divorce).
- Is unemployed/retired.
- Has expressed a wish to commit suicide.
- Evidence of plans to end their life.
- Previous suicide attempts.
- A family history of suicide.

Violence/aggression

- Evidence of previous violent incidents and acts (possible previous criminal convictions or admission to secure settings).
- A tendency towards dangerous behaviour.
- Has committed impulsive acts.
- Expressing a wish to harm others.
- Access to, and or use of, weapons.
- Has identifiable paranoid delusions relating to others.
- Experiences 'command hallucinations'.

- Has an interest in violent fantasies.
- Evidence of sexually inappropriate behaviour.

Self-harm

Often self-harm occurs in the form of repeated or focused self-injury to specific parts of the body. In particular, damage to the skin in the form of cutting or burning may be noticeable. However, often as a result of shame self-harm can occur secretively to areas of the body which are not visible and may be focused on the upper legs or genitalia. Self-harm can take numerous different forms including the breaking of bones, hair pulling, insertion of needles or objects beneath the skin and eating disorders (Noonan 2005).

Neglect

Neglect might be noticeable over a period of time by the person stopping their behaviours or not acting as they might normally. For example, a person who was very tidy and house-proud no longer cleans their home. Other areas where neglect may be evident include:

- Not meeting the need for hydration adequate to maintain health.
- Not meeting the need for nutrition suitable to maintain health.
- Not meeting the need for elimination (going to the toilet).
- Not maintaining hygiene.
- Not changing clothing or wearing inappropriate clothing and not dressing appropriately to the season of the year.
- Living in accommodation which does not have a suitable supply of water, heating and light and suitable sanitation and hygiene (an appropriate kitchen and toilet).
- Experiencing financial difficulties (Morgan and Wetherell 2005).

The framework shown in the next panel provides a structure within which we can identify how a particular risk is active within the person's life, and also the likelihood of the risk occurring. Where relevant to the individual, the areas of risk outlined above can be mapped against each of the headings in the framework on the next page to provide a comprehensive examination of how risk is relevant to the person.

Risk assessment framework: applying theory to practice

Context   Significant changes to an individual's circumstances affect their predisposition to risk. Yet while for one person inpatient admission may lead them to be more likely to self-harm, another person may feel more secure and reassured.

Environment   The person's surroundings are influential in affecting their mood and behaviour but also influence their exposure to hazards, for example, violence or abuse.

Predictability   If the person has a previous history of risk-related behaviour, does the risk form a pattern? Alternatively, does the person appear to present a predisposition to risk-related behaviour?

Evidence and research   Demographic factors are important. For example, males under 35 are at risk of using violent methods of suicide (University of Manchester 2006). While characteristics of mental health problems are useful indicators of potential risk, people with bipolar disorder frequently behave impulsively and are *also* at risk of suicide.

The above factors ought to be cross-referenced in order to be able to view the person accurately in their circumstances. It is also worth remembering the person's risk profile will change over time and therefore it is necessary to frequently review the risk assessment in order for it to remain relevant (Morgan and Wetherell 2005).

Effective risk assessment also depends on *communication* with the service user in order to identify what is a concern for the person and how it affects them. The risk assessment will only be accurate if the person with a mental health problem participates in an open and trusting relationship with the mental health nurse and engages willingly in the process.

While it may not always be feasible in the clinical environment to carry out a comprehensive risk assessment, it is desirable for the mental health nurse to have:

- read the service user's notes and case history in detail, including any previous risk assessments;
- the opportunity to discuss risk with the service user; often this will form part of the overall nursing assessment;

- a discussion concerning possible areas of risk with the service user's carer, husband/wife or significant other; again this may form part of the overall nursing assessment;
- knowledge of whether any other professionals are involved in the person's care and if so to discuss their level of risk with those professionals.

Having considered the process by which risk is identified we will progress to explore how risk is managed in the mental health setting.

Risk management in mental health nursing interventions

Risk management concerns the actions taken to address and minimize risk based on the information emerging from a risk assessment. It may be felt that this involves regarding service users with suspicion or as a source of threat. Yet it is important to remember that in accordance with our duty to care as registered professionals it is our obligation to assess risk, while often as a result of the effects of mental illness people do not prioritize or actively seek to place themselves at risk (NMC 2008). Even within a risk management framework the role of the mental health nurse is still therapeutic. The scenario below outlines a positive example of practice carried out by a student.

Scenario: Paul

Paul is a 24-year-old third-year mental health student nurse. He has been placed on an adult mental health inpatient unit for adults aged 16–70. The unit is a ward for service users who have agreed to be admitted and are informal admissions, as well as people who are compulsorily detained under the Mental Health Act 2007. Paul has been on the unit for two months, and, while finding it challenging, has enjoyed the experience. He has worked frequently with his mentor who was satisfied that Paul was a highly competent student.

Three weeks ago John was admitted. John is 28 years old with a long history of schizophrenic illness and drug misuse. He had a council flat, but many of his friends and acquaintances also lived there, often making lots of noise and playing loud music late at night, and in spite of repeated warnings John did not ask them to leave and was evicted for antisocial behaviour. He then lived in various squats in the locality and was recently found by police wandering, confused and in a dishevelled state and agreed to be admitted to the unit voluntarily.

Paul had not worked directly with John before although he noted that he would often be pleasant in conversation with the staff, but could change rapidly and become threatening and argumentative, making personal remarks and appear to be close to violent behaviour.

Paul was working a late shift and allocated to be John's keyworker for the first time under the supervision of his mentor. Shortly after handover Paul went and spoke to John and advised him he was his keyworker for the shift. He tactfully enquired what John's plans were for the afternoon. John replied that he was not sure but was a bit bored on the unit.

Shortly after this, John approached Paul and asked if he could have individual time. The unit operates a policy where 45 minutes' individual time is allocated for service users with their keyworkers per shift. Paul was surprised, as John had never made use of individual time before, but John went on to explain that he had no money as his benefit was due the next day and as it was raining and cold he could not go out, so wanted to talk.

Paul mentioned to his mentor that John has asked for individual time, which was unusual. Paul's mentor agreed that it was, but in discussion it was decided that Paul would provide John's individual time.

Paul advised the other staff where he would be and then found a small interview room and sat opposite the window but still closer to the door than John; he was visible from the main lounge on the unit where at least one member of staff was permanently situated. Paul also had a personal alarm which he had tested at the beginning of the shift to ensure it was working.

Paul felt nervous and not sure how he could help John. John began speaking immediately. Paul had read John's notes and knew of his mental health history and family background, but much of what John told him was not in his notes. John stated he had never known his father but his mother had remarried a soldier and the family had frequently moved around, often to foreign countries with his stepfather's postings. John explained that was why he liked to wear military-style clothes and boots. John had two step-siblings but they had never got along. John was bullied at school and as the family kept moving never settled. He left school with no qualifications and moved back to where he had been born, losing contact with his family. He then explained how he began to experience the onset of his schizophrenic illness, came to use drugs and began stealing to finance his drug use; as a result he got into trouble with the police.

After an hour John stopped talking. He said he wanted to go and read the newspaper before tea. John shook Paul's hand and thanked him for letting him talk.

After the meeting Paul felt there were some issues he wished to discuss. He made a brief but detailed entry into John's case notes and asked to speak to his mentor before the end of the shift.

When meeting with his mentor Paul explained he was initially anxious about John's potential for aggression as he had found him intimidating when observing him on the unit, but this anxiety was also due to a lack of personal confidence in his professional role and doubts over his inexperience and whether he had the therapeutic skills to be able to help John. In hindsight Paul felt the meeting with John had been an excellent learning experience and an opportunity to build his confidence, yet had also been a positive therapeutic experience for John. Paul was glad he had agreed to continue with the meeting and not allowed his doubts to take precedence.

The mentor reflected to Paul that sometimes it just helps to listen, and that John obviously felt Paul was someone who could listen. Paul related the practical measures he had taken to risk manage the situation. His mentor felt that Paul had shown good presence of mind to take these actions and had assessed the situation correctly. He asked Paul how he would have acted if John had suddenly become hostile or aggressive, and on thinking about this Paul remembered often seeing the other staff remain calm and use an even tone of voice, but continue to use open body language, to try and help where possible, but to observe trust policy and the rules of the unit.

● Write down a list of the measures Paul took to assess the risk John presented.

Place your notes in your professional portfolio.

It is important when implementing risk management interventions that we reflect afterwards on whether they have been successful and whether we managed the situation appropriately, and what were the most effective choices of action. Evaluation can be through reflecting individually, with colleagues and mentors or other team members. Handovers, team meetings, ward reviews and multidisciplinary meetings also provide useful forums at which to discuss these issues.

Reflecting on such events allows feelings of anxiety to be worked through but also successes and achievements to be appreciated. Furthermore, the majority of mental health nursing occurs within teams and conscious effort needs to be invested to build good communication, trust and support, and positive regard. It is only through discussions which reflect on and evaluate practice that we can explore ideas and approaches, share information and also develop effective team approaches to care.

It is worth considering different levels of risk interventions which can be regarded as spanning three areas, as shown below.

Types of risk management

Preventative

This is the most proactive form of risk management and involves acting to avert potential risk situations from developing. An example might be when working with a community mental health team arranging appointments with a service user who has a known history of violence and illicit drug use on trust premises and while there are other staff in the building.

Interventionist

In this form of risk management actions are taken to de-escalate a situation where a risk is beginning to become apparent. An example would be where an argument is occurring between two service users on an inpatient unit and neither party is willing to admit they are wrong and both are becoming increasingly angry. The staff might intervene by taking the individuals to one side in order to calm down.

Post-incident response

It is necessary to regard all incidents as opportunities to learn and inform future practice. An example might be on an inpatient unit where a service user has engaged in self-harm and at the end of the shift in handover the ward team reflect on the experience and identify how they might have approached the situation differently. It is important to retain a balanced view, to work as a team and support one another to promote positive teamwork and avoid a blaming culture. In some cases debriefing after critical incidents will be planned some weeks afterwards to allow the staff to reflect (Morgan and Hemming 1999).

Practice-based risk assessment in mental health nursing

In this section of the chapter we will discuss practice-based risk assessment. In practice settings the assessment of people's mental health needs often occurs in hectic circumstances where a number of different events are occurring simultaneously. Mental health nurses utilize a high level of complex skills involving time management, prioritization, of tasks, communication, negotiation, teamwork, management of staff and accessing support, together with awareness and involvement of the skills and knowledge of other team members.

From a student perspective, gaining an understanding of how mental health teams work is essential in developing an understanding of practice-based risk assessment and helps to identify how to provide safe and effective care for service users (RCN 2002).

Scenario: James

You are a student placed on an adult mental health unit which cares for a maximum of 15 male and female adults aged 16–70, with a mix of service users, some admitted voluntarily and others detained under a section of the Mental Health Act 2007.

James is a 24-year-old male and the younger of two brothers. He never knew his father although his mother told them he had been violent and an alcoholic. When James was 14 his mother died of bowel cancer and having no close family or relatives the brothers fended for themselves. James left school with no qualifications and went to work in a factory. When his older brother left home to live with his girlfriend, James remained living alone in the family's council-owned home.

James became interested in martial arts and engaged in a number of competitive events and won competitions and championships. Eventually he tired of the discipline required in training and gave up four years ago.

Lacking interests and friends James felt low in mood and took to habitually drinking large quantities of alcohol, taking drugs and avoiding contact with people. James began to hear voices telling him people were plotting against him and that there was a conspiracy between television companies, the media and the government. To warn other people about this, James painted a message on the front of the block of flats where he lived. When he also went round telling his neighbours they laughed at him, and James began to believe they were also part of the plot and became suspicious of them as well.

Council officials called on James to discuss the message he had painted on the wall of the flats. James believed they were a part of the conspiracy and threw them out. He argued with contractors who were removing the message from the wall and the police were called. The police brought James to the mental health inpatient unit where you are placed as a student. While James did not resist he was highly suspicious and confused about what was happening to him.

- Which aspects of James's story have particular relevance with regards to risk?
- Reflect on, and then write down, how the ward team might begin to engage with James.

Place your notes in your professional portfolio.

Communication of risk

Throughout this chapter it has been emphasized that risk assessment should not occur in isolation but be integrated within all mental health nursing activity. Communication is a crucial element which links together mental health nursing interventions and effective risk assessment. Sharing assessment of risk with other multidisciplinary staff will ensure that care is consistent. Through discussion all of the members of a team will be aware of the existence of particular kinds of risk, the threat posed and methods of managing the risk. Good communication also allows sudden changes and new developments to be communicated within the team.

Promoting a culture of preventative risk management allows for the early detection of danger and through recording 'near misses' swift action can be taken to learn from mistakes and avoid their recurrence in the future. Where an incident has occurred, support can then be accessed and appropriate action taken.

Effective risk assessment depends on the observations of the assessor. If the actions of an individual cause you to experience concern, anxiety or fear, what is it about their behaviour which leads you to feel this way? Interpreting our own feelings and intuitions is an important part of self-awareness. Alternatively it is often helpful for two people to conduct a risk assessment in order to discuss their views and arrive at a conclusion. Very experienced mental health nurses are able to articulate their impressions accurately and succinctly.

Scenario: Andy

Cassie is a first year mental health nursing student on placement at a day hospital. She has been on the placement for three weeks and attended a number of group sessions. One service user called Andy, who attends regularly, asks if he can mention something to Cassie confidentially.

Caught unawares, Cassie is unsure what to say and before she can reply Andy tells Cassie he has a gun at his home. Cassie asks for more information but at that point someone comes into the room and Andy ends the conversation.

- What response should Cassie make to Andy when he asks if she can keep his disclosure confidential?
- What should Cassie do when Andy reveals he has the gun?
- Write down the different options and then identify which you think is the most appropriate and why.
- Discuss this dilemma with your mentor.

Place your notes in your professional portfolio.

The notion of risk as inextricably bound up with the role of the mental health nurse ought to mean that risk assessment is not a dispassionate appraisal of the service user's propensity to self-harm or harm others. Risk assessment can perform a positive role and be used to encourage the person with a mental health problem to take control and influence their own lives.

Positive risk

Positive risk-taking is identified as good practice in mental health nursing (DoH 2004). A key role of the mental health nurse is to promote autonomy, social inclusion and to actively encourage the person with a mental health problem to use their capacity to make decisions in their lives and view risk assessment from a positive perspective. One method of achieving this goal is to make the person aware of their choices of action in certain situations. In this respect the power and responsibility for choice lie with the person. However, this requires their having the capacity to make rational choices which are not impaired by their mental illness.

The scenario below considers the promotion of positive risk-taking in an acute setting and the questions which follow draw your attention to a range of mental health nursing issues.

Scenario: Stephanie (I)

Stephanie is 35 years old and until recently appeared to have had a happy and successful life. She did well at school and gained a university degree, then married at 22 and had a successful job with a bank.

However, seven years ago Stephanie revealed that she had experienced sexual abuse from the father of a school friend when she was a teenager. She explained that she was reminded of the abuse after reading of the death of the friend's father in a road accident in the local newspaper, having not thought about it for a number of years. Following her disclosure of the abuse her relationship with her husband deteriorated, eventually breaking down and they separated four years ago. Stephanie became very withdrawn and was diagnosed with depression. Having taken a long time off work she felt unable to return and lost her job.

Stephanie tried unsuccessfully to commit suicide with an overdose of pills. In spite of input from a community psychiatric nurse and supportive friends, on returning home from hospital, Stephanie began cutting herself with knives and on several occasions has been taken to the A&E department with severe self-inflicted lacerations.

Recently a friend found Stephanie at her home having taken an overdose of prescribed medication and with severe cuts to her wrists. Stephanie was assessed by a mental health liaison nurse at the A&E department and reluctantly agreed to an informal admission to an inpatient mental health unit. In her admission interview she stated that she felt there was no purpose in living but that she had no plans to end her life. On admission, through agreement with the staff, her belongings were checked and any knives and sharp objects removed. Stephanie also agreed with the staff that she would not self-harm, and if she experienced a wish to do so would speak to her allocated nurse. It was agreed she would be cared for on general level of observations (rather than, for example, one-to-one observations).

During her first night on the unit Stephanie was found in her room having made severe cuts to her wrist and stomach with a blade removed from a pencil sharpener she had brought onto the unit.

- Read the scenario again and consider how we distinguish self-harming behaviour from suicidal behaviour. Refer to suitable books, journals, websites and other sources of nursing knowledge, and identify how these types of behaviour differ, are similar, or overlap. Write down your findings and reference any sources of literature you used to support the points made.
- Are there any differences in the predisposing risk factors to suicide and self-harm?
- Has the understanding you have gained of self-harming and suicidal behaviour changed your understanding of Stephanie's case?
- Write down what changes might be made to Stephanie's care plans after the recent incident of self-harm and identify the rationale(s) for these.
- How has Stephanie been involved in collaboration on her care? Does the care she has received empower her? Write down your opinion and explain the reason(s) why.
- Finally, reflect on this scenario. Imagine you are a student mental health nurse placed on the inpatient mental health unit to which Stephanie has been admitted and have received the early shift handover after the most recent incident of Stephanie self-harming. Consider your emotions and feelings about the scenario as a person and professional, then identify outcomes and changes which can be made to Stephanie's care in order to manage risk and promote her mental health.

Now place your notes in your professional portfolio.

In the above scenario the positive risk of Stephanie agreeing to notify staff if she experienced a wish to self-harm was not successful. However, this is no reason to assume that positive risk-taking is not effective and ought to be abandoned. Below we will find out what happened next in Stephanie's case.

Scenario: Stephanie (II)

Following the incident of self-harm Stephanie was placed on Section 2 of the Mental Health Act which lasts for 28 days and is for the purposes of assessment of the person's mental health. She was maintained on close observation and did not engage with staff. On some occasions she was noted to bang her head and scalded herself with hot tea in one instance. At the ward review after a week of close observation Stephanie refused to speak or make eye contact. After two weeks of close observation she was referred to be assessed by a specialist self-harm unit in another area which functions as a therapeutic community.

While waiting for the assessment, in discussion with her keyworker Stephanie agreed that if the close observation was withdrawn she would not self-harm. The ward team discussed the situation with the psychiatrist and unit manager and it was agreed for the close observation to be withdrawn.

Stephanie did not self-harm when the close observation was withdrawn. The referral to the therapeutic community was withdrawn and eventually she was discharged and went back to her home and continued to be supported by a community psychiatric nurse and to attend the day hospital.

The length of time during which people may be severely unwell can be a protracted period. Yet recovery is not a static concept but varies from person to person. What constitutes significant evidence of recovery will differ for each individual.

Therefore the role of the mental health nurse is to offer continued support and interventions which are flexible to the person's need, while nevertheless promoting and considering their safety and well-being. In spite of the professional knowledge of the nurse it is important to remember that in many cases the person with the mental health problem is the only one who can make the choice to bring about change to their circumstances and improvement in their mental health.

Conclusion

In this chapter we have considered risk assessment and risk management as concepts within nursing and applied them to the practice placement setting. A characteristic of risk in a practice-based profession such as nursing is that professional training will not equip students with all the answers to all the situations they will encounter because they are so many and varied. As people we are expert at assessing risk in our daily lives and it is important to reflect on how these skills can be used in our practice. Together with these skills a

number of tools and aspects of knowledge can assist you to understand situations from a risk perspective and to focus on the person at that point in time as a unique individual. Working with practice mentors will develop your skills and understanding to arrive at a professional perspective on risk while also becoming aware of the expectations of risk assessment and management on professionals by trusts and employers.

As we have identified, risk assessment is not something which should be seen as separate from nursing care. There is a danger that health care professionals may become preoccupied with calculating risk. We can become victim to the misconception that documenting risk removes the danger it imposes or make only very safe decisions which limit the capacity for the person's mental health to improve.

Instead the principles of mental health nursing applied to risk are to promote empowerment and social inclusion and the making of independent choices by people with mental health problems. Often risk assessment involves balancing these considerations against the potential and actual levels of risk. Effective risk assessment requires working responsibly and accountably, yet also the application of skill and experience, and for there to be clear and logical rationales supporting our interventions and actions.

References

DoH (Department of Health) (1999) *National Service Framework for Mental Health: Modern Standards and Service Models*. London: DoH.

DoH (Department of Health) (2004) *The Ten Essential Shared Capabilities: A Framework for the Whole of the Mental Health Workforce*. London: DoH.

DoH (Department of Health) (2006) *Mental Health Bill, 2006: Summary Guide*. London: DoH.

DoH (Department of Health)/Welsh Office (1999) *Code of Practice: Mental Health Act, 1983*. London: HMSO.

Morgan, S. and Hemming, M. (1999) Balancing care and control: risk management and compulsory community treatment, *Mental Health and Learning Disabilities Care*, 3(1): 19–21.

Morgan, S. and Wetherell, A. (2005) Assessing and managing risk, in I. Norman and I. Ryrie (eds) *The Art and Science of Mental Health Nursing: A Textbook of Principles and Practice*, pp. 208–40. Maidenhead: Open University Press.

NMC (Nursing and Midwifery Council) (2008) *Standards of Conduct, Performance and Ethics for Nurses and Midwives*. London: NMC.

Noonan, I. (2005) Therapeutic management of attempted suicide and self-harm, in I. Norman and I. Ryrie (eds) *The Art and Science of Mental Health Nursing: A Textbook of Principles and Practice*, pp. 747–69. Maidenhead: Open University Press.

Royal College of Nursing (RCN) (2002) *Helping Students Get the Best from their Practice Placements: A Royal College of Nursing Toolkit*. London: RCN.

Salter, M. and Turner, T. (2008) *Community Mental Health Care: A Practical Guide to Outdoor Psychiatry*. London: Elsevier Churchill Livingstone.

University of Manchester (2006) *Five Year Report of the National Confidential Inquiry into Suicide and Homicide by People with Mental Illness: Avoidable Deaths*. Manchester: University of Manchester.

Mental health nursing and the law

5

James Trueman and Richard Khoo

Learning objectives

By the end of this chapter you will have:

- Gained an understanding of the current legislation relevant to mental health nursing.
- Developed an insight into issues of consent and treatment for mental health problems.
- Gained an appreciation of how issues of legality are present in decision-making in the practice area.

Introduction

This chapter will focus on the law concerning mental illness. It is important to know about the law and mental health as in many clinical settings we will be working with people whose mental health conditions make this a relevant considera-tion. The law regarding mental illness is also very specific and so understanding how and in what circumstances it applies will avoid infringing the person's rights. There are also certain legally required expectations on us as mental health nurses. These include always working to empower the person yet also advocating on their behalf and making them aware of their rights to be able to make informed choices.

This chapter will focus on recent developments in the legislation concerning mental health, examining the most common legislation you are likely to encounter in mental health nursing set-tings: the Mental Health Act 1983 (amended 2007), the Human Rights Act 1998 and the Mental Capa-city Act 2005. The discussion then considers how decisions are made in the practice setting. A brief conclusion is then provided summarizing the issues discussed.

Practice-focused scenarios and examples are used to demonstrate the professional and ethical complexities of the issues being discussed. It is necessary to point out that this chapter covers the law concerning *England and Wales* and does not include Scotland which has for many years enacted its own mental health legislation.

Background

For hundreds of years there has been provision within the law for the care of the mentally ill. Periodically there have been developments and revisions of this legislation, often in response to public pressure to redress abuses, yet also to reflect changing views and opinions within society about how the mentally ill should be treated.

It is worth remembering that not everyone receiving mental health services is subject to mental health legislation. Often on open inpatient units there are people who are voluntary or informal admissions alongside people who are formally detained under the Mental Health Act 1983. The Mental Health Act is used where the person does not agree that they have a mental health problem and will not accept treatment for their mental illness. In these circumstances the person might, after assessment by appropriately trained mental health professionals, be deemed to require compulsory mental health care.

An important point to remember is that more restrictions apply to people who are formally detained than those who are informally admitted. For example, a person who is an informal admis-sion can discharge themselves at any time, while people detained under the Mental Health Act can only be discharged with the agreement of the appropriate health care professional. Therefore if we are to practice effectively and within the law we need to be aware of the person's status with regards to the law and the conditions which apply.

The reason why this chapter discusses three major pieces of legislation relating to mental health is that each Act serves a very specific purpose with regards to a different aspect of mental health.

When does the Mental Health Act apply?

The Mental Health Act 1983 applies when a person with a mental health problem refuses to accept necessary treatment for their mental health. It also applies in circumstances where a person presents a risk to their own well-being and/or others or is vulnerable as a result of their mental illness. The purpose of the Act is not to punish the person but to ensure they receive appropriate care and treatment which as a minimum requirement prevents further deterioration of their mental health. A further consideration is to protect the person's rights and independence and wherever possible the least restrictive option will be chosen.

The Human Rights Act 1998 was created to protect universal liberties and the freedom of the individual. The Act applies to numerous areas of society and citizenship. However, there is a particular relevance to mental health where in some instances it is necessary to deprive a person of their liberty due to mental illness for the purposes of providing them with mental health care. Increasingly the focus of the Mental Health Act 1983 has emphasized encouraging people who are compulsorily detained against their will to apply for independent tribunal reviews of these decisions to promote transparency and accountable decision-making.

Finally the Mental Capacity Act 2005 focuses on how people make decisions concerning health care. Often where people are experiencing a severe mental health problem, identifying their wishes and choices in advance of a time when they cannot express a preference is an important principle which this Act has been introduced to protect.

The Mental Health Act 2007

The 1983 Mental Health Act was amended by a further Act passed in 2007 and which came into force in 2008. The main changes it introduced are outlined below.

- Previously there were four categories of mental disorder. These were: mental illness; mental impairment; severe mental impairment; and psychopathic disorder. This has now been replaced by a single definition of mental illness that simply states that it is: ' . . . any disorder or disability of mind'.
- A new 'treatability test' has been introduced, creating a principle of 'appropriate treatment' based not necessarily on improving health but on preventing the disorder worsening. This concept is crucially important as, for example, some people with personality disorders were previously denied care due to a lack of effective treatment being available for their condition and this is now no longer the case.
- Supervised Community Treatment Orders (CTOs) now make it possible to manage the care of people with mental health problems living in the community. Within the provisions of a CTO the person could be subject to recall to hospital if it is deemed necessary. However, if the person's mental health improves sufficiently, the order can be revoked.
- The range of practitioners who can implement the legislation has been broadened from psychiatrists and approved social workers (ASWs) to include any mental health care professionals with appropriate training.
- All people under the age of 18 in inpatient mental health services must be accommodated in an age-appropriate setting subject to their needs.
- All people compulsorily detained under the Mental Health Act 1983 are to be advised, encouraged and supported in exercising their right to an independent review by the Mental Health Review Tribunal.
- Under the provisions of the Mental Health Act 2007 it is now required that information on how to access the advocacy service is provided to all detained patients.

- Additional new safeguards have also been introduced concerning the use of electro-convulsive therapy (ECT). For those who are under 18 a second appointed doctor's approval is required whether or not the person consents to ECT and regardless of whether they are an informal admission or detained under the Mental Health Act 1983.
- A civil partner can be named as the person's next of kin in the same way a spouse was previously recognized. People can also apply to a court to displace their nearest relative and nominate their own choice of replacement.
- Finally, a person with parental responsibility will not be able to override the consent or refusal of consent made by a child aged 16 or 17 with regard to their wish to be admitted to hospital.

The Human Rights Act 1998

The Human Rights Act came into force in 2000 and incorporates most of the provisions of the European Convention on Human Rights within English law. The Human Rights Act protects our basic human rights in a number of articles. There are four articles with particular relevance to the care and treatment of people with a mental health problem. These are:

- Article 2 – the right to life.
- Article 3 – the prohibition of torture.
- Article 5 – the right to liberty and security.
- Article 8 – the right to respect for private and family life.

We will now discuss how each of these articles relates to mental health.

While every person has the right to a safe health care environment which would not place their life at risk, Article 2 has also been used to secure legal protection for the participant in an assisted suicide – for example in the case of Dianne Pretty. In this case it was argued that her inability to end her life was a breach of Articles 2 and 3. However, in this case the court determined these Articles as referring to the *preservation of a person's life and dignity* and not their right to their own death.

Within mental health care it is sometimes necessary to detain someone against their wishes

for their own well-being or due to the risk they present to others. This many appear to contradict Article 5. However, for a compulsory detention under the Mental Health Act to be lawful the following conditions must be met:

- it must be undertaken in accordance with domestic law, such as the Mental Health Act 1983;
- a true mental disorder must be established by a competent authority based on objective medical opinion;
- the mental disorder must be of a kind or degree which warrants compulsory detention;
- the detention is only allowed to continue for as long as the mental disorder persists.

Article 5 also contains another very important element. This requires that an individual has the right to have their deprivation of liberty reviewed by a court speedily. In our case this means that hearings such as the Mental Health Review Tribunals must be conducted rapidly.

Scenario: Steven

Steven is detained under Section 3 and has appealed to a Mental Health Review Tribunal, although primarily for administrative reasons his hearing has been postponed twice. He has now been waiting six weeks and will have to wait another two before he will be able to have his hearing.

It is likely that such a delay would be considered a breach of Steven's rights under Article 5 of the Human Rights Act as recent case law has determined that the practice of listing all hearings for eight weeks' time represents a breach of the speediness requirement in Article 5.

Article 8 has implications such as the decision to restrict visits from family members to people in inpatient units, particularly from children. Such visits would generally be allowed if it was decided that it was in the interests of the child and that the decision to allow the visit was regularly reviewed.

A decision not to allow the child to visit should only be taken exceptionally and would need to be supported by clear evidence of concerns.

The Bournewood safeguards

The Bournewood case has had important implications for mental health services and is outlined below.

The Bournewood case

L was a 49-year-old man with autism who lacked capacity. Following an episode of severe agitation L was admitted to Bournewood Hospital for about three months in 1997. Initially he was compliant and as he had not resisted admission was not detained under the Mental Health Act 1983 but accommodated in his own 'best interests' under the Common Law doctrine of 'necessity'. L brought legal proceedings against the managers of the hospital, claiming he had been unlawfully detained.

Following lengthy legal proceedings in the English courts, the European Court of Human Rights heard the case. L alleged that his rights under Article 5 of the Human Rights Act 1998 had been violated as he had been detained as an informal patient and access to a review of the legality of detention did not exist under these terms.

The court found in L's favour and decided that there had been a breach of Article 5 and that L had been unlawfully detained. Yet furthermore within the existing law there were *insufficient safeguards* for him to be detained. This case led to changes to the Mental Capacity Act (2005) brought about by the measures included within the Mental Health Act (2007) and known as the *Bournewood safeguards*. These measures only apply to a select group of people who are:

- over 18 years old and in a hospital or care home;
- experiencing a disorder or disability of the mind;
- lacking the capacity to give consent to the arrangements made for their care.

For whom such care amounts to a deprivation of liberty but is considered after an independent assessment to be necessary and a proportionate response in their best interests to protect them from harm.

The Bournewood case brought to light the need for legislative measures to protect such individuals but also to allow mental health services to provide the necessary level of care within the law.

In some cases it is necessary for mental health services to require the powers to deprive the person of their freedom in order to protect their well-being. Where a deprivation of liberty application is made it is necessary to seek authorization and this involves a range of stringent procedures as set out below.

Bournewood: deprivation of liberty

Deprivation must be:

- in the person's best interests;
- necessary to prevent harm;
- a proportionate response to the risk of harm.

Deprivation is not:

- related to treatment;
- permitted where a valid and applicable advanced directive exists;
- where it would conflict with a valid decision by an attorney or a deputy.

The Mental Capacity Act 2005

The Mental Capacity Act 2005 resulted from a concern that there should be legislative guidance in the care and treatment of people who lack the mental capacity to be able to provide informed consent to care or treatment. The Act came into force in 2007 as a statutory framework intended to empower and protect people who may not be able to make their own decisions. The Act also enables people to plan ahead for a time when they may lose their capacity. Examples include where a person is experiencing a dementia-type illness or recurrent bouts of severe depression. The person can make their wishes known when they may not be able to express them at the specific time their opinion is required.

The Mental Capacity Act 2005 is based on five principles:

1. That there should be a presumption of the person having mental capacity unless we are aware of evidence to the contrary.
2. Individuals should be supported to make independent decisions.
3. People retain the right to make eccentric or unwise decisions.
4. The law operates in the person's best interests.
5. Where the person is not able to make a choice, the least restrictive intervention should be chosen.

Mental capacity

A person lacks *capacity* if in relation to a certain matter at the time they are unable to make a decision because of an impairment or disturbance in the functioning of the mind or brain which may be temporary or permanent. The person is considered unable to make a decision if they are unable to understand the relevant information and retain it for use in the decision-making process or to communicate their decision.

If a person is able to retain the information relevant to a decision for only a short period of time this does *not* prevent them from being regarded as able to make the decision. It is also required that any reasonable foreseeable con-sequences or risk is included in the information provided to the person in order for them to be able to make an informed choice freely and without interference.

Scenario: Samantha

Samantha has dementia and is often very confused. She lives in a care home where a number of her day-to-day decisions are made for her. She has recently started a relationship with Clive who is another resident and the staff think that the relationship may be sexual.

Samantha's son Kevin is unhappy about this development and tells staff that his mother is being taken advantage of as she is unable to consent to this relationship. The staff are unwilling to intervene as Samantha and Clive appear very fond of each other.

In this situation Samantha has the capacity to consent to a sexual relationship if she can understand the nature and likely consequences of the relationship. She must make the choice herself and then communicate her decision to those around her. The demand for the staff to intervene may need to be acted upon if there are doubts over Samantha's capacity or she is considered to be vulnerable within the relationship.

There are two further provisions in the Mental Capacity Act 2005 to protect vulnerable people:

- The Independent Mental Capacity Advocate (IMCA) is a newly-created role and an individual appointed to support a person who lacks capacity but has no one to represent their interests. The IMCA can make representations about the person's wishes, bring to the attention of the health care services all of the factors affecting the person's circumstances and challenge decisions made on behalf of the person if necessary.
- A new criminal offence has been created of *ill treatment and neglect*. Allegations of this offence will generally be dealt with by the police and/or adult services under adult

protection procedures. The penalty for this offence may be a fine and/or sentence of imprisonment for up to five years.

Across the UK there is a small but significant group of people who cannot be assessed as having mental capacity and neither accept nor refuse treatment. In many cases these people have high levels of need for care and support. Section 5 of the Mental Capacity Act 2005 provides statutory guidance for interventions that would otherwise be considered a civil wrong or crime in other circumstances. Examples include the use of the person's money to buy essential items for their use or the giving of an injection against the person's will. These considerations protect the rights of this vulnerable group of people while also providing legal sanction for their care.

Restraint is defined in Section 6 of the Act as the use or threat of force where the person lacking capacity resists and is only permitted to prevent harm to the person lacking capacity. In addition it should only be used in *proportion* to the circumstances of the situation.

The Mental Capacity Act 2005 also allows for decisions to be made by the person about their future care which we will discuss next.

Advance decisions, advance statements and lasting power of attorney

Within the Act three mechanisms are identified. The first two involve decisions known as *advance decisions* and *advance statements*. The third is the appointment of another person to make decisions on the person's behalf when they are no longer capable and is called the *lasting power of attorney*. We will explain each of these in turn.

Advance decisions

An advance decision is a person's refusal of future treatment. It does not have to be written down but, if expressed verbally, nursing notes documenting the decision can, for example, become the written record. By whichever medium advance decisions are expressed, these decisions are generally legally binding if the criteria shown apply.

Advance Decision: refusal of treatment

An advance decision may be regarded as legally binding if:

- the person making the decision was 18 or older when it was made and had the necessary mental capacity;
- it specifies in lay terms the treatment which is refused and the particular circumstances in which the refusal is to apply;
- the person making the decision does not later withdraw it while still in possession of mental capacity;
- the person did not later appoint a lasting power of attorney to make the decision;
- the person making the decision has not done anything clearly inconsistent with the wishes expressed in the decision.

Advance decisions are the same as if a person refuses consent at the moment it is requested. If the advance decision does not relate to the circumstances currently being experienced, it generally would not have the same legal standing but can still be taken into account. Circumstances in which advance decisions are outweighed by other viewpoints are:

- if the person is being treated under the Mental Health Act 1983 and the decision at issue relates to mental health treatment;
- where a doctor considers that the treatment is necessary to sustain life.

However, in some cases an advance decision is a refusal of life-saving treatment. In order to be legally binding it must:

- be in writing;
- be signed;
- be witnessed;
- include a statement making clear that the advance decision applies to a situation where the person's life is at risk.

The scenario below provides a practice-based illustration of an advance decision.

Scenario: Sam

Sam is a patient known to community mental health services. Prior to his contact with the service he made a signed and witnessed advance decision to refuse any treatment to keep him alive by artificial means. A few years later he suffered serious injuries following a fall from a multi-storey car park (which may have been attempted suicide). Sam was paralysed from the neck down and only able to breathe with artificial ventilation. Initially he was conscious and able to agree to treatment. He participated in a rehabilitation programme. However, some months later he lost consciousness. His advance decision refusing treatment was found although he had never mentioned it.

In the above scenario Sam's verbal consent to treatment and participation in rehabilitation places doubt on the validity of the advance decision as it is inconsistent with his actions prior to his lack of capacity. Therefore the staff would be justified and acting within the law in continuing to provide treatment and care.

Advance statements

Advance statements express a general treatment preference, for example, 'I would like to have drug X' rather than a refusal such as, 'I *do not* want to have drug Y'. These are not legally binding but subject to the 'best interests test' where if the health care team feel it is to the benefit of the person to have what they are requesting they may comply. However, the health care staff are not obliged to and could provide an alternative which they believe better meets the person's best interests.

How would you feel?

Imagine you were in a situation where you are aware of what you do want and what you do not want, but are unable to communicate that to people around you. How would you feel if those making decisions for you were doing so in a way that did not meet your personal beliefs, because they did not know them? Now imagine how you might feel if you had taken the opportunity to express to someone or write down these desires, and you knew they were being used by those making decisions about you now.

Lasting power of attorney

A lasting power of attorney (LPA) enables another nominated person to make decisions on behalf of the person when they lose mental capacity. These will include decisions regarding the person's health and welfare. Court-appointed deputies with more limited powers are appointed by the Court of Protection where a person lacks capacity and they have not arranged for their own LPA.

Implementing mental health legislation

Having considered the legal provisions concerning mental health we now progress to look at how these are implemented in nursing practice.

Mental health nurses are frequently very much involved with applying the Mental Health Act 1983 when working with people who are compulsorily detained in inpatient areas. An example is whether to allow a person under a section of the Mental Health Act 1983 to go for a walk unescorted. At the other extreme is whether to restrain a person who appears to be beginning to become aggressive and a threat to others.

Decisions should be made based on individual need and circumstances and therefore the same situation occurring with different people can lead to another choice of action. Especially in emergencies, choices need to be made quickly to prevent harm either to the person or to others. Often in inpatient areas decisions are arrived at by the multidisciplinary team working as a group to incorporate differing perspectives and views, and share accountability.

While decisions concerning the imposition of sections of the Mental Health Act 1983 reside with specially trained health care professionals in inpatient settings, mental health nurses will nevertheless be involved in the process of assessing people under the Mental Health Act 1983 and providing views and opinions.

The decision about whether to detain a person due to their mental health does not relate to single interventions. Instead a range of factors are taken into account. These include:

- the severity and degree of the person's mental health problem;

- the potential and likely risk the person presents to their own well-being and that of others;
- the balance of the loss of personal rights and freedom of being under a section of the Mental Health Act 1983 against the likely benefit of treatment and care to the person;
- whether it would be in the person's best interests;
- the availability of appropriate treatment options;
- delivering necessary treatment in the least restrictive setting.

All of these factors reflect the particular perspective of mental health professionals as concerned with benefiting the person's mental health.

Reaching important decisions

- Consider a time when you have made a decision which you believed would have a significant impact on a range of people, for example, joining your course.
- What factors were involved in your decision? These may be internal, such as to do with your own confidence, or fear and apprehension of the unknown. Or they may be external factors such as financial issues or needing to move to a different place as a result of making the decision.
- On a piece of paper write down the headings 'Advantages' and 'Disadvantages' and then list all the reasons involved in the decision under the appropriate heading.
- Read the lists and consider how you arrived at the final decision and what account you took of each of the advantages and disadvantages. Write down your thoughts.
- As this refers to a decision you have taken, that decision was made in spite of the disadvantages. How did you appraise the disadvantages and then decide to make the decision anyway? Write down your thoughts.

When you have finished, place your notes in your professional portfolio.

In assisting us to understand decision-making in mental health nursing Fletcher (1997) uses a simple 'three approaches' process offering a guide to how we reach decisions about people with mental health problems. He refers to these three approaches as *legalism*, *situationism* and *antinomianism*.

In *legalism* we come to our decision by reference to rules and regulations and this involves not only the *spirit* but also the *letter* of the law. Principles are not merely guidelines to behaviour but directives to be followed. In practice, failing to abide by these rules and regulations could attract sanctions.

Situationism is when we reach our decision guided by the ethical maxims and expectations of the community and based on what is perceived as good conduct and behaviour. The *community* is broader than the health care community and involves the public as a whole. In contrast with legalism, situationism is derived from ethics. Ethics is the principle used to provide rational answers to problems and there is an expectation that mental health care professionals will do what is right and reach decisions based on clinical judgement which can be rationally explained.

Scenario: David

David is an elderly gentleman in his seventies. He has been an informal patient on the ward for a few months. His wife died about a month before his admission. He is diagnosed as suffering from dementia. David often talks about going home to see his wife and would at times make attempts to leave the ward. He has been known to wander off occasionally but never far away. David is sometimes reluctant to come back to the ward with the nurses but he can be persuaded to do so, although there will be times when he needs to be held by his arms to lead him back.

This scenario demonstrates that while it would be unlawful to prevent David from leaving the ward, the consequences of letting him do so would pose a greater risk. The community would expect the nurse to act in a manner that befits their role and to act in a manner that would prevent harm occurring to David. It would appear that only persuasion and the benign use of force are necessary to return David to the ward. Situationism is in part seen in natural law as it accepts reason as a tool to assist in exercising clinical judgement where the good outcome is as important as the process, as long as we are able to provide reasons that are acceptable to the community.

In reality it is unlikely that the health care professional would consciously ignore the rule of law. Instead they would balance what is right with what is demanded as a rule. In David's case the consequence of non-intervention could be fatal. If this problem persists the best course of action is to consider whether a mental health assessment ought to be carried out to determine whether a detention order would be more appropriate.

Antinomianism is when we make a decision often without forethought for legality or ethical maxims for guidance. This is due mainly to the situation being unique or when we are confronted with a situation that demands our immediate attention. The situation itself is used to provide the ethical solution or reason for intervention. This instinctive aspect of our work occurs frequently in mental health nursing. Fletcher (1997) claims that the process of knowing what to do or what is right when needed is borne out of knowledge based on experience of similar situations and linked with our emotions.

Conclusion

This chapter has provided an outline of the main legislation you are likely to encounter in the practice setting and will need to consider.

Student mental health nurses need to be aware of the fundamentals of mental health legislation and their accountability in order to be able to practice competently and effectively. While it is crucially important to practice in accordance with the law, increasingly the legislation itself has emphasized that the nurse's role in mental health nursing is more than simply enacting the law. Instead, mental health nurses have a specific role in working to empower and advocate for the person and always promote their best interests and rights. At times these competing considerations may appear to be conflicting. Yet it is important to reflect on these issues if we are to provide appropriate help for the individuals with whom we work.

References and Further Reading

Bartlett, P. and Sandland, R. (2007) Mental Health Law: policy and practice, 3rd edition. Oxford: Oxford University Press.

Bermingham, V. (2002) Tort in Nutshell, 6th edition. London: Sweet & Maxwell.

Bowen, P. (2007) Blackstone's Guide to The Mental Health Act 2007. Oxford: Oxford University Press.

DCA (2006) A Guide to the Human Rights Act 1998: Third Edition. London: Department of Constitutional Affairs.

DCA (2007) Mental Capacity Act 2005 Code of Practice. London: TSO.

Department of Health (1999) Review of the Mental Health Act 1983: Report of the Expert Committee. London: Department of Health.

Department of Health (2008a) Reference guide to the Mental Health Act 1983. London: TSO.

Department of Health (2008b) Code of Practice: Mental Health Act 1983. London: TSO.

Department of Health / NIMHE (2008) Supervised Community Treatment: A Guide for Practitioners. London: NIMHE.

Dimond, B. (2005) Legal Aspects of Nursing. Harlow: Longman.

Dimond, B. (2008) Legal Aspects of Mental Capacity. Oxford: Blackwell Publishing.

Fennell, P. (2007) Mental Health: The New Law. Bristol: Jordans.

Fletcher, J. (1997) Situation Ethics: The New Morality. Louisville: Westminster John Knox Press.

Garwood-Gowers, A., Tingle, J. and Lewis, T. (2001) Healthcare Law: The Impact of the Human Rights Act 1998. London: Cavendish Publishing.

Jones, R. (2008) Mental Health Act Manual, 11th edition. London: Sweet & Maxwell.

Jones, R. (2008) Mental Capacity Act Manual, 3rd edition. London: Sweet & Maxwell.

Ministry of Justice (2008) Mental Capacity Act 2005: Deprivation of liberty safeguards: Code of Practice to supplement the main Mental Capacity Act 2005 Code of Practice. London: TSO.

TSO (1999) Reform of the Mental Health Act 1983: Proposals for Consultation: Cm 4480. London: TSO

6

Mental health promotion

Tim Schafer

Learning objectives

By the end of this chapter, you will:

- Have gained an understanding of the concepts and practical application of mental health promotion, mental health and mental illness prevention.
- Appreciate the various ways in which stigma, discrimination and social exclusion affect people with mental health problems.
- Understand a conceptual map of mental health promotion and how it contributes to practice.

Introduction

In this chapter we begin by briefly discussing the emergence of health promotion. We then move on to look at several concepts including an understanding of the concept of mental health promotion, mental health and positive mental health before looking at the notion of mental illness prevention. The chapter then considers the many and varied ways in which stigma, discrimination and social exclusion can disadvantage people with mental health problems before outlining a conceptual map of mental health promotion. We will end with a conclusion summarizing the issues which have been discussed.

Throughout the chapter there are examples of interventions you can apply in your practice placements and which add to your emerging understanding of the role of the mental health nurse. There are also frequent references to current national and local mental health promotion campaigns that you may want to learn more about.

Background

For many years after its introduction in 1947 there was a focus on acute interventions in severe illness in the NHS. However, it became apparent that in many cases people had predisposing risk factors and the potential for developing ill health and diseases that were preventable at an earlier stage. By focusing health resources and activity on the wider public, people would live longer and enjoy better health, and health services could become more than a 'sickness service'.

Through nurses and health care staff carrying out initiatives that raise public awareness, and by promoting healthier lifestyle choices and people's awareness of health, the risk of experiencing illness can be reduced. Our prospects for a better quality of life will also be enhanced and the burden on acute services will be lessened.

Over the last 30 years health promotion has become highly prominent as an essential component of a comprehensive health service, yet it emerged as a specialist area developed out of public health. In the nineteenth century, due to the sudden growth of massive cities, the environment in many areas of the country was hazardous to people's health. A series of general public health measures – for example, introducing clean water and sanitation systems – eradicated illnesses such as cholera and typhoid and enhanced people's lives and health. The effectiveness of public health measures is well established and still continues in the form of vaccinations to prevent diseases – for example, measles, mumps and rubella.

In contrast with the universal and physical illness-specific measures within public health, the work of health promotion targets more specific areas and groups within the population. Within the UK there are numerous health promotion campaigns being carried out at any one time. As health care professionals we are obliged to consider all aspects of health and be aware of up-to-date events and changes. Recent prominent health promotion campaigns include:

- smoking cessation;
- consuming alcohol during pregnancy;
- healthy eating;
- tackling obesity;
- binge drinking.

Health promotion campaigns

- Consider a news article or leaflet promoting positive health-related activity. It may be on an area of health related to the list above or another aspect.
- Think about how the message is conveyed. What techniques are used? For example, are there positive visual images or written facts? Or are there warnings about the potential health risks and long-term damage of certain activities? Write down your thoughts.
- Place yourself in the role of the person to whom the leaflet is targeted. What effect do you feel the message will have? For example, will you ignore it? Will you think about the information? Might you change your behaviour as a result? Write down your response is and consider the reasons why.

When you have finished, place your notes and the leaflet or article in your professional portfolio.

Definitions and concepts

One definition is that: 'Mental health promotion is both any action to enhance the mental well being of individuals, families, organisations and communities, and a set of principles which recognise that how people feel is not an abstract and elusive concept, but a significant influence on health' (Friedli 2000).

Mental health promotion is an activity we carry out as part of our everyday practice in our roles as healthcare professionals and often we do not realize we are engaging in this activity. At other times we will be actively seeking information about health promotion activities, as one student explains below.

A mental health student's insight into information-gathering in health promotion ...

While working on a presentation assignment, we had to gain information on services available in our area. This was incredibly difficult and a number of services almost seemed obstructive in giving simple information. I could not help but reflect on how I would feel if I needed this information for myself or a loved one. It seemed to me an indicator of how hard it could be to get access to services even when you know they exist. How hard must it be to access services when you are not sure what is out there.

On the next page is a list of brief practice-based scenarios that will help you develop an understanding of different types of health promotion activity.

Practice scenarios

1 A mental health nurse works with users of a local mental health day centre in setting up and manning a stall in a local shopping centre for World Mental Health Day. They hand out leaflets on mental health conditions and what the centre offers.

2 A mental health nurse provides support and encouragement to a person with a mental health problem regarding their wish to return to employment.

3 A mental health nurse talks to a relative of a person with a psychotic illness allowing him to express his fears and frustrations and offers advice on how to relate to the person without arguing. The nurse also provides information about a local carers support group.

4 A counsellor helps a person with a mental health problem to develop practical strategies to get better sleep through measures such as taking no caffeine after 6.00 p.m. and carrying out relaxation exercises.

5 A health visitor leads a discussion with an antenatal group about promoting healthy and fulfilling attachment between mother and baby in the first years.

6 A practice nurse encourages a person with a long-standing mental health problem to have annual checks for blood glucose and to check their blood pressure regularly with a home testing kit.

7 A mental health nurse supports a person with a mental health problem who is making a complaint to his housing association about the behaviour of another family who live nearby. They often call him 'nutter' and keep shouting that he should be 'locked up in a loony bin'.

8 You write to the BBC to complain about a recent programme because you felt it gave an unbalanced assessment of the risks that people with mental health problems pose to society.

9 A community psychiatric nurse (CPN) talks with a group of sixth-formers about how they can combat exam stress and negotiate the stresses of university life.

10 A mental health nurse works with a person who has a mental health problem to examine how her 'negative automatic thoughts' makes her over-sensitive to criticism from her partner and children.

11 A mental health nurse discusses healthy eating with a person who is on long-term medication for a bipolar depressive illness.

12 A mental health nurse arranges for and accompanies a group of people with mental health problems on a country walk to the local forest.

Write down which of the above scenarios you think is health promotion activity and why. When you have finished, place your notes in your professional portfolio.

All of the above could be classified as mental health promotion as each one has a positive influence on mental well-being. Example 10 refers to 'negative automatic thoughts'. This is where the person experiences recurrent self-critical thoughts and is a term used in the psychological therapy cognitive behavioural therapy (CBT). While the intervention could be described as therapy through promoting psychological balance, the CBT still represents mental health promotion.

The government has issued guidance suggesting that mental health promotion should focus on strengthening individuals, strengthening communities and reducing structural barriers to mental health (DoH 2001). Next we will explain these terms and provide examples of health promotion activities.

- *Strengthening individuals* by increasing emotional resilience through interventions designed to promote self-esteem, life and coping skills. For example, communicating, negotiating, relationship and parenting skills: Practice Scenarios 2, 4 and 10.

- *Strengthening communities* by increasing social support, social inclusion and participation, improving community safety, neighbourhood environments, promoting child care and self-help networks, developing health and social services which support mental health, promoting mental health within schools and workplaces. For example, through anti-bullying strategies and mental health strategies: Practice Scenarios 3, 5 and 9.
- *Reducing structural barriers to mental health* through initiatives to reduce discrimination and inequalities and to promote access to education, meaningful employment, housing, services and support for those who are vulnerable: Practice Scenarios 1, 7 and 8.

Features of mental health promotion

We will now consider the various features of mental health promotion and examine five principles on which it is based. These are:

1. Mental health promotion involves very varied interventions.
2. Mental health promotion works at different levels.
3. Mental health promotion is 'everyone's business'.
4. Mental health promotion takes place in a variety of settings and contexts.
5. Mental health promotion has ethical dimensions.

Characteristics of mental health promotion

1 *Mental health promotion is varied:* it can be found in a one-to-one session between a nurse and a client, or in an expensive national campaign to combat negative attitudes and stigma.

2 *Mental health promotion works at different levels:* mental health promotion works at different levels involving various stakeholders. These include:

- Individuals
- Couples
- Families
- Local groups
- Communities
- Disadvantaged or stigmatized groups
- Geographical regions
- Whole populations

3 *Mental health promotion is 'everyone's business':* mental health promotion is not a task that is exclusive to mental health nurses or mental health professionals. The scenarios in the panel on page 79 show how practice nurses and health visitors make a crucial contribution to mental health through their role in, for example, promoting positive parenting skills and improved physical health. There is a wealth of evidence about the impact of mental health on physical health and vice versa. For example:

- people with mental health problems have higher rates of physical illness and poor dental health;
- people with mental illness experience worse treatment in A&E departments (Phelan *et al.* 2001; Disability Rights Commission 2006);
- most mental disorders carry with them an increased risk of premature death (Thornicroft 2006).

4 *Mental health promotion takes place in a variety of settings and contexts:* the majority of mental health promotion takes place outside mental health services through various forms of health care, for example, housing departments, social services and educational establishments. Any activity or process that leads to an improvement in mental health could be said to be mental health promoting. Making time to listen to and support a friend in distress is as important as promoting a society that values difference and encourages equality of opportunity.

5 *Mental health promotion has ethical dimensions:* the following definition, taken from the WHO report on the *Prevention of Mental Disorders* (2004), and originally given in Hosman and Jane-Llopis (1999: 16) highlights some of the values implicit in mental health promotion:

> Mental health promotion activities imply the creation of individual, social and environmental conditions that enable optimal psychological and psychophysiological development. Such initiatives involve individuals in the process of achieving positive mental health, enhancing quality of life and narrowing the gap in health expectancy between countries and groups. It is an enabling process, done by, with and for the people.

Mental health promotion is not just about promoting the mental health of individuals but also about creating an environment that enhances the mental health of the whole community.

Positive mental health

So far in this chapter we have taken for granted that 'positive mental health' or mental health exists and is observable, measurable and real. However, in the exercise below we will examine what we understand as mental health.

Positive mental health

Together with other students from your group or with friends or family members, each write down as many features of positive mental health you can think of. Aim to write at least 10 points or features that make a person mentally healthy. When you have all finished, share your lists with each other.

Next discuss:

- What features did you all agree on, and why?
- What features did you differ on, and why?
- Do you think that other groups – for example, people from a different culture, gender, occupation or religion – would have come up with the same lists as you?
- Reflect on the exercise and write down your thoughts.

When you have finished, place your notes together with the list of 10 points or features that you wrote down in your professional portfolio.

Although the list will vary from person to person, among the answers you may have written are:

- to be able to feel and experience a sense of happiness and well-being;
- feeling valued by others through having positive family relationships, healthy and loving relationships with partners and friends and good relationships with colleagues and acquaintances;
- feeling that we have a role in life and that we can make a contribution which has a value within society and provides us with a sense of identity and purpose;
- feeling mentally stimulated and learning new things;
- to have the opportunity to reach our potential and achieve our goals;
- a good work/life balance and the opportunity to engage in recreational activities which we enjoy and find rewarding;
- having a sense of personal freedom and the ability to choose what we do;
- having enough money to live on, enough food to eat and somewhere to live;
- to feel safe and secure;
- to enjoy physical and mental health.

The characteristics above do not appear in terms of relative importance to each other but in the order in which they were identified in a brainstorming exercise. However, it seems surprising to realize that if they were to be listed in terms of importance they would probably appear in the reverse order to how they are here. Without basic resources such as our health, safety and security, somewhere to live, enough food to eat and enough money to pay our bills, our mental health and well-being would most likely suffer. This demonstrates that there are a number of aspects of mental health that we do not appreciate when present but suffer the lack of when absent. It also appears that mental well-being is comprised of a number of characteristics.

There are many different understandings of mental health which are all influenced by individual experiences and expectations as well as differing beliefs about medicine, religion and culture (Friedli 2003). Seedhouse (2002) casts doubt on the idea of mental health as a concept and instead views it as composed of value judgements and abstract ideas as opposed to the description of anything specific. Instead the physical, mental, social and spiritual world are inextricably united and it is impossible to identify what is mental health separate from the whole. To appreciate the difficulty of identifying mental health as a specific entity, in completing the above exercise you may have found the problem of avoiding identifying what is positive mental health by saying what it is not. For example, that positive mental well-being is achieved by the absence of bullying, harassment or abuse.

However, similar to our exercise other writers have sought to identify what mental health is. It will be interesting to see which of the 'definitions' below appeared in your list.

- Agency and the degree of influence an individual feels s/he has over their life.
- The capacity to learn, grow and develop.
- Feeling loved, trusted, understood and valued.
- Interest in life.
- Autonomy and being able to think and acting on one's own.
- Self-acceptance and self-esteem.
- Optimism and hopefulness.
- Resilience and the ability to persist and bounce back from setbacks.

Some other indicators identified in the health promotion literature include the following (Schafer 2000; Seedhouse 2002; Svedberg *et al.* 2007):

- well-being;
- the ability to cope and solve problems;
- sense of self and identity;
- maturity;
- being able to fit in with other people;
- ability to love;
- wanting to be part of things;
- empowerment.

There are many research instruments that can be used to measure an individual's positive mental health, such as the general health questionnaire (GHQ), self-esteem questionnaires, community integration questionnaires and empowerment questionnaires. However, there are fewer instruments to measure mental health at the neighbourhood or community level.

Neighbourhood and community

Think of your own neighbourhood or community. What are some of the features of it that affect mental well-being?

- Write down at least five features.
- Which three features do you think have the most important impact on mental well-being, and why?

When you have finished, place your notes in your professional portfolio.

Your responses to the exercise on neighbourhood and community will vary depending on your individual circumstances and values, beliefs and culture, and the issues specific to the area in which you live. If you live in a neighbourhood that is beset by vandalism and crime, then safety may be at the top of your list. In contrast, if you live in a rural area where many shops, post offices and local facilities have been closed down, then the availability of more services which promote the life of the community may be your priority.

The Audit Commission (2002) has developed a series of quality of life indicators concerning neighbourhoods and local environments which are relevant to mental health, shown in the next panel.

Quality of life indicators relevant to mental health

- The percentage of residents satisfied with their neighbourhood as a place to live.
- The quality of the natural environment and surroundings.
- The cultural, recreational and leisure services available.
- Opportunities to participate in local planning and decision-making.
- The percentage of residents who consider their neighbourhood is getting worse.
- The percentage of residents concerned about noise.
- The amount of parks and green spaces per 1000 head of population.

Another approach to classifying communities is through the use of social capital indicators. These include factors such as:

- feeling safe;
- trusting other unfamiliar community members;
- access to social support;
- employment and meaningful activity;
- support for parents.

Mental health nurses focus their health promotion work at the level of the individual or family, but they also need to think creatively about how they can influence the community or neighbourhood in which they work or live. Examples include working with housing and employment agencies, linking people with mental health problems with community groups and self-help groups and developing or participating in mentoring systems to help people back into further and higher education.

Mental illness prevention

So far in this chapter we have explored features of mental health promotion and seen how it is based on ideas of mental health and well-being as opposed to notions of illness, disease and deficit. We will next consider the similarities and differences between mental health promotion and mental illness prevention.

The science of illness prevention has been enormously successful in the area of physical

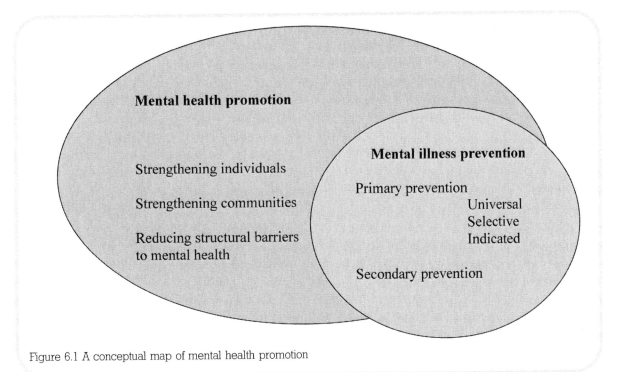

Figure 6.1 A conceptual map of mental health promotion

health in eliminating and reducing communicable diseases such as smallpox, tuberculosis and many others. In recent decades illness prevention has also been applied with some success to mental illnesses and diseases.

The aim of illness prevention is distinct from mental health promotion as it is defined within the limits of the biomedical disease-orientated model, because mental health promotion is concerned with enhancing well-being and factors that go beyond symptoms, illnesses and disorders. However, health promotion and health prevention are also sometimes identical.

Figure 6.1 maps the elements of health promotion and prevention.

The scenarios that we considered earlier in the chapter (see p. 79) all have an element of illness prevention. It could be argued that as the majority of them involve working with people who have already developed a mental illness, this contradicts the notion of illness prevention. However, the interventions carried out serve to prevent the further deterioration or relapse of the person's mental health. Scenarios 6 and 11 relate to diabetes and so demonstrate the mental health nurse working to prevent the person becoming physically unwell.

It will be helpful in developing our understanding of mental health prevention to explore the different levels of prevention. A traditional public health approach to preventive medicine distinguishes between primary, secondary and tertiary prevention.

Levels of illness prevention in mental health

- *Primary prevention:* targets the 'non-clinical' population to prevent the occurrence of illness. Examples include the use of relaxation tapes and relaxation methods to reduce anxiety and stress, as well as engaging in exercise to promote mental health and well-being (Mental Health Foundation 2005).
- *Secondary prevention:* focuses on people who are already unwell and aims to reduce the length, frequency or intensity of the illness. Examples include CBT-based 'self-help' books and leaflets for people with mild depression or the input of early intervention from psychosis services to reduce the severity of illness through early detection and treatment.
- *Tertiary prevention:* aims to reduce or prevent the negative consequences associated with illness. An example of this would be the development of an occupational and leisure programme for someone with a severe and enduring illness such as bipolar disorder or schizophrenia.

There are also several subdivisions of illness. These are *universal prevention, selective prevention* and *indicated prevention* (Mrazek and Hagerty 1994).

Preventative, selective and indicated mental illness prevention

- *Universal prevention strategies* are applied to a whole population regardless of whether any subgroups are at an increased or lesser risk of susceptibility to the mental health problem. An example of this is the government campaign to encourage responsible drinking within the recommended limits. In addition to the potential physical effects of the excessive use of alcohol, it can lead to depression and even to people developing dementia-type illnesses such as Korsafoff syndrome. Other universal mental health prevention strategies include prenatal care, parenting programmes, universal child benefit payments and restrictions on the purchasing of painkillers in supermarkets.
- *Selective prevention strategies* focus on individuals, groups or communities within the larger population who have an increased risk of susceptibility to a mental health problem. An example is in

Scenario 5 where a health visitor is working with an antenatal group concerning attachment with the baby in the first years. New mothers are at a high risk of developing postnatal depression (PND). In some cases difficulty in bonding with the baby can be caused by or lead to PND. By working with expectant mothers the health visitor can support them in developing an understanding of what is healthy attachment with the baby, help them to recognize where there are problems and enable them to access help at an early stage. By running a group the mothers may develop a supportive network as well, which constitutes a prevention measure as lack of social support can also lead to depression after childbirth.

● *Indicated prevention* identifies high-risk individuals who are showing either detectable signs of a mental health problem or who have a biological predisposition to mental illness. In the case of Huntington's disease, for example, unfortunately some people are genetically predisposed to acquiring the illness. Other instances of selective mental health prevention strategies are extra family support for vulnerable people such as young single mothers and socially isolated families. Another example is doctors completing a brief depression screening tool for people with diabetes or coronary heart disease as both conditions are associated with a higher incidence of depression.

Stigma, discrimination and social exclusion

An important role of mental health promotion is to reduce stigma, discrimination and social exclusion.

Stigma

Stigma can be defined as the possession of a perceived 'discrediting characteristic'. Often people in a minority group within society have characteristics which make them different, which are exaggerated within popular perception to produce a stereotyped image. Often these perceptions reflect a misunderstanding of the person and their culture. Groups that are the subject of stigma are often seen as a threat or challenge to society and are subjected to hostility, isolation from society or abuse for no other reason than they are different.

Many groups have been stigmatized throughout history. Your answers to the exercise next will depend on the background and life experiences of the people within your group, but it might be a surprise to discover just how frequently and in what ways people experience stigma. Often people who have not been subjected to stigma do not appreciate the fear, anxiety and distress it can cause.

While it is often believed that stigma is on the decline, many people with mental health problems

Stigma

● With other students in your group, discuss the concept of stigma.
● Can you identify any groups of people in history and/or within your knowledge and experience who have been stigmatized?
● What characteristics about this group led them to be stigmatized?
● How did this happen and in what ways were these people disadvantaged?
● Write down your thoughts on this exercise.

When you have finished, place your notes in your professional portfolio.

are deeply affected. Someone who hears voices may perceive themselves as unworthy or bad in accordance with the stigma which they believe attaches to them. This could lead to:

● delays in seeking help;
● low self-esteem;
● self-isolation and withdrawing from friendships and social circles;
● avoiding work and family commitments.

One approach to reduce stigma is through the 'pride' movements. These emerged in the 1990s with 'Gay Pride', probably the most prominent, and which has been extremely successful in reshaping popular perceptions and challenging the stigma around homosexuality. Today, being gay is not a source of stigma and is increasingly being incorporated in the law to reflect how society's views have changed. In mental health we now have a movement known as 'Mad Pride' that aims to promote a more balanced understanding of people with mental health problems and challenge negative attitudes.

Another important approach to dealing with stigma is self-help and mutual aid groups. A large number of self-help groups have developed, often on the basis of a diagnosis. Examples include depression alliance groups, manic depression Fellowship groups, 'rethink' self-help groups and many others. Some have a campaigning aspect to them and work through websites, publications, charity work and events to promote improved public attitudes and better resources, laws and policies.

For many people a crucial aspect to self-help/mutual aid is the sharing of personal stories, anecdotes and experiences of recovery with others who have known similar distress. Anybody reading this who has attended self-help/mutual aid groups will be familiar with the newcomer's relief upon the realization that they are not the only person in the world who has faced these problems and the sense of hope that these groups can instil. Mutual aid promotes hope and a sense of usefulness. Borkman (1999) introduced the term 'helper/helped' to describe how people can discover through self-help that their problems and experiences, far from being a curse, place them in an ideal position to help others.

There are also a wide range of self-help fellowships based on the enduring Alcoholics Anonymous (AA) model such as Narcotics Anonymous (NA), Overeaters Anonymous (OA) and Co-dependents Anonymous (CODA). These groups are in some ways a very 'pure' form of self-help in that the sole objective is to help those with alcoholism or other addictions to recover with the help of other alcoholics or addicts. These groups are not involved in campaigning and have developed and flourished for nearly 70 years without a hierarchical structure or any professional or medical involvement.

Discrimination

Discrimination is defined as being treated negatively due to prejudice. With regard to this concept the focus shifts to the role and attitudes of other people rather than the person with a mental health problem, although these beliefs have an impact on that person. For example, a person who is unable to find meaningful employment after recovering from a mental health problem may perceive the discrimination as evidence that she or he is now worthless or flawed. Experiencing discrimination can lead to increased isolation, social problems, a reduced sense of self-worth and attempts to 'self-medicate' through drug or alcohol use. This could also be perceived by employers as evidence that the stigma of mental illness is correct and people with mental health problems do not deserve equal opportunities in the workplace.

Social exclusion

The origins of social exclusion are in the New Labour period in British politics from 1997 to the present day. The idea emerged from a belief that a healthy society is characterized by high levels of participation in social, cultural and political activities involving people from all sectors of society. Social exclusion proceeds on the premise that people with mental health problems are not involved and do not receive the same opportunities within society as other people.

A definition of social exclusion

The Social Exclusion Unit of the UK government was set up in 1997 and was superseded by the Social Exclusion Task Force in 2006. Its website (www.cabinetoffice.gov.uk/social_exclusion_task_force/context.aspx) states that:

> Social exclusion is about more than income poverty. It is a short-hand term for what can happen when people or areas have a combination of linked problems, such as unemployment, discrimination, poor skills, low incomes, poor housing, high crime and family breakdown. These problems are linked and mutually reinforcing. Social exclusion is an extreme consequence of what happens when people don't get a fair deal throughout their lives, often because of disadvantage they face at birth, and this disadvantage can be transmitted from one generation to the next.

● To what extent do you think the emphasis on social exclusion and inclusion is worthy or ethical? Write down your thoughts and place them in your professional portfolio.

The question at the end of the last panel may seem unusual. Clearly not many people will argue *against* giving others a fair deal and tackling discrimination. Surely any mental health promoting policies that help people into employment, ease access to education and tackle poverty have got to be good. However, some people may be concerned that social inclusion becomes the predominant consideration above personal choice. Not everybody *wants* to be politically active, surrounded by friends or to go to the pub or the gym. Not everybody wants to work. The rise of social exclusion and inclusion in our language and culture signals a renewed emphasis on equality of opportunity and a more tolerant attitude to societal differences but it should be consensual and we should avoid making inclusion compulsory. Personal choice and empowerment also matter.

The effects of stigma, discrimination and social exclusion

There is an increasing amount of research to identify the impact of stigma and discrimination on people experiencing mental health problems. It is important to remember that stigma, discrimination and social exclusion are problems arising from the reaction of others and not a direct consequence of the experience of mental illness. For some people the detrimental impact of stigma, discrimination and social exclusion is greater than the effect of the mental health problem itself (Sartorius and Schultze 2005). The mental health survivors movement in the 1980s and 1990s in the UK began from the premise that people not only had to survive their own mental distress but also the response of society.

Actions Speak Louder

The Mental Health Foundation (MHF) report, *Actions Speak Louder: Tackling Discrimination Against People with Mental Illness* (Thornicroft 2006) provides a thorough review of the evidence.

● Download a copy of the report which is available from http://www.mentalhealth.org.uk/publications/.
● Read through Sections 2 and 3 of the report.
● Write a list of the areas where people with mental health problems are disadvantaged.

When you have finished, place your notes in your professional portfolio.

The next panel presents a summary of the problems and disadvantages people with mental health problems experience as a result of social exclusion.

The experience of social exclusion

People with mental health problems:

- can experience discrimination, negative attitudes and exclusion from their families;
- sometimes experience abuse and hostility from neighbours;
- lose friends as a result of their illness;
- feel they cannot be totally honest with friends, family and employers;
- often find difficulties developing intimate relationships;
- are less likely to marry or remain married;
- have poorer-quality intimate relationships;
- are more likely to lose custody of their children;
- experience difficulties gaining and remaining in meaningful employment;
- are more likely to be unemployed despite being keen to work;
- often say they have been dismissed from employment;
- feel they have been denied employment;
- are discriminated against at work far more than in other areas;
- have reduced leisure and recreation opportunities;
- may have difficulties travelling and obtaining travel insurance;
- find it harder to get loans, mortgages and other financial services;
- cannot sit on a jury and have limited voting rights;
- receive poorer health care in a variety of settings and ways;
- are more likely to suffer from diabetes and coronary heart disease;
- are likely to die younger than those without mental health problems.

The list above, while not being exhaustive, provides a good outline of the wide range of disadvantages people with a mental health problem are confronted with as a result of social exclusion. If you have not experienced a mental health problem this provides an insight into how mental illness can affect your life, often in varied and unexpected ways.

In terms of employment, less than 4 in 10 employers say they would employ someone with a mental health problem (SEU 2004). This is far fewer than the proportion that would employ people with physical health problems, the long-term unemployed or lone parents. There are also disturbing levels of negative attitudes in the community affecting the ability of people with a mental health problem to take part in community life. The children of people with a mental health problem are also more likely to be teased and bullied in school (SEU 2004).

Housing is another area of disadvantage for people with mental health problems (Meltzer *et al.* 2002), who are:

- one and a half times more likely than other people in society to live in rented housing and with higher uncertainty about how long they can remain in their current home;
- twice as likely than other people in society to say that they are very dissatisfied with their accommodation or that the state of repair is poor;
- four times more likely than other people in society to report that their health has been made worse by their housing.

We found in our discussion about what constitutes mental health that many of the most basic attributes of life such as safety, a secure home and sufficient food and money to pay bills are under-appreciated but important aspects of mental health and well-being. Yet as a result of stigma, discrimination and social exclusion access to all of these basic requirements is made harder for people with mental health problems. While the introduction of social inclusion has made progress in allowing us to identify the needs of people with mental health problems, more needs to be done to pave the way towards promoting genuine inclusion.

Are attitudes to people with mental health problems improving?

The government has carried out a series of national surveys of attitudes to mental health that have been completed on a three-yearly basis since 1993. In some areas attitudes have improved but overall we are a society less well disposed to mental illness than we were in 1993 (see 'Attitudes to Mental Illness' online at

www.dh.gov.uk/en/Publicationsandstatistics/ Publications/PublicationsStatistics/DH_076516). Compared to the first survey in 1993 we are now more likely to think that:

- people with mental illness do not deserve our sympathy;
- people with mental illness are a burden on society.

We are less likely to think that:

- people with mental illness have for too long been the subject of ridicule;
- we need to adopt a more tolerant attitude to people with mental illness in our society;
- we have a responsibility to provide the best possible care for people with mental illness.

As health care professionals in mental health we are obliged to challenge stigma, discrimination and social exclusion and promote a positive image of mental health.

National campaigns to promote mental health

There are a variety of national campaigns that promote knowledge and tackle stigma, discrimination and social exclusion. Here are some examples.

- SHIFT is an initiative run by the Care Services Improvement Partnership (CSIP) that aims to tackle discrimination at work and help employers to meet their responsibilities under the Disability Discrimination Act 2005. Details of the programme can be found at http://www.shift.org.uk.
- Moving People is a Lottery and Comic Relief funded collaborative campaign that aims to challenge prejudicial attitudes and combat discrimination through a programme of local and national projects. Many projects involve encouraging mental health service users to exercise in order to promote physical and mental health. More details can be found at http://www.movingpeople.org.uk.
- Look up other websites, for example, MIND and the Mental Health Foundation, and find out what campaigns are currently ongoing.

You may think that mental health promotion is beyond the scope of mental health nurses or other practitioners but in many ways the day-to-day work and practice of mental health nursing are an ideal setting to challenge discrimination and promote social inclusion.

- Discuss with your peers how the mental health nurse can promote mental health through challenging stigma, discrimination and exclusion.

Although we can support national campaigns and share information with colleagues and the people with mental health problems we work with, we need to challenge discrimination and social exclusion in practice. As a student mental health nurse you will come across negative attitudes from all sorts of people in all sorts of settings. As health care professionals we need to adopt a constructive and assertive approach to highlighting and challenging negative and stigmatizing attitudes and behaviour.

A model for mental health promotion

Finally in this chapter we suggest a model of mental health promotion which offers a useful framework for locating health promotion within your practice.

The *settings approach* has been developed by MacDonald and O'Hara (1998) and is based on the assumption that no one practitioner, group or organization is able to meet the requirements for Standard 1 of *The National Service Framework for Mental Health* (DoH 1999). Instead, mental health promotion requires an interprofessional and col-laborative approach which is adaptable to different social settings and environments. Mental health promotion should aim to include the following elements:

- *The micro level* of individuals.
- *The meso level* of family, workplaces, peer groups, community groups and small neighbourhoods.
- *The macro level* of wider systems that shape our thinking and behaviour and govern many aspects of our lives. This level would also include policy, law, culture, religions and the media (DoH 2001).

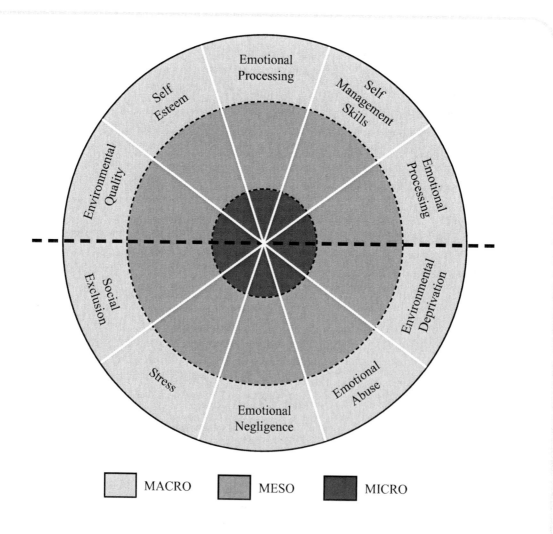

Figure 6.2. Ten elements of mental health promotion and demotion (DoH 2001)

The elements above the horizontal dotted line in Figure 6.2 are factors that promote mental health and those below are factors that make it worse. Importantly, the model also considers demoters to mental health as not all health promotion activity improves mental health. For example, promoting problem-solving and stress management skills is very good but will be more health promoting if underlying stresses are also addressed.

All of the scenarios that appeared earlier in the chapter (see p. 79) fit into this framework but here we will explain the levels of intervention and provide an example of each.

● *Micro level* interventions could, for example, be providing appropriate training and/or promoting individual self-worth and self-confidence.

● *Meso level* interventions might involve working with an employer to promote positive attitudes and reasonable allowances for the person's mental health problem within the workplace.
● *Macro level* interventions could involve campaigning for people to be able to return to work gradually without losing out financially.

The 'ten elements map' (Figure 6.2) encourages mental health nurses and other practitioners to look beyond the individual and the often narrow remits within individual professional roles. It also encourages us to think about promoting the strengths and positive qualities of people with mental health problems rather than focusing on problems and deficits. Much of the mental health nurse's work involves mental health promotion.

'Everybody's business'

As we have learned in this chapter, mental health promotion is 'everybody's business'. Often it is believed that mental health promotion has to be on a large scale and is a specialist discipline. However, mental health promotion is an integral part of the role of anyone working with people with mental health problems and can be carried out in individual relationships and specific interventions or with groups over a period of time.

● Look at Figure 6.2 and think about what you have read in this chapter.
● Identify a mental health promotion initiative you can carry out within your placement and discuss this with your practice mentor.
● Carry out the activity and then evaluate it. Discuss it with anyone who was involved, your practice mentor and other students.
● Write down your reflections on how the health promotion activity went and what you have learned.

This initiative can be something which has been carried out before or a new idea. Examples include a themed group on an inpatient unit concerned with, say, healthy living, exercise, healthy eating, gardening, music or reading, or in any setting, on an individual or group basis, working with people who have mental health problems to learn about the medication they take for their mental health.

A working example is Jane, who is a second-year mental health student nurse and went with her mentor Sue to visit Julie, who is experiencing postnatal depression and the mother of an 18-month-old boy called Daniel. In common with many people in modern society Julie is an older mother, having had her first child at 34. Previously she was a personnel manager in a large company and had a highly responsible job. She never thought she would struggle as a mother. Julie feels that she is a 'bad mother' for not coping and that she is 'mental' and weak and letting everyone down. Julie is engaging in *self-stigmatization*. Jane is much younger than Julie but suggests to her that many new mothers experience postnatal depression and this is not necessarily a sign of weakness. Instead Julie is undergoing a massive transition to the role of a new mother. In fact Julie is a good mother and is aware that although Daniel is very demanding, she manages very well. Julie thinks about Jane's comments and reappraises her view of mental health. As a result she shares her experiences of postnatal depression with friends and family and is no longer embarrassed about her experience.

Conclusion

In this chapter we have discussed several concepts concerning the promotion of mental health including mental health and mental illness prevention. We then considered the effects of stigma, discrimination and social exclusion as these add significantly to the problems of people who are already experiencing mental health difficulties. Finally we looked at a conceptual map of mental health promotion. While it is commonly perceived that mental health promotion is beyond the remit of students, change will only occur as a result of a concerted effort and as the accumulation of small changes. It is necessary for us all to contribute to promoting mental health and to convincing society that people with mental health problems can make a valid contribution.

References

Audit Commission (2002) *Voluntary Quality of Life and Cross-Cutting Indicators: Indicators Handbook,* www.audit-commission.gov.uk.

Borkman, T.J. (1999) *Understanding Self-help/mutual-aid: Experiential Learning in the Commons.* New Brunswick, NJ: Rutgers University Press.

DoH (Department of Health) (1999) *The National Service Framework for Mental Health: Modern Standards and Service Models.* London: DoH.

DoH (Department of Health) (2001) *Making it Happen: A Guide to Delivering Mental Health Promotion.* London: DoH.

Friedli, L. (2003) *Making it Effective: A Guide to Evidence-based Health Promotion.* London: Sainsbury Centre for Mental Health.

Hosman, C. and Jane-Llopis, E. (1999) Mental health promotion, in *The Evidence of Health Promotion Effectiveness: Shaping Public Health in a New Europe.* Brussels: ECSC-EC-EAEC.

MacDonald, G. and O'Hara, K. (1998) *Ten Elements of Mental Health, its Promotion and Demotion:*

Implications for Practice. Glasgow: Society of Health Education and Promotion Specialists.

Meltzer, H., Singleton, N., Lee, A., Bebbington, P., Brugha, T. and Jenkins, R. (2002) *The Social and Economic Circumstances of Adults with Mental Disorders.* London: The Stationery Office.

Mental Health Foundation (2005) *Up and Running? Exercise Therapy and the Treatment of Mild or Moderate Depression in Primary Care,* www.mentalhealth.org.uk/publications.

Mrazek, P.J. and Hagerty, R.J. (eds) (1994) *Reducing Risks for Mental Disorders: Frontiers for Preventive Intervention Research.* Washington, DC: National Academy Press.

Sartorius, N. and Schultze, H. (2005) *Reducing the Stigma of Mental Illness. A Report from the Global Programme Against Stigma of the World Psychiatric Association.* Cambridge: Cambridge University Press.

Schafer, T. (2000) Towards a participatory model for the evaluation of the empowering therapeutic environment, *Mental Health and Learning Disabilities Care,* 3(7): 233–7.

Seedhouse, D. (2002) *Total Health Promotion: Mental Health, Rational Fields and the Quest for Autonomy.* Chichester: Wiley.

SEU (Social Exclusion Unit) (2004) *Mental Health and Social Exclusion.* London: ODPM, www.cabinetoffice.gov.uk/social_exclusion_task_force/publications.aspx.

Stewart-Brown, S. (2002) Measuring the parts most measures do not reach, *Journal of Mental Health Promotion,* 1(2): 4–9.

Svedberg. P., Svensson, B., Arvidsson, B. and Hansson, L. (2007) The construct validity of a self-report questionnaire on health promotion in mental health services, *Journal of Psychiatric and Mental Health Nursing,* 14: 566–72.

Thornicroft, G. (2006) *Actions Speak Louder: Tackling Discrimination Against People with Mental Illness.* London: Mental Health Foundation.

WHO (World Health Organization) (2004) *Prevention of Mental Disorders: Effective Interventions and Policy Options.* Geneva: World Health Organization.

Section 2
Mental health and illness over the lifespan

Child and adolescent mental health

7

Steven Walker

Learning objectives

By the end of this chapter you will have gained:

- An understanding of the importance of theories of human growth and development.
- An insight into risk and resilience factors in young people.
- An appreciation of the assessment of children and adolescents.
- An insight into analysing information and its significance, and identifying appropriate interventions.

Introduction

This chapter focuses on mental health problems in children and younger people. It will help you to develop skills to engage with individuals, families, carers and other professionals in this increasingly influential area of nursing practice and health care.

We will discuss the major theories and models of human growth and development to place the mental health needs of younger people in context. Risk and resilience factors are also highlighted as an important consideration in assessment, focusing on both the strengths as well as the difficulties of the individual, the family and the community. In addition, this chapter will help you to understand the importance of assessment. Finally, we consider working in partnership with children and adolescents, their families and other agencies, and the identification of appropriate models and methods of intervention to effectively address needs.

Scenarios will be used to illuminate and enhance the learning outcomes and provide opportunities for you to reflect on your learning experience.

Background

Recent evidence indicates that 10 per cent of young people up to the age of 18 years in Britain have a mental health problem, with a higher prevalence among those living in inner-city environments. One in five young people has a mental health problem which, although less serious, still requires professional support (Audit Commission 1998; ONS 2001). It has also been estimated that young people's mental health services only reach a minority of the population who require help, which means that a large number of young people are not receiving the support and help they need.

The World Health Organization (WHO) estimates that one in five of the world's youth under 15 are experiencing a mild to severe mental health disorder and a large number remain untreated as services to help them simply do not exist (WHO 2001). Figures have consistently shown that boys express their problems through external actions and behaviour, for example, in the form of aggression or delinquency. In contrast, girls respond to their problems internally and may become depressed and anxious or engage in self-harming behaviour (Dogra *et al.* 2002).

Definitions and distinctions

Mental health among young people can be described as: 'a relative state of mind in which a person ... is able to cope with, and adjust to, the recurrent stress of everyday living' (Anderson and Anderson 1995: 86). A multidisciplinary group (HAS 1995) has agreed that mental health in younger people is indicated by:

- a capacity to enter into and sustain satisfying personal relationships;

- a continuing progression of psychological development;
- an ability to play and learn so that attainments are appropriate for age and intellectual level;
- a developing sense of right and wrong;
- the degree of psychological distress and maladaptive behaviour being within normal limits for the young person's age and context.

Mental health problems can be understood as 'abnormalities of emotions, behaviour, or social relationships sufficiently marked or prolonged to cause suffering or risk to optimal development in the child or distress or disturbance in the family or community' (Kurtz 1992: 22).

However, who decides what is abnormal? The mental health worker, a parent or the child? How is the notion of 'sufficiently marked or prolonged' measured and against what standard?

Mental health problems are a disturbance of function in one area of relationships, for example, in mood, behaviour or development, of sufficient severity to require professional intervention. A *mental health disorder* is either a severe problem which is persistent or the simultaneous occurrence of a number of problems in the presence of a number of risk factors.

It is important to try to understand the emotional world of young people if we are to effectively assess their need(s) and offer appropriate interventions to meet them. We need to appreciate the vocabulary, perceptions and culture of emotional and behavioural difficulties that young people employ and engage in. For example, younger children describe emotional problems using physical descriptors such as 'my tummy hurts' when they are anxious. Equally, stigma and pride prevent many teenagers from discussing mental health difficulties and their distress is often apparent through aggressive or antisocial behaviour.

A psychosocial approach will adopt a holistic viewpoint which seeks to assemble the important information about a young person and incorporate their internal and external context. Values and principles of empowerment are at the heart of good practice in assessing the mental health of young people.

Prevalence and problems

Research shows that 1 in 17 adolescents in the UK have harmed themselves, representing 200,000 11–15-year-olds (Walker 2005). At the other end of the age spectrum there are increasing numbers of young children under 7 who are excluded from school due to uncontrollable behavioural problems. The increased rate of suicide over the last 30 years in young people is a major cause for concern and a stark indicator of the mental health of this group within society (McClure 2001). Table 7.1 shows the prevalence and range of specific problems affecting young people at different ages and those indicating a gender bias.

Factors associated with suicide in young people include depression, severe mental illness and personality disorder. In many cases substance misuse, particularly with regard to alcohol also occurs as a pre-emptive activity before suicidal behaviour. The recent sharp increase in suicide among 15- to 19-year-old males coincides with the trend reflecting a large increase in the use of alcohol and drugs among young people (Appleby *et al.* 1999). Recent evidence confirms for example that suicide is of particular concern in marginalised and victimised adolescent groups including gay, lesbian and bisexual youth. Research suggests that despite the rhetoric of anti-discriminatory policies and professional statements of equality, heterosexist and homophobic attitudes continue to be displayed by some nurses (Morrison and L'Heureux, 2001). This can further reinforce feelings of rejection, confusion and despair in troubled young people. Other evidence warns against a narrow definition of sexual-minority adolescents that pathologises their behaviour or wrongly assumes a higher risk of self-harming behaviour (Savin-Williams, 2001). Similar discriminatory attitudes are well documented against black and other ethnic minority young people contributing to their emotional vulnerability and risk of developing serious mental health problems.

Disrupted relationships due to family breakdown and social exclusion through unemployment are also factors strongly associated with suicide in young males. There is an assumption that the gender disparity in rates of suicide in young people

Table 7.1 Prevalence of specific child and adolescent mental health problems (ONS 2005)

Mental health problem	Prevalence
Emotional disorders	4.5–9.9% of 10-year-olds
Major depression	0.5–2.5% of children, 2–8% of adolescents
Conduct disorders	6.2–10.8% of 10-year-olds
Tic disorders	1–13% of boys, 1–11% of girls
Obsessive compulsive disorder (OCD)	1.9% of adolescents
Hyperkinetic disorder (ADHD)	1 in 200 of all children
Encopresis (faecal soiling)	2.3% of boys, 0.7% of girls aged 7–8 years
Anorexia nervosa	0.5–1% of 12–19-year-olds
Bulimia nervosa	1% of adolescent girls and young women
Attempted suicide	2–4% of adolescents
Suicide	7.6 per 100,000 15–19-year-olds
Alcohol abuse	29% of all 13-year-olds drink weekly
Cannabis	3–5% of 11–16-year-olds have used
Heroin and cocaine	Less than 1%
Hallucinogens	Increase reported

(three males to one female) reflects the changing roles of men and women in contemporary society.

Poverty is a factor strongly associated with mental health problems among young people. The prevalence for any mental disorder ranges from 16 per cent among young people living in families with a gross weekly household income of under £100 to 9 per cent among those within families in the £300–£399 weekly income range. Only about 6 per cent of young people in families earning £500 per week or more will suffer a mental health problem (ONS 2001). Using this data it has been calculated that in a primary school of 250 pupils there will be 3 children who are seriously depressed, 11 suffering significant distress, 12 who have phobias and 15 with a conduct disorder. In a typical secondary school with 1000 pupils there will be 50 who are seriously depressed, 100 experiencing significant distress, and 5–10 girls with an eating disorder. Many of these young

people will be exhibiting defensive behaviour such as aggression, poor attention and disruption in the classroom combined with poor attendance. They will almost certainly be seen as troublesome rather than suffering from a mental health problem and unfortunately will not receive much needed help and support.

Studies show that problems beginning in early childhood and which remain untreated are likely to persist into later childhood and young adulthood (Mental Health Foundation 2001). Evidence suggests that with conduct disorders and attention deficit hyperactivity disorder (ADHD) it is difficult to prevent the development of later antisocial activity. Young people with emotional disorders tend to be helped with a greater degree of success (Sutton 2000). Some of the more common disorders of mental health found in young people are shown in the next panel.

Mental health disorders in children and adolescents

- Emotional disorders (phobias, anxiety states, depression).
- Conduct disorders (stealing, defiance, fire-setting, aggression, antisocial behaviour).
- Hyperkinetic disorders (disturbance of activity and attention, ADHD).
- Developmental disorders (autism, speech delay, poor bladder control).
- Eating disorders (infant eating problems, anorexia nervosa, bulimia).
- Habit disorders (tics, sleeping problems, soiling).
- Somatic disorders (chronic fatigue syndrome).
- Psychotic disorders (schizophrenia, manic depression, drug-induced psychoses).

Definitions and prevalence

- Consult your friends, neighbours, relatives and/or partner about their perceptions of the behaviour and emotional world of young people.
- Now consider these impressions in relation to the data on prevalence and causation (Table 7.1) and explain the differences.

Place your notes in your professional portfolio.

Developmental theories

Recent advances in genetic research have concluded that to regard nature and nurture as separate and independent is an oversimplification. The answer to what shapes the mental health of young people is both nature *and* the environment or rather the interplay between the two.

Theories provide a framework for discussion and thought to guide and inform the selection of assessment and intervention methods and models. This will be helpful in case conferences, legal issues and writing reports and care plans. Sometimes it is helpful to acknowledge that there is no clear-cut explanation or that there are multiple interpretations for a young person's emotional and behavioural problems.

Nurses with a holistic perspective utilize theoretical concepts to add to their framework of explanation. The combination can be powerful, adding weight to professional arguments, and provide authority for interpretations. However, such theories can also be burdensome and confusing and so should always be used cautiously. It is necessary for the chosen theoretical preference to be identified and acknowledged, and a plan developed which can proceed consistently within that premise.

Key elements of some of the theories relating to human development and the growth of young people are summarized below (for more detail, see Walker 2003). They have been simplified and should be seen as part of a wide spectrum of potential in the genesis of mental health problems in young people rather than deterministic factors. The summaries should be adapted to every individual situation encountered and always considered against the white, Eurocentric perceptions they embodied when first constructed.

Developmental theories

Erikson's psychosocial stages of development

The five stages of Erikson's developmental model which pertain to childhood and adolescence are as follows.

- *Year 1:* the infant requires consistent and stable care in order to develop feelings of security. The child begins to trust the environment but can also develop suspicion and insecurity. Deprivation at this stage can lead to emotional detachment throughout life and difficulties forming relationships.
- *Years 2 and 3:* the child begins to explore and seeks some independence from parents/carers. A sense of autonomy develops but improved self-esteem can combine with feelings of shame and self-doubt. Failure to successfully negotiate this stage may lead to difficulties in social integration.
- *Years 4 and 5:* the child explores the wider environment and plans and initiates new activities but fears punishment and guilt as a consequence. Successful negotiation of this stage results in a confident person while problems can produce deep insecurities.
- *Years 6 to 11:* the older child begins to acquire knowledge and skills to adapt to surroundings and develops a sense of achievement but these can be inhibited by feelings of inferiority and failure if efforts are denigrated.
- *Years 12 to 18:* the individual enters the stage of personal and vocational identity formation with heightened self-perception but with the potential for conflict, confusion and strong emotions. (Erikson, 1968)

Freud's psychosexual stages of development

- *Year 1:* the oral stage during which the infant obtains their principal source of comfort from sucking the breast milk of the mother, and gratification from the nutrition.
- *Years 2 and 3:* the anal stage when the anus and defecation are the major sources of sensual pleasure. The child is preoccupied with body control with parental/carer encouragement. Obsessional behaviour and over-control later in childhood could lead to problems as this stage of development.
- *Years 4 and 5:* the phallic stage with the penis as the focus of attention. In boys the Oedipus complex and in girls the Electra complex are generated through desires to have a sexual relationship with the opposite sex parent. The root of anxieties and neuroses can be found here if successful transition to the next stage is prevented.
- *Years 6 to 11:* the latency stage which is characterized by calm after the storm of the powerful emotions which occur before.
- *Years 12 to 18:* the genital stage where the individual becomes interested in opposite-sex partners as a substitute for the opposite-sex parent, and as a way of resolving the tensions from the Oedipus and Electra complexes. (Freud, 1955)

Bowlby's attachment theory

The following stages represent the process of healthy attachment formation. Mental health problems may develop if an interruption occurs in this process, if care is inconsistent or there is prolonged separation from the main carer.

- *Months 0 to 2:* this stage is characterized by pre-attachment and undiscriminating social responsiveness. The baby is interested in voices and faces and enjoys social interaction.
- *Months 3 to 6:* the infant begins to develop discriminating social responses and experiments with attachments to different people. Familiar people elicit more response than strangers.

- *Months 7 to 36:* attachment to the main carer is prominent with the child showing separation anxiety when carer is absent. The child actively initiates responses from the carer.
- *Years 3 to 18:* the main carer's absences become longer, but the child develops a reciprocal attachment relationship. The child and developing young person begins to understand the carer's needs from a secure emotional base. (Bowlby, 1971; 1982)

Piaget's stages of cognitive development

- *Years 0 to 1.5:* the sensory-motor stage is characterized by the infant exploring their physicality and modifying reflexes until they can experiment with objects and build a mental picture of things around them.
- *Years 1.5 to 7:* the pre-operational stage when the child acquires language, makes pictures and participates in imaginative play. The child tends to be self-centred and fixed on her or his thinking, believing they are responsible for external events.
- *Years 7 to 12:* the concrete operations stage when a child can understand and apply more abstract tasks such as sorting or measuring. This stage is characterized by less egocentric thinking and more relational thinking: differentiation between things. The complexity of the external world is beginning to be appreciated.
- *Years 12 to 18:* the stage of formal operations characterized by the use of rules and problem-solving skills. The child moves into adolescence with increasing capacity to think abstractly and reflect on tasks in a deductive, logical way.

A more recent view of personality development lists five factors that combine elements of the older more classic ways of understanding a child or adolescent together with notions of peer acceptability and adult perceptions (Hampson 1995; Jones and Jones 1999).

1 *Extroversion:* includes traits such as extroverted and introverted, talkative and quiet or bold and timid.
2 *Agreeableness:* is based on characteristics such as agreeable and disagreeable, kind and unkind, selfish and unselfish.
3 *Conscientiousness:* reflects traits such as organized and disorganized, hard-working and lazy, reliable and unreliable, thorough and careless, practical and impractical.
4 *Neuroticism:* is based on traits such as stable and unstable, calm and angry, relaxed and tense or unemotional and emotional.
5 *Openness to experience:* includes the concept of intelligence, together with level of sophistication, creativity, curiosity and cognitive style in problem-solving situations. (Piaget, 1952)

The influence and impact of developmental theories

- Re-read the information above on developmental theories and select one or more that fit with your beliefs about the influences on people.
- Now use it/them to construct and write down your own personal developmental process and make an assessment of yourself at age 13.

Place your notes in your professional portfolio.

Factors of risk and resilience

Evidence suggests that the child and young person's characteristics and the environment are influential in their developing mental health problems (Dulmus and Rapp-Paglicci 2000). Table 7.2 illustrates the risk factors commonly identified as indicators of potential mental health problems in young people.

Table 7.2 Factors that are known to increase the risk of mental health problems in children and young people (Audit Commission 1998)

Child risk factors	Family risk situations	Environmental risk factors
Genetic influences	Overt parental conflict	Socioeconomic disadvantage
Low IQ and learning disability	Family breakdown	Homelessness
Specific developmental delay	Inconsistent or unclear discipline	Disaster
Communication difficulty	Hostile and rejecting relationships	Discrimination
Difficult temperament	Failure to adapt to a child's	Other significant life events
Physical illness, especially if chronic and/or neurological	changing developmental needs	
Academic failure	Abuse – physical, sexual and/or emotional	
Low self-esteem	Parental psychiatric illness	
	Parental criminality, alcoholism, and personality disorder	
	Death and loss, including loss of friendships	

The rise in drug and substance misuse, alcohol consumption and the widening socioeconomic inequalities between the rich and poor within society have created fertile potential for risk factors to proliferate (Townsend 1993). The risks presented to young people from parents with mental health problems are also well known but surprisingly there is a lack of liaison between adult and child and adolescent mental health services to improve services to all family members (Howe 1999; Parsloe 1999; Hetherington and Baistow 2001). Risk assessment in the protection of young people focuses on the likelihood of a parent harming a young person in the future and this usually takes place after an incident has happened with the aim of preventing further harm (Parsloe 1999).

Risk

- Spend 5 to 10 minutes reflecting on examples from your practice experience where you have come into contact with a family.
- Reflect on and write down the general and specific developmental factors which may lead to children and young people being at risk.
- Would this list contain different risk factors if a colleague from a different agency or organization undertook this activity?

Place your notes in your professional portfolio.

When exploring the record of potential risk you compiled in the last exercise, it is worth remembering that this is a *potential* list. Some children and families live through and survive emotional, physical or financial trauma with their lives intact while other families may not be able to endure relatively minor changes in family circumstances.

How people manage can be due to a number of resilience factors an individual or family may have. Werner (2000: 116) defines resilience as 'an end product or buffering process that does not eliminate risks and stress but that allows the individual to deal with them effectively'.

She goes on to identify three mechanisms which enable these protective factors to occur. *Compensation* offers a framework where stress and protective factors counterbalance each other and personal qualities and support outweigh stress. *Challenge* serves as a protective mechanism highlighting the strength that a moderate amount of stress can add to levels of competence. Finally *immunity* is where the protective developmental factors of the young person or their environment moderate the impact of the stress and the young person adapts to the changing environment with less distress. These factors are not mutually exclusive but work together or in sequence depending on the age and stage of the child's development.

While there are a number of specific protective factors, these may vary over time depending on the age and resources of the young person. They include (Corby 1987; Werner 2000; Buchanan 2002):

- low distress;
- low emotionality;
- sociability;
- good self-help skills;
- average intelligence or above;
- impulse control;
- strong motivation;
- keen interests or hobbies;
- positive self-image;
- self-confidence;
- independence;
- good communication skills;
- good problem-solving skills;
- reflective learning style;
- assertion;
- positive values;
- supportive peer group.

Resilience factors in the mental health of young people

- Self-esteem.
- Sociability and autonomy.
- Family compassion and warmth.
- Absence of parental discord.
- Social support systems.
- Encouragement of personal effort and coping.

Scenario: Josh

Josh is 7 years old and at school his behaviour has deteriorated. Josh has become aggressive towards other children and his schoolwork has worsened. He appears to have difficulty concentrating.

Josh's teacher spoke to his parents who could not think of anything which could be causing him concern. However, on reflecting at home they realized he had become more prone to emotional outbursts, was easily upset and often anxious when being left at school or parties even though he always knew his parents would return to collect him.

Josh's behaviour continued to deteriorate and he started to resist going to school. His parents went with Josh to see their family doctor who referred him to Child and Adolescent Mental Health Services (CAMHS) for assessment.

A mental health nurse assessed Josh and his family. It seemed that the family were in debt due to an increase in their mortgage and lately Josh's parents were arguing often. Josh ate meals at different times to his parents and they did not spend much time together. The mental health nurse visited regularly and worked with the whole family. The nurse suggested the family should do more activities together and consciously build family relationships through eating together and spending time in one another's company.

Josh's behaviour has now improved and returned to normal while his parents say they feel less stressed and their relationship has improved.

Often mental disturbance in children and adolescents is not identified or under-reported. Difficult behaviour is attributed to maladjustment or 'bad' behaviour when in fact a mental health problem may be the cause.

Mental health problems frequently occur in young people who cause concern to staff working in education, social services or youth justice. The ability of teachers, social workers and probation officers to identify mental health problems in children and young people is crucial. Responding in a timely and appropriate manner to the early signs of mental health problems makes an enormous difference to the chances of interventions being successful. However, barriers remain to the development of a better understanding of mental health difficulties between professionals in all agencies who come into contact with young people.

Barriers between agencies involved in the health care of young people

- A widespread reluctance to 'label' a child or young person as mentally ill.
- A poor appreciation of specialist child psychology and mental health services.
- Priorities which are set within the statutory framework of the Mental Health Act 1983, 2007, Children Act 1989 and Education Act 1993 conflicting.
- Lack of knowledge and close working between agencies.

How a young person deals with adversity either actively or reactively and the ability to remain positive is a function of self-esteem and self-efficacy. Features such as secure, stable and affectionate relationships, success, achievement and temperamental attributes all have a positive role. However, Rutter (1985) suggests that protection does not lie in the buffering effects of supportive factors, while the evidence points towards the importance of developmental links. The quality of a young person's resilience to developing mental health problems or emotional and behavioural difficulties is influenced by early life experiences but does not determine later outcomes.

Effective assessment should take account of individual characteristics, the family and the broader environment in order to be effective in helping young people escape from adversity. Organizing services across the spectrum of multi-agency provision in partnership between CAMHS professionals and parents offers the opportunity of involving dormant protective factors to interrupt the causal chain of negative events (Little and Mount 1999). A progressive, preventive environment that promotes the young person's emotional well-being is preferable to reacting afterwards to the consequences of neglect or abuse. Individual factors regarded as promoting resilience are listed in the next panel.

Factors that help promote resilience

- An even and adaptable temperament.
- A capacity for problem-solving.
- Physical attractiveness.
- A sense of humour.
- Good social skills and supportive peers.
- A sense of autonomy and purpose.
- Secure attachment to at least one parent.
- Links with the wider community.

Consider the above list, and then answer the questions below.

- What details do you know about a child or young person you have come across in practice?
- In relation to that child, can you think of three risk factors and three resilience factors?
- Weigh them up and decide whether the balance falls towards risk or resilience.

Place your notes in your professional portfolio

The Common Assessment Framework

Government guidance indicates that the Common Assessment Framework (CAF) should be used at the first sign of emerging vulnerability of young people and act as a marker for referral to another agency or specialist service. The concept of the CAF is to provide a shared approach to an initial needs assessment for use by statutory or voluntary sector staff in education, early years, health, police, youth justice or social work. This will reduce the number of assessments experienced by young people and their families and prevent their being asked the same questions multiple times as well as promoting better communication between health care professionals from different agencies.

The CAF is expected to contribute to a change in culture across the workforce involved with the mental health of young people (DfES 2005).

Advantages offered by the CAF

- General guidance on its use.
- A common procedure for assessment.
- A methodology based on the Framework for the Assessment of Children in Need and their Families (DoH 2001a).
- A focus on child development and communication skills with children, carers and parents.
- Gaining consent.
- How to record findings and identify an appropriate response.
- How to share information when a child moves between local authority areas.
- An explanation of the roles and responsibilities of different agencies and practitioners.

The process of the CAF

Staff in adult services and agencies, and not just those directly involved in working with children and young people, need to be aware of the CAF. The assessment should be completed with the full knowledge, consent and involvement of the young person and their parents, be centred on their care and action-focused, and form part of an ongoing process.

- *Preparation:* the health care professional will discuss the process with the young person and their family and gain an understanding of the issues and what can be done to help and communicate with other health care professionals already involved. If a health care professional decides a common assessment would be useful, then the agreement of the young person and their parent(s) is sought as appropriate.

- *Discussion*: the health care professional meets with the child or young person and their family and completes the assessment with them. Use is also made of any information which is already known and existing assessments are updated. A picture of the strengths of the young person and their family can be gained and their needs ascertained. It is important that actions are agreed to be carried out by the health care service, other agencies and the young person and their family and that these are written down.

- *Service delivery*: actions need to be delivered, coordinated and monitored. The young person and family may also be responsible for carrying out some actions. The health care professional may, for example, make referrals or negotiate access to other services using the CAF to demonstrate evidence of the need or of direct interventions with the family. Progress also needs to be monitored and evaluated. Where the young person or family needs services from a range of agencies, a coordinator needs to be appointed as the central point for contact. The elements of the CAF are listed in the next panel.

Elements of the CAF

Development of the baby, child or young person

- *General health:* health conditions or impairments which significantly affect everyday life functioning.
- *Physical development:* includes mobility and level of physical or sexual maturity or delayed development.
- *Speech, language and communications development:* the ability to communicate effectively, confidently and appropriately with others.
- *Emotional and social development:* the emotional and social response the baby, child or young person gives to parents, carers and others.
- *Behavioural development:* lifestyle and the capacity for self-control.
- *Identity:* the growing sense of self as a separate and valued person, self-esteem, self-image and social presentation.
- *Family and social relationships:* the ability to empathize and build stable and affectionate relationships with others, including family, peers and the wider community.
- *Self-care skills and independence:* the acquisition of practical, emotional and communication competencies to increase independence.
- *Understanding, reasoning and problem-solving:* includes the ability to understand and organize information, reason and solve problems.
- *Participation in learning, education and employment:* the degree to which the young person has access to and is engaged in education and/or work-based training and, if not, the reasons why this is the case.
- *Progress and achievement in learning:* the young person's educational achievements and progress including social relationships and skills in recreational activities.
- *Aspirations:* the ambitions of the child or young person and whether they are realistic and they are able to plan how to meet them. There may be barriers to their achievement because of other responsibilities within the home or family.

Parents and carers

- *Basic care, ensuring safety and protection:* the extent to which the baby, child or young person's physical needs are met and they are protected from harm, danger and self-harm.
- *Emotional warmth and stability:* the provision of emotional warmth in a stable family environment, giving the baby, child or young person a sense of being valued.
- *Guidance, boundaries and stimulation:* enabling the child or young person to regulate their own emotions and behaviour while promoting their learning and intellectual development through encouragement, stimulation and social opportunities.

Family and environmental factors

- *Family history, functioning and well-being:* the impact of family situations and experiences.
- *Wider family:* the family's relationships with relatives and other people.
- *Housing, employment and financial considerations:* the environment in which the family live including amenities, facilities, employment and income.

Social and community resources

- *Neighbourhood:* the wider context of the neighbourhood and its impact on the baby, child or young person; availability of facilities and services.
- *Accessibility:* the proximity and transport links to schools, day care, primary health care, places of worship, transport, shops, leisure activities and family support services.
- *Characteristics:* levels of crime, disadvantage, employment, substance misuse or trading.
- *Social integration:* includes the degree of the young person's social integration or isolation, peer influences, friendships and social networks.

Using the CAF

- While student nurses are unlikely to be involved in these assessments it is a good learning opportunity to observe a health care professional carrying them out.
- Review the above material and write down those elements with which you are less familiar.
- Discuss these with other students, health care professionals on your placement and read more about these issues to help you understand them and integrate an awareness of them into your practice.

Place your notes in your professional portfolio.

Assessment is often mistakenly regarded as a one-way process done by nurses to service users with the purpose of gathering information. However, it is more helpfully viewed as an interactive process and the way it is conducted can positively influence the outcome of the assessment. Simply engaging with a child in some basic drawing or play activity to gain an understanding of them can begin to change the child's behaviour. Interpretation of the child's emotional and behavioural state therefore needs to take account of the potential impact of the assessment process.

Intervention

It is more likely in practice placements that you will experience your mentor working with families. In these settings your interventions ought to be focused on benefiting the mental health and well-being of the whole family, which includes the parents and children. It is helpful to reflect on the issues, the decisions involved and the consequences of delivering therapeutic interventions with young people and their families, as reflected in the following scenario.

Scenario: Sonali

Sonali is 32 years old and married to Anwar. They have two children, Kamisha aged 7 and Anil aged 5. After Anil's birth Sonali became very depressed and required inpatient admission to an adult mental health unit. As the family are very private, securing Anwar's support for Sonali's admission involved a large amount of work and development of trust between the family and the mental health services.

The admission was brief but since then Sonali has received regular visits and support from Jaswinda, a female mental health nurse with a community mental health team (CMHT).

Jaswinda has noticed that Sonali's mood has deteriorated recently. Sonali has become pregnant for the third time, and during a visit Sonali revealed to Jaswinda that she has not taken her antidepressant medication for some time as she was concerned this would affect her ability to have children.

Jaswinda visits Sonali's home with Kala, a third-year mental health nursing student who is two months into a three-month placement and has visited Sonali with Jaswinda on two previous occasions. On leaving the house Jaswinda asks Kala what she observed at the home which she felt was significant. Kala noticed the house seemed less clean and tidy than before and there were piles of washing lying about. Also that Jaswinda was heavily pregnant and seemed tired and low in mood. Her facial expressions lacked animation and seemed 'mask' like.

Jaswinda was concerned and spoke to Anwar who has a large extended family. He arranged that Sonali would receive support at home in managing domestic tasks but also that she had company in the home and was not left alone. Sonali was successfully delivered of a third child.

Every intervention should have a purpose and be part of the agreement established with the young person and their family and other key individuals and health care professionals. The seemingly routine task of an assessment is an intervention in its own right and provides the opportunity to gain a greater understanding of young people and their situations in a therapeutic way. The assessment meeting can be used to establish a helping relationship as the basis for initiating change rather than being an administrative task.

The choice of intervention available in mental health work with young people is broad because of the variety of psychological and social factors affecting young people. Before embarking on any one form of intervention it is necessary to reflect on the ethical questions raised by the choices made and the potential consequences. For example, individual counselling or therapy may succeed in helping a young person to develop a sense of self but alienate them from their family. While family therapy may result in the improvement of a child with emotional difficulties, their relationship with their siblings may be adversely affected or problems may be exposed in the marriage/partnership (Sharman 1997). A child who is bottling up their feelings may learn to express them in counselling but then come into conflict with their community because an expectation of their culture is to develop self-control and the containment of emotions.

A student comments on their experience of finding health promotion resources for adolescents with Aspergers ...

I have recently been researching the services available for 16–18-year-olds with Aspergers syndrome. Due to it being a mild form of autism there seem to be no services. This is the age where people may need extra support, for example, looking for a job or going to college. However, I found this website about the support group SAFE (Supporting Aspergers Families in Essex) who explain that they have experienced the same difficulties as my family have and are working to develop services for people and families affected by Aspergers syndrome. Hopefully I will be able to attend one of their monthly meetings.

What I found most interesting is that Essex has one of the largest populations of people with Aspergers syndrome in the country, but it is still poorly understood by health, education and social services. I have also looked at the primary care trust website and read quite a few of their meeting notes and reports where some of them touch on how they need to improve child and adolescent mental health services. The draft commissioning intentions discuss how they should have a clearer point of access, especially those with low to moderate emotional and behaviour problems, which I found very interesting.

Each interventionist approach comes with its own set of assumptions and the potential for unintended consequences. While the same intervention could be given to two children with the same problem, only one of them may benefit. It is important to acknowledge potential ethical dilemmas and reflect upon these before proceeding with any course of action. The crucial point is to ensure the most effective intervention is offered for the appropriate problem with the right child.

Preventive practice

Evidence demonstrates conclusively that one of the biggest risk factors in developing adult mental health problems is a history of untreated or inadequately supported childhood mental health problems (DoH 1998, 2001b; Howe 1999). Therefore it is imperative that our work addresses this growing problem and offers a distinct contribution to preventive practice and the government's health improvement programme. Early intervention is often synonymous with preventive practice and nowhere is this more the case than in child and adolescent mental health work (Walker 2001a, 2001b).

Initiatives to prepare young people for potential difficulties can be carried out in various settings, not just the health services. These include schools, youth clubs and via resources such as telephone helplines, internet discussion groups and campaigns, to reach out to children and young people before they reach a crisis.

One of the most significant preventive approaches is helping children and young people cope with the stresses faced in modern society. Every generation has to negotiate the manifestations of stress within their culture, and relying on approaches used by former generations is not useful. This is challenging to nurses who will naturally draw from their own experiences as an instinctive resource and may find this does not coincide with the very different world views and values of a new generation of children and young people.

A good starting point is to understand the different levels of stress experienced by young people. Stress is a broad concept embracing a diverse range of experiences. The key is to ensure that the young person can independently categorize their level of stress. For example, whether bereavement is an acute or moderate stress or parental separation/divorce is a severe and longer-lasting stress. What helps is enabling the young person to focus on what can be done to improve the situation rather than concentrating on negative feelings (Rutter and Smith 1995).

Empowering practice

Services geared towards the needs of specific age groups of children, young people or adults are determined by the type of help offered and whether it is perceived as family or individual support (Walker 2001a). While age is one factor, the type of problem and degree and duration will also be relevant in the decision on the type of help which is offered to the child or young person. Nurses working to empower children and young people will strive to find or offer themselves as the most acceptable and accessible type of intervention resource. However, dilemmas can be encountered where some parents and/or young people express rigid views about what they want which contradict the evidence of what can help.

For example, a parent might insist on a child receiving individual counselling to address troublesome behaviour while all of the evidence points towards couple/marital counselling. In specialist settings your offer of help may be rejected because parents insist on a consultation with a psychiatrist even though this may reinforce their beliefs that their child is the one with the problem. This may inhibit engaging with them in a partnership approach which widens their field of vision from scapegoating a child who may be simply displaying the symptoms of familial/marital or environmental stress. These beliefs and perceptions are rooted in a number of factors such as professional status, wanting the best for the child and being driven by deep feelings of guilt, anxiety, fear and anger. Using a holistic model will enable you to respectfully address these issues in an empathic manner and with unconditional positive regard (Rogers 1951).

Scenario: Lewis

Lewis, aged 8, was referred to the child and family consultation clinic at CAMHS with frequent episodes of bed wetting at night (nocturnal enuresis). A meeting was arranged with a mental health nurse who works with CAMHS. On attending assessment the mother expressed great distress and embarrassment about the situation and wanted medication which she had read about on the internet.

During the assessment the nurse discovered that the parents were arguing and in financial trouble and the male partner had begun drinking heavily just before the onset of the problem. Rather than seeking a prescription for medication the nurse encouraged the parents to attend counselling sessions in which they could discuss their relationship problems and work on solutions. After several sessions and a period of more harmonious behaviour they reported that Lewis's enuresis had stopped.

Characteristic of a psychosocial model is to understand the person as well as their problem(s). This means adopting a framework that accepts the notion of the inner and outer worlds of the service user which may be in conflict and cause repetitive, self-destructive behaviour (Walker 2005). For example, a person may have a low sense of self-esteem due to receiving repeated and sustained parental criticism when young and engage in a series of relationships with partners who are abusive. Their mental picture of their identity leads them to make choices which are detrimental.

The psychosocial model offers another resource for the person whose anxiety, defence mechanisms and personal difficulties are hampering their attainment of fulfilling relationships with others and hindering effective development. Recognition of the feelings underlying these behaviours offers a source of material with which to work. Practice based on a psychosocial model therefore (Stepney and Ford 2000):

● concentrates on the present rather than the past;
● helps the person establish equilibrium between their inner emotional states and the pressures they face in the outside world;
● uses the service user's relationship with the nurse actively.

Reflective practice

Reflective practice is an essential element of working with people in a helping role. Practicing reflectively fosters self-awareness of the feelings generated in the helping relationship between the nurse and the service user. Supervision or professional consultation in the area of child and adolescent mental health is a crucial component of reflective practice. Student nurses need to work closely with and seek regular supervision, guidance and feedback from, their practice mentor.

Analysing and planning

In developing a deeper understanding of difficulties with a view to deciding on an intervention, you can draw on a range of theories and methods. Differing solutions can be arrived at by viewing situations with the aid of these theories. Forming alternative understandings and explanations is a good habit to acquire, and the most desirable practice is where an interpretation is helpful to both you and your client in developing solutions and where it is supported by a sound rationale.

Maintaining a perspective which considers the consequences of using particular theories and encourages the young person and their family to develop their own theories about their situation will empower them and enhance your practice. You will need more than one model of assessment and intervention to be able to meet the many varied situations which can be encountered. Having a grasp of different models of practice should enable you, together with the young person and their family, to select the most appropriate.

Integrating knowledge, skills and values in analysing information and being able to weigh its significance and priority as a basis for effective planning is a demanding task. O'Sullivan (1999) suggests that sound planning relies on the elements outlined in the next panel being taken into account in the decision-making process.

Skills and knowledge in planning care

- *Being critically aware and taking context into account:* knowledge of legal requirements and agency procedures is critical to planning what is possible and permissible. Statutory obligations have to be balanced against our endeavour to take a holistic perspective of the situation.
- *Involving the client to the highest feasible level:* there are four levels: being told; being consulted; being a partner; and being in control. A key skill is to identify the level of involvement most appropriate to the particular situation.
- *Consulting with all stakeholders:* there could be numerous stakeholders involved in working with a particular service user. Some will have more systematic contact but only general knowledge of the client. However, they could be just as valuable as someone with limited contact but who has specialized knowledge. A range of perceptions can either enhance the clarity of a situation or produce a disparate and confusing picture.
- *Being clear in your thinking and aware of your emotions:* a heightened element of self-awareness is always useful. Over-reacting to a situation on the basis of tiredness, stress, the day of the week or false information needs to be guarded against. Equally, under-reacting to a risky situation because of feelings of pity, empathy or over-optimism can contribute to an escalation of risk factors.
- *Producing a well-reasoned 'frame' of the decision situation that is consistent with the available information:* through framing processes you can shape the information into a picture of the situation, plan goals and create a set of options. Listing key factors and considering the weight to give to each requires knowledge, experience and the capacity for short- and long-term predictions of the consequences of various interventions.
- *Basing your course of action on a systematic appraisal of the options:* the plan could be based on the principle that a statutory duty overrides the traumatic impact of the subsequent intervention. Or an option is chosen based on risk assessment and an awareness of the available resources to support the intervention.

Strategies for integration

Learning arises as a result of the four-stage process of concrete experience, reflective observation, abstract conceptualization and active experimentation. You can use this model to describe and facilitate the application of your knowledge and theory to practice. The following points can guide you in this process:

- guard against the false belief that practice does not need the support of theory;
- research-minded practice can help integrate theory and practice;
- the *critical incident technique* is a way of analysing a situation where strong emotions are raised and interfere with the ability to function effectively then or in the future;
- developing a group approach for narrowing the gap between theory and practice can be very effective;
- planning intervention in your work and the decision-making process includes thinking about the situation being addressed.

In health and social care some professionals believe in practice based on intuitive wisdom derived from years of experience. Others advocate the use of objectivity offered by detailed assessment and clear analysis of all the factors in a situation. As with many polarized debates, the desire to simplify in order to heighten differences can obscure the valuable contribution of each approach. Intuition can be unreliable while analysis is not inevitably technical, but both can offer equally useful ways of thinking.

Methods and models of practice

The following methods and models of practice are not unique to working with young people or an exclusive list. They have been chosen from the range of modern methods and models available to aid clarity in selecting the most appropriate interventions in child and adolescent mental health work (Milner and O'Byrne 1998; Dogra *et al.* 2002).

Systemic practice

Using a systemic model in mental health practice with young people is characterized by the key notion that young people have a social context which influences their behaviour to a greater or lesser extent and affects their perception of their problem. An important factor is the family and this has led to the practice of family therapy. It offers a broad framework for intervention enabling the mapping of all the important elements affecting families as well as a method of working with those elements to effect beneficial change. Key features are listed below.

Features of systemic practice

- Convening family meetings to listen to everyone connected to an individual's problem (e.g. at a family group conference).
- Constructing a geneogram (family tree) with a family to help identify the relationships and dynamics.
- Harnessing the strengths of families to support individuals in trouble.
- Using a problem-oriented style to energize the family to find their own solutions.
- Assisting in the development of insight into patterns of behaviour and communication within the family system.
- Adopting a neutral position as far as possible in order to avoid accusations of collusion.

Many professionals use this model to help guide their practice. It is useful to clarify situations where there is multiprofessional involvement and can help in establishing boundaries and identifying who does what in often complex, fast-moving and confusing situations. It also helps to avoid the assumption that the individual young person is the main focus for intervention.

Some families experience difficulty appreciating the interconnectedness of the problems of young people with wider influences. This model is a way of viewing the position, role and behaviour of individuals within the context of the whole system, but can appear to be abstract, culturally insensitive and disempowering. The model also has the potential to undermine the importance of individual work and avoid locating responsibility in child abuse situations.

Psychodynamic practice

This model offers a concept of the mind and the mechanisms by which it works, providing an understanding of why some children behave in seemingly repetitive, destructive ways. It is a 'one-to-one' helping relationship involving advanced listening and communication skills. The psychodynamic model provides a framework to address profound disturbances and inner conflicts in children and adolescents concerning issues of loss, attachment, anxiety and personal development.

Features of the psychodynamic model

- It is a useful way of attempting to understand seemingly irrational behaviour.
- The notion of defence mechanisms is a helpful way of assessing male adolescents who have difficulty expressing their emotions.
- The model acknowledges the influence of past events/attachments and can create a healthy suspicion about surface behaviour.
- The development of insight can be an empowering experience to enable children and young people to understand themselves and take more control over their own lives
- The model has influenced a listening, accepting approach that avoids being directive.
- It can be used to assess which developmental stage is reflected in the young person's behaviour and to gauge the level of anxiety/depression.

Criticisms of the psychodynamic model are that it originated from a medical model of human behaviour and relies on expert opinion without taking very much account of the person in their socioeconomic context. It is not considered an appropriate way of working with some ethnic minority groups and on its own cannot adequately explain the effects of racism.

Cognitive behavioural practice

This model is based on the key concept that all behaviour is learned and is therefore amenable to be unlearned or changed. The cognitive behavioural approach offers a framework for assessing the pattern of behaviour in young pepole and a method for altering their thinking, feelings and behaviour. The model aims to help the person become aware of how their thoughts and emotions are linked and enables them to acquire new life skills. Using this approach you would decide on the goals/new behaviours to be achieved in collaboration with the client, and these goals would be clear and capable of measurement.

Characteristics of the cognitive behavioural approach

- The ABC formula can be used to establish the antecedents (A), the behaviour (B) and the consequences (C) of the problem.
- The model focuses on what behaviours are desired and reinforces them.
- Interventions involve modelling and rehearsing desired behavioural patterns.
- Behavioural and cognitive approaches are combined to produce better results.
- The young person is gradually desensitized to the threat or phobia they are experiencing.

The cognitive behavioural model offers a systematic, scientific approach and framework with which to structure practice and interventions. The approach goes some way towards encouraging participatory practice and empowers the person by providing them with useful techniques to overcome their problems. The model also has a focus on both social and individual factors.

Usually it is only the immediate environment of the young person that is examined, and this technique is not as value-free as it claims. The scientific nature of behavioural assessment depends on assumptions about certainty. In practice, there is also is often a tendency to rush to a solution after a limited assessment where the theory is adapted so that the individual client changes to accommodate their circumstances rather than the other way round.

Task-centred practice

Task-centred work is the most popular base for contemporary assessment and intervention practice but it may be that it is used as a set of activities rather than a theoretically-based approach from which a set of activities flows.

Key features of task-centred practice

- This approach is based on client agreement or service user acceptance of a legal justification for action.
- The aim is to move from problem to goal and from what is wrong to what is needed.
- It is based on tasks which are central to the process of change and build on the strengths of the service user.
- The approach is time-limited and preserves client self-esteem and independence as far as possible.
- It is a highly structured model of practice using a 'building block' approach so that each task can be agreed and success measured by moving from problem to goal.
- The approach serves as a basic method for use with the majority of children and young people.

In the task-centred model the problem is always defined by the client and therefore their values, beliefs and perceptions are respected. This approach encourages young people to select the problem they want to work on and engages them in task selection and review. It lends itself to a collaborative and empowering approach by enabling you to carry out your share of tasks and review them alongside the client's. Setting time limits and dates for task reviews allows progress to be regularly monitored, aids motivation and promotes optimism.

While the task-centred approach to practice has the capacity to provide empowerment, it can sometimes prohibit active measures by nurses to ensure this is the case. Although ostensibly value-free and intrinsically non-oppressive it is necessary to continually reflect on practice to make this explicit. The coaching role could be open to abuse or be used in an authoritarian manner. The emphasis on simple and measurable tasks may focus attention on concrete solutions that obscure the potential advocacy role of practice. Finally, the approach requires a degree of intrinsic cognitive ability and motivation in the young person that in some cases will be lacking.

Crisis intervention

Crisis theory is concerned with situations where a person finds themselves much more dependent on external sources of support than at other times in their life. It has three distinct phases. *Impact* is where a threat is recognized. Then *recoil* occurs, which is an attempt to restore equilibrium, but failure can leave the person feeling stressed and defeated. Finally *adjustment/adaptation* or *breakdown* occurs where the person begins to move to a different level of functioning.

Crisis is usually precipitated by interrelated factors. It is helpful to view crisis as a stage of *disequilibrium* where tension and anxiety have risen to a level which overwhelms the individual's coping mechanisms. However, rather than regarding crisis as the failure of the individual to manage, it is instead more useful to regard it as providing the opportunity for significant interventions at times when stakeholders are more likely to engage with your strategy.

Characteristics of crisis intervention

- Crisis intervention uses ideas from psychodynamic theory in understanding the way each person can be helped to gain insight into their functioning and discover ways of coping better.
- This approach is used in conjunction with risk assessment and risk management techniques.
- Crisis intervention is short-term in nature.

- Crisis interventions focus on relating a client's internal crises to external changes.
- It can help in cases of bereavement, loss, reactive depression and trauma.
- It is based on the notion that people can return to their previous level of functioning depending on the nature of the problem and the quality of help provided.

Conclusion

Increasingly the mental health of children and adolescents is recognized as being a priority in mental health services. In recent years there has been an emphasis on the development of a community-based network of services and identifying mental health problems as early as possible has become a priority. Health services endeavour to provide a flexible approach and work in partnership with other agencies. Nowhere is this more vital than in services for children and adolescents, because identifying mental health problems as soon as possible reduces the extent and severity of longer-term mental ill health.

Children and adolescents have a particular perspective and viewpoint of life which radically changes as they progress through developmental stages. As adults we can only attempt to guess at what the world looks like to a child or adolescent and what is important to them. Therefore we need to listen carefully to their needs, understand their specific and individual views and take their concerns seriously. As health care practitioners we need to develop solutions which often involve the views and perspectives of the whole family and are flexible to individual situations and circumstances.

Unlike other age groups within society children and adolescents are often involved with compulsory or statutorily regulated education or care services, ranging from nurseries and preschools to infants school, primary school, senior schools and further education colleges. Working to overcome barriers between agencies is a necessity if we are to offer effective multi-agency solutions for children and adolescents with mental health problems.

References

Anderson, K. and Anderson, L. (eds) (1995) *Mosby's Pocket Dictionary of Nursing,* London: Mosby.

Appleby, L., Cooper, J. and Amos, T. (1999) Psychological autopsy study of suicides by people aged under 35, *British Journal of Psychiatry,* 175: 168–74.

Audit Commission (1998) *Child and Adolescent Mental Health Services.* London: HMSO.

Bowlby, J. (1971) *Attachment and loss.* Harmondsworth: Penguin

Bowlby, J (1982) *Attachment: Vol. 1.* New York: Basic Books.

Buchanan, A. (2002) Family support, in D. McNeish, T. Newman and H. Roberts (eds) *What Works for Children? Effective Services for Children and Families.* Buckingham: Open University Press.

Corby, B (1987) *Working with Child Abuse.* Buckingham: Open University Press.

DfES (Department for Education and Skills) (2005) *Common Assessment Framework.* London: HMSO.

Dogra, N., Parkin, A., Gale, F. and Frake, C. (2002) *A Multidisciplinary Handbook of Child and Adolescent Mental Health for Front-line Professionals.* London: Jessica Kingsley.

DoH (Department of Health) (1998) *Modernising Mental Health Services: Safe, Supportive and Sensible.* London: HMSO.

DoH (Department of Health) (2001a) *Children Looked After in England: 2000/2001.* London: HMSO.

DoH (Department of Health) (2001b) *Framework for the Assessment of Children in Need and their Families.* London: HMSO.

Dulmus, C. and Rapp-Paglicci, L. (2000) The prevention of mental disorders in children and adolescents: future research and public policy recommendations, *Families in Society: The Journal of Contemporary Human Services,* 8(3): 294–303.

Erikson, E. (1968) *Identity, youth and crisis.* New York: Norton.

Freud, S. (1955) "Three essays on the theory of sexuality" Standard Edition of the Complete Psychological Works of Sigmund Freud, Vol. 10. London: Hogarth Press.

Hampson, S.E. (1995) The construction of personality, in S.E. Hampson and A.M. Coleman (eds) *Individual Differences and Personality.* London: Longman.

HAS (Health Advisory Service) (1995) *Together We Stand: Thematic Review on the Commissioning, Role and Management of Child and Adolescent Mental Health Services.* London: HMSO.

Hetherington, R. and Baistow, K. (2001) Supporting families with a mentally ill parent: European perspectives on interagency cooperation, *Child Abuse Review,* 10: 351–65.

Howe, D. (ed.) (1999) *Attachment and Loss in Child and Family Social Work.* Aldershot: Ashgate.

Jones, D. and Jones, M, (1999) The assessment of children with emotional and behavioural difficulties: psychometrics and beyond, in C. Cooper (ed.) *Understanding and Supporting Children with Emotional and Behavioural Difficulties.* London: Jessica Kingsley.

Little, M. and Mount, K. (1999) *Prevention and Early Intervention with Children in Need.* Aldershot: Ashgate.

McClure, G. (2001) Suicide in children and adolescents in England and Wales 1970–1998, *British Journal of Psychiatry*, 178: 469–74.

Mental Health Foundation (2001) *Turned Upside Down.* London: Mental Health Foundation.

Milner, J. and O'Byrne, P. (1998) *Assessment in Social Work Practice.* London: Macmillan.

Morrison, L. and L'Heureux, J. (2001) *Suicide and gay/lesbian/bisexual youth: implications for clinicians*, Journal of Adolescence, 24, 39–49.

ONS (Office for National Statistics) (2001) *Child and Adolescent Mental Health.* London: HMSO.

ONS (Office for National Statistics) (2005) *Child and Adolescent Mental Health Statistics.* London: HMSO.

O'Sullivan, T. (1999) *Decision-making in Social Work.* London: Macmillan.

Parsloe, P. (ed.) (1999) *Risk Assessment in Social Care and Social Work.* London: Jessica Kingsley.

Piaget, J.P. (1952) *The origins of intelligence in children.* New York: International Universities Press.

Rogers, C. (1951) *Client-centred Therapy.* Boston, MA: Houghton Mifflin.

Rutter, M. (1985) Resiliance in the face of adversity, *British Journal of Psychiatry*, 147: 598–611.

Rutter, M. and Smith, D. (1995) *Psychosocial Disorders in Young People.* London: Wiley.

Savin-Williams, R. (2001) *A critique of research on sexual minority youth*, Journal of Adolescence, 24, 5–13.

Sharman, W. (1997) *Children and Adolescents with Mental Health Problems.* London: Bailliere Tindall.

Stepney, R. and Ford, S. (2000) *Social Work Models, Methods and Theories.* Lyme Regis: Russell House.

Sutton, C. (2000) *Child and Adolescent Behaviour Problems.* Leicester: BPS.

Townsend, P. (1993) *The International Analysis of Poverty.* Hemel Hempstead: Harvester Wheatsheaf.

Walker, S. (2001a) Developing child and adolescent mental health services, *Journal of Child Health Care*, 5(2): 71–6.

Walker, S. (2001b) Consulting with children and young people, *The International Journal of Children's Rights*, 9: 45–56.

Walker, S. (2003) *Working Together for Healthy Young Minds: A Multidisciplinary Workbook.* Lyme Regis: Russell House Publishers.

Walker, S. (2005) *Culturally Competent Therapy: Working with Children and Young People.* Basingstoke: Palgrave Macmillan.

Werner, E. (2000) Protective factors and individual resilience, in *Handbook of Early Childhood Interventions*, 2nd edn. Cambridge: Cambridge University Press.

WHO (World Health Organization) (2001) *World Health Day, Mental Health: Stop Exclusion, Dare to Care.* Geneva: WHO.

Mental health services in the community

8

Geoffrey Amoateng and Nick Wrycraft

Learning objectives

By the end of this chapter you will have:

- Gained a brief overview of the historical background leading to the emergence of care in the community.
- Developed an understanding of the *National Service Framework for Mental Health* and the role of the Care Programme Approach (CPA).
- Gained an appreciation of the network of mental health services in the community, and in inpatient areas as a result of the *National Service Framework for Mental Health*.

Introduction

Over the last 50 years the mental health services have transformed considerably from long established inpatient institutions to being based in the community. It is important for student mental health nurses to understand how and why these changes have occurred and so the chapter commences by very briefly outlining the background to the emergence of care in the community.

Wherever mental health nursing students work in practice settings they will encounter the *National Service Framework for Mental Health* (DoH 1999) and the Care Programme Approach (CPA), and so we will discuss their origins and the role they perform in mental health services. The chapter then considers the range of mental health services in the community-based network in accordance with the *National Service Framework for Mental Health* 1999.

Throughout the chapter scenarios and examples of mental health problems will be presented to illustrate the clinical and professional complexities involved.

A mental health student's insight into placement in a community mental health team ...

The placement was in the community and a chance to work with service users first hand. My mentor was very laid back, and had been in the job for many years. She instantly made me feel at ease, offering me cups of tea for which I was very grateful as this was the first time I had ever worked in an office environment. It was actually the first time I had worked anywhere in the last six years. I was given my own desk with two drawers, a phone, and a lamp on a flexi-arm that never stayed up and had my own pigeon hole for my mail. This really helped me settle in and made me feel like I was part of the team. My desk was my comfort zone.

The history of mental health services

Some form of care and control has existed for people who have a mental illness for at least 800 years in the UK, with the first institution, the Bethlem hospital, founded in London in 1247 (Jones 1993; Norman and Ryrie 2005). Yet in spite of existing for so long, services for the mentally ill through the centuries have been slow to develop.

One reason for this is that the causes of mental illness are not well understood. Through the centuries there have been numerous different and competing theories concerning the origins of mental illness, ranging from religious fervour or possession to moral iniquity (Jones 1993). While some doctors claimed a medical and scientific basis to mental illness, until the seventeenth century their knowledge was very limited and there was a lack of successful treatment options.

People with mental health problems were a source of fear and apprehension and presented a challenge to society. Often the mentally ill were physically restrained or kept under lock and key and out of sight. Asylums were established to discreetly remove the mentally ill from public view and minimize embarrassment to their families and disruption to society.

By the eighteenth century, through pressure to regulate the system and prevent illegal detention, a network of state-run institutions were in existence across the country. Generally these functioned as self-contained communities with little contact or communication with the world outside. Frequently conditions were harsh with little difference between the treatment of the mentally ill, criminals and the poor (Jones 1993).

As discussed in Chapter 1, the practice of what was to become mental health nursing was steadily evolving during the institutional era. In spite of the bleak image of this period for mental health services, there are a number of positive examples of health care staff working effectively with service users. However, until the latter part of the twentieth century large mental health institutions continued to be the main source of mental health service provision.

In the period following the Second World War a rapid sequence of events unfolded with important and far-reaching consequences. The spirit of optimism which prevailed following years of hardship and austerity signalled the end of the institutional era. Several factors have been identified as instrumental in bringing about this change and are summarized below.

Influences on the development of mental health services post-1945

- *Developments in medication:* in 1953 a new class of psychiatric drugs called phenothiazenes became available. The effect was to transform mental hospitals from intimidating environments designed to contain aggression and distress to institutions which permitted staff to work more proactively with patients and offer the possibility of life within the community due to the better management of psychiatric symptoms.

- *Changes in treatment and philosophy of care:* before the Second World War large-scale institutions reinforced a sense of order and equilibrium within society which disempowered patients. From working with traumatized soldiers, psychiatrists in the Second World War increasingly recognized the therapeutic effect of 'talking treatments'. In the post-war era, groups and therapeutic communities were established to treat large numbers of soldiers psychologically traumatized by their experiences. The innovative work of figures such as Bion and Foulkes fundamentally altered mental health care but was also very successful and adopted and then further developed by other psychiatrists. Many former servicemen found work in the mental health services and sought to change the antiquated institutionalized ways of working (Nolan 1993).

- *Legal and organizational issues:* in 1947 mental health services and facilities came under the auspices of the newly-created NHS rather than local authorities. The long overdue review of the mental health legislation and the Mental Health Act (1959) led to psychiatrists becoming responsible for detaining people for reasons of their mental health as opposed to magistrates. This represented an important shift in the perception of mental illness as located within a specialist health-focused service as opposed to being a matter of public order.

- *Economic factors:* as a consequence of becoming part of the NHS it soon became apparent that the existing mental health service provision was inadequate (Coppock and Hopton 2000). Many of the buildings dated from the nineteenth-century Victorian and Edwardian eras and were in dire need of repair and maintenance, and due to overcrowding patients often slept in beds inches apart or in corridors (Jones 1993). By the mid-1950s it was clear to the government that a programme of inestimable investment was necessary simply to maintain many of the buildings which were outdated for use as modern hospital facilities (Jones 1993).
- *Public perceptions:* mental health institutions became increasingly unpopular in the post-war era and in 1961 the UK government embraced a policy to abolish them. In the same year Foucault, Goffman, Laing and Szasz, authors from different countries, all published very different but unanimously highly critical accounts of mental hospitals (Jones 1993).

The transition from an inpatient system to care in the community took over three decades to achieve as there was no clear plan for a service model for care in the community. Unfortunately, successive governments of different political persuasions between the 1960s and the 1990s regarded the closure of mental hospitals as an opportunity to save money for the public purse rather than as an alternative method of service provision (Coppock and Hopton 2000).

The National Service Framework for Mental Health

In response to the long evident need to review the provision of mental health services in the community the *National Service Framework* (NSF) *for Mental Health* was published in 1999 after a major consultation exercise. The NSF represented the first national strategy for mental health services and was significantly supported with a commitment of funding and resources to support the implementation of the changes it proposed (DoH 1999, 2000).

The goals of the NSF were to provide services which were:

- *safe:* to protect the public and care for those with mental health problems at the time care was needed;
- *sound:* to ensure service users and carers were able to access a full range of services appropriate to their needs and when needed;
- *supportive:* working together with service users, their families, carers and significant others to build healthier communities.

To meet these goals seven standards were proposed (DoH 1999).

- *Standard 1:* health and social services should promote mental health and work with individuals and the community, combat discrimination against mental health problems and promote social inclusion.
- *Standard 2:* service users contacting their primary health care team with a mental health problem regarded as commonly occurring in the population should receive an assessment, have their mental health need(s) identified and be offered appropriate further assessment, treatment and care, or if necessary referral to specialist services.
- *Standard 3:* any person with a mental health problem which is regarded as commonly occurring in the population should have access to services suitable to meet their mental health needs 24 hours a day, 7 days a week, 365 days a year and NHS Direct ought to be available for first level advice and referral to specialist helplines or local services.
- *Standard 4:* all mental health service users registered on the CPA should receive care which engages them to the optimum, and strives to reduce risk or crisis; receive a copy of a written care plan which states the action(s) to be taken by the service user, their carer and the care coordinator in the event of a crisis and advising the GP on how to respond. The care plan should be regularly reviewed by the appointed care coordinator and the service user ought to

have access to services which are available 24 hours a day, 365 days a year.

- *Standard 5:* every service user who is assessed as requiring a period of care which involves them being away from their home should have access to a suitable hospital or alternative bed or place as close to their home as possible, and in the least restrictive environment to protect both the service user and the public. On their discharge they should receive a written copy of an agreed care plan identifying the care and rehabilitation which is to be provided, the care coordinator and the action(s) to be taken in a crisis.
- *Standard 6:* individuals who provide regular and a significant levels of care for a person on CPA ought to receive an annual assessment of their caring and physical and mental health needs and a copy of their own written care plan which is carried out in discussion with them
- *Standard 7:* local health and social care organizations should prevent suicides by promoting mental health among individuals and communities (cross-referenced with Standard 1); provide effective primary mental health care (cross-referenced with Standard 2); ensure people with mental health problems are able to access local services through a primary care team, help lines or A&E (cross-referenced with Standard 3); ensure people with a severe and enduring mental illness are provided with a care plan which is specific to their needs and provides access to services 24 hours a day, 365 days a year (cross-referenced with Standard 4); provide safe hospital facilities for service users requiring inpatient admission (cross-referenced with Standard 5); facilitate the carers of people with severe mental health problems to access support to allow them to continue in the caring role (cross-referenced with Standard 6). Also to: support prison staff in preventing the suicide of prisoners; ensure staff are competent in assessing the risk of suicide and that adequate audit systems are in place to learn and implement necessary changes

The standards were also grouped into five areas, which are outlined in the panel below.

Standards of the NSF

- *Standard 1:* mental health promotion; to combat discrimination and social exclusion associated with mental health problems.
- *Standards 2 and 3:* primary care and access to services for those with a mental health problem.
- *Standards 4 and 5:* the care of those with severe mental illness.
- *Standard 6:* concerns individuals who are carers for people with mental health problems.
- *Standard 7:* outlines actions to accomplish the government's target of reducing suicides.

The NSF sets out the basis for recovery by emphasizing the sharing of information, empowerment, partnership, community-based care, family support and health promotion. The standards provide guidance on promoting mental health and social inclusion, better access to primary care, written care plans and home treatment wherever possible.

The concept of *recovery* first emerged in the NSF, which proposed a new vision for mental health and began to talk about principles and values in mental health care. The key principles and values of a recovery-focused approach now inform mental health nursing practice in all areas of care and mental health services, including the education and preparation for practice of mental health professionals. These values are crucial to what we do as mental health nurses because they recognize the necessity of valuing the aims of the service user, working in partnership, offering meaningful choice, promoting social inclusion and being optimistic about the possibilities of positive change (DoH 2007a).

The CPA

The CPA was introduced in 1990 (DoH 1990), nearly a decade before the NSF (DoH 1999) as part of a range of measures by the Conservative government including the commissioning of the

Griffiths Report to make recommendations to reform the mental health services (Coppock and Hopton, 2000). The intention of the CPA was to specifically address shortcomings repeatedly identified by a number of inquiries, including the lack of adequate communication and consideration of planning and risk management in the care of service users in the community (Morgan and Wetherell 2005; Salter and Turner 2008).

The CPA provides a unified system of documentation for users of mental health services. While this might appear to be a basic and obvious goal, the multi-agency nature of care in the community requires significant coordination. For example, a service user who attends a day hospital, has a CPN and is in receipt of social care and has a named social worker requires coordination and regular multidisciplinary reviews of their care to be arranged by *one person*. The CPA provides a process by which this can be achieved.

The CPA acts to link together the aspects of care in the community. Among the measures by which this is achieved is an obligation on health care professionals to develop care plans based on assessed needs. There is an appointed, named CPA care coordinator, regular reviews of care are required and services are responsible for ensuring service users, their carers and significant others receive adequate support in the community (DoH 2007b; 2008; Salter and Turner 2008). All service users who are in contact with the specialist mental health services are subject to the CPA and currently two different levels apply. The criteria for these are identified in the panel below (DoH 2008).

Levels of CPA

- *Standard support:* which applies to people who receive care from just one agency, maintain their mental health and retain contact with the services.
- *Enhanced support:* where the person has contact with a range of agencies but is perceived to be at a higher level of risk, and more likely to disengage with services.

New guidance is currently being introduced and to avoid unnecessary bureaucracy, the CPA criteria will be revised and only apply to those who would otherwise be on enhanced CPA (DoH 2008). It has been suggested that the CPA focuses resources on adult service users while the mental health care needs of older adults, adolescents and children are not catered for. However, different issues regarding risk and vulnerability are applicable to these age groups. The specialist mental health services for older adults, children and adolescents apply the same standards of care to those with whom they work as the health care staff who work with adults.

The CPA has generated enormous debate and discussion, not only among mental health nurses and health care professionals but among service users and their carers, independent groups and organizations with a stake in mental health services. In the panel below you will find a summary of the practical advantages and disadvantages of the CPA (Salter and Turner 2008).

Advantages and disadvantages of the CPA

Advantages	*Disadvantages*

Advantages

- Organizes care; defines responsibility; allows for agreed review times.
- Involves multidisciplinary input: medical, social care, voluntary and family.
- Care is documented.
- Resources are targeted at serious mental illness.
- Can be audited and used to identify local health needs.

Disadvantages

- Time-consuming with planning meetings and the documenting of needs and plans.
- Some disciplines do not participate; large meetings can intimidate service users.
- High level of paperwork; can replicate other documentation.
- Focuses on risk assessment and can promote defensive practice.
- Responds to government targets rather than service users' care needs.

The scenario below considers the experience of a service user, and how the CPA is used to assess and meet their needs and plan their care.

Scenario: Steven

Steven is 19 years old and lives with his father, stepmother, older brother Paul, who is 21, and three stepbrothers and sisters who are aged 7, 5 and 4.

Although always a quiet person, after starting to attend college Steven increasingly isolated himself and stayed in his room all the time. He played computer fantasy games or wrote in a journal, often late into the night, and eventually formed a routine of staying awake all night and sleeping all day. Steven seemed far less friendly, often irritable and out of character, and appeared to be suspicious of others.

He was found acting strangely in a shop which sold fantasy computer games, speaking to computer screens. The police were called and he was taken to a psychiatric unit and agreed to be admitted informally.

Steven spent eight months on the inpatient unit. Initially he was silent for long periods of time and resistant to and suspicious of the staff, but eventually was able to speak about the issues which were affecting him. He appeared to be experiencing auditory hallucinations and had difficulty separating reality from his own thoughts. At his psychiatrist's request he reluctantly commenced using antipsychotic medication, but found this to be helpful in reducing his symptoms and his mood improved.

Eventually Steven was discharged from the unit. He has attended the day hospital twice a week for the last six months and began to work as a volunteer at a youth project as well as engaging on a programme attending a local gym and swimming. Recently Steven has repeatedly expressed a wish to live independently and is looking at adverts for flats to rent in the local paper. Phil, who is a mental health nurse and Steven's keyworker based at the day hospital, decided to call a CPA review of Steven's care.

Phil met with Steven to explain the planned CPA review and discuss his progress and current goals. Steven explained he felt he was managing well. However, living at home with his family was difficult as he has no privacy, and while he liked his family's company, at the same time he wanted more independence. Steven also complained of feeling drowsy and lethargic and was concerned he was gaining weight as a side effect of his anti-psychotic medication. He felt if the dose was reduced he might feel more alert and lose weight.

The CPA meeting was attended by the psychiatrist, Phil, Steven and his dad. The coordinator from the youth project and Steven's family doctor did not attend. Steven's trainer from the gym sent his apologies but wanted to feed back to the meeting that Steven's attendance and hard work were good but he sometimes complained of feeling drowsy and seemed lethargic at times, perhaps due to the effects of the medication. In the CPA meeting while Steven was subdued and quiet his dad made a number of points on his behalf, also agreeing Steven often seemed lethargic and might benefit from a reduction in his medication.

The psychiatrist expressed concern at reducing the medication now as Steven was also considering moving out of home and he may be making too many changes too quickly.

Concerning Steven's wish to live alone his dad explained that Steven's brother Paul also wanted to move out and perhaps they could jointly rent a flat. As the two brothers had a good relationship Paul might be able to not only be some company but detect early on whether Steven's mental health was deteriorating.

Phil suggested Steven might benefit from being assessed by an occupational therapist who could ascertain how good he was at daily skills of self-care and identify any deficits. Steven admitted he was not very good at cooking but had enjoyed the cooking group when he had tried it at the day hospital.

At the end of the CPA meeting it was agreed that:

- Steven would look for a flat to rent with his brother;
- Steven would continue on his current dose of medication and for this to be reviewed in one month;

The CPA raises ethical questions of how the mental health services engage with service users. There has been much discussion regarding the necessity of services working with service users in the community who are unwell but reluctant to engage and the need for services not to infringe on people's human rights by compelling them to remain in contact (Coppock and Hopton 2000).

Frequently mental health nurses mistake the CPA for a model of nursing, which it is not. Nursing models provide theories, belief and knowledge and represent an understanding of what is actually nursing (Pearson *et al.* 1996). In contrast the CPA lacks an underpinning ideology and is instead a *framework of standards* and *system for communication*.

While the CPA is now widely used throughout specialist mental health services, uptake has been greatly assisted by the increasing use of computers in the following ways:

- it was possible to introduce a standard form

with specific fields requiring compulsory completion;
- automated reminders can be sent to staff regarding discharge follow-ups and cases due for review;
- activity levels can easily be monitored.

It could be argued that there is a danger the CPA will become the driving purpose behind the work of nurses instead of working with the service user. Although the CPA provides a uniform approach across different disciplines, mental health assessments have become generic as they can be carried out by a health care practitioner from any one of a range of disciplines and the profession-specific skills of health care practitioners have in this respect become obsolete.

However, as we have said, the CPA is not a model of health care but a process of documentation and in order to be able to use it effectively professional training is necessary to guide our observations. Furthermore, the government guidance emphasizes that the implementation of the CPA ought to be in accordance with the person-centred and empowerment-focused principles of *The Ten Essential Shared Capabilities* (DoH 2004a, 2008).

The network of mental health services in the community

In this part of the chapter we will discuss in more detail the range of different mental health services for adults which have been developed as a result of the NSF.

Primary care: NSF Standard 1

Primary care is the universal availability of essential health care to individuals and families in the community and forms an integral part of the national health system. It is the first level of contact between health services and individuals, families and community, bringing health care as close as possible to where people live and work. It is locally provided and focused on individual and local needs. In the UK the NHS provides health care which is available to all and free at the point of source.

Before the NSF, specialist or secondary mental health services existed separately from GP services in primary care with limited contact and communication. However, Standards 1 and 2 of the NSF proposed a stronger relationship between primary and secondary services through a commitment to improve mental health promotion and the development of mental health services available within primary care.

A review of progress on the standards of the NSF in 2004 (DoH 2004b) found there to be only limited evidence of success regarding Standard 1. In response to Standard 2 there was a significant effort to train 1000 specialist mental health workers called graduate workers to provide mental health expertise for service users in primary care and to work with other primary care health staff and carry out mental health promotion activities (NICE 2003; NIMHE 2003, 2004a, 2004b). Unfortunately, graduate workers were never trained in sufficient numbers to have a nationwide impact and the target was never met (Rushforth 2005;

Harkness and Bower 2006). However, the Layard Report (Layard 2004) not only repeated the need for mental health expertise to be available in primary care but suggested the training of many more mental health workers in primary care. As a result a new wave of training has been commissioned on a nationwide scale to improve access to psychological therapies (DoH 2007a, 2007b).

Nationally, the provision of mental health services in primary care is variable. Many GPs work with their own patients concerning mental health issues. Yet this depends on the personal interest and skills of the GP. Commissioned counselling services or therapists are also frequently used and available for referrals within GP practices. In some cases community psychiatric nurses (CPNs) are employed by primary care trusts to work as therapists with people who experience mental health problems in the community and liaise with GPs. Alternatively CPNs from community mental health teams (CMHTs) liaise with local primary care services. An example is of a CPN who facilitates a group for new mothers at a health visitor clinic to discuss their mental health and provide support.

While steps have been taken to develop mental health services in primary care settings the established divisions between primary care and secondary mental health services have endured to the detriment of mental health services in primary care. Many people who are sensitive to the stigma relating to mental illness do not access help, while those who do seek help or are identified as having a mental health problem need a variety of different services, and these depend in turn on local provision in the area. Specialist mental health services continue to work only with a small sector of the population who they become involved with by direct referral.

Consistent with mental health promotion it is necessary to ensure that mental health services are convenient and easy to access. This is an area of weakness within the current system of provision and further development is necessary if we are to contribute to improving the nation's mental health.

Secondary care

Secondary care services are provided by mental health trusts, and have an important role in promoting social and vocational opportunities for people with severe and enduring mental health problems. The support people receive can influence their success in retaining their current occupation, and impact on their self-confidence and future aspirations.

Standards 3, 4 and 5 of the NSF refer to the specialist mental health services and include a long-term plan for the organization and development of mental health services, proposing a model comprising of the areas of service provision outlined in the next panel.

NSF range of services

Inpatient care	Inpatient care is still an important part of the service but as one of a range of different options.
Crisis resolution teams	The introduction of crisis resolution teams focused on managing crises in the community. Through being supported in the home environment the service user and their family avoid the trauma of being required to go into hospital.
Early intervention teams	Early intervention teams were created to work with service users identified as being future high users of services. An advantage is the early identification of mental health problems, and working with people when they are younger reduces the level and extent of service use the person requires later in their life (Zengeni 2008).
Assertive outreach	Assertive outreach teams were created to work with service users with severe and enduring mental health problems who are in need of continuing support and contact with the mental health services but are at risk of disengaging.

Alongside the newly-created teams were:

- *CMHTs:* these have existed since the 1950s, and before the NSF were the major national providers of specialist mental health services in the community. CMHTs continue to be the focal point of adult mental health services. They support people with complex mental health problems and their families in the community when their needs cannot be met by their GP, primary care or generic social services.
- *Substance misuse teams:* under the previous Mental Health Act 1983 substance misuse and addiction were not regarded as constituting a mental health problem. The new Mental Health Act (DoH 2006) has widened the definition of mental illness to include substance misuse. Traditionally substance misuse teams have regarded their work as separate from mental health services and a distinct specialism.
- *Criminal justice and court diversion teams:* often experienced mental health nurses attend court and where necessary carry out mental health assessments of people appearing before the magistrates. They also work on a short-term basis with people going through the court process who have a mental health problem. There is an overlap with substance misuse teams where people have a substance misuse problem and are going through the criminal justice system receive input from a substance misuse worker to rehabilitate and avoid further offending.

While the NSF created a range of new and different specialist teams, the intention was for these to collectively represent a cohesive, interlinked mental health service network within the community with the CPA providing the administrative system holding the services together.

In the panel below are three scenarios which illustrate the role performed by each of the three new community-based roles created by the NSF.

A mental health student's insight into placement in a community mental health team ...

I arrived early and no one seemed to know I was coming, even though I had phoned the week before to confirm. I was seated at a desk that looked like a filing cabinet had been emptied all over it. After an hour or so the student coordinator came in and told me I was not expected. She then went round the office asking if anyone was prepared to take a first-year student. Most were not. Eventually I was moved to sit at another desk until lunchtime, when I first met my new mentor.

At the end of the placement I had been truly accepted as a member of the team and was even presented with a leaving gift. I now count many of the team among my friends, which was not how I felt at the end of my first day.

Scenarios: implementation of the NSF

Crisis resolution

Amanda is 38 years old and married to Phil who is 42. They have a son called Darren who is 17 and is using illegal drugs. Amanda is a senior carer in a residential care home while Phil works as a handyman for the same employer. Recently the home was taken over by a large company which introduced a number of changes. Phil now has to work longer hours while Amanda's job has changed requiring her to take greater responsibility and manage more staff. The couple also have a large mortgage and due to a recent rise in interest rates their monthly payments significantly increased. The couple already have sizeable debts. Amanda has experienced a rise in anxiety to the point where she feels unable to concentrate and in a permanent state of agitation and panic. She consulted her GP who phoned the mental health services and the crisis resolution team became involved. Amanda was commenced on medication to assist with her anxiety. The team carried out a CPA assessment of Amanda and discussed her situation and concerns with her and Phil. Over the next few weeks the team maintained contact with Amanda daily by phone or visit and Amanda's anxiety gradually reduced.

Early intervention

Ayisha is 17 years old and studying at sixth form college. In spite of always achieving well Ayisha is often in trouble, seen as disruptive, makes few friends and dislikes college. She has missed a significant amount of attendance and is regarded as surly and a difficult student when she does attend. She has been isolating herself at home and her relationship with her mother has also deteriorated and they argue often. There are concerns that she is expressing paranoid thoughts and feeling that other students at college are talking detrimentally about her. Ayisha's mother works full-time, is a single parent, having been bereaved of her husband some 10 years ago, and has a history of depression which has deteriorated to paranoid psychosis several times in the past. On one occasion she spent some time in an inpatient mental health unit.

Ayisha's mother has remained well for the last three years due to keeping up with her medication and she regularly sees a CPN and consultant psychiatrist at six-monthly outpatient appointments. Following a referral from Ayisha's GP a mental health nurse trained in family therapy and specializing in early intervention assessed and worked with Ayisha and her mother over a three-month period. From the assessment it seemed Ayisha was experiencing depression and some paranoid ideas which while having a basis in truth disproportionately influenced her thinking.

The CPN felt Ayisha's low mood and isolation created a vicious circle whereby, due to her paranoid feelings, she isolated herself more and therefore felt lower in mood and in turn more paranoid. Through working with Ayisha and her mother their relationship improved significantly. The CPN attended a meeting with Ayisha and her mother at the college to discuss her concerns. The college was very supportive and since then Ayisha's attendance has improved. The CPN felt that Ayisha's problems might have been detected earlier through increased cooperation between the college and the health services. Often disruptive behaviour is seen as disobedience rather than an indication of a mental health problem and in Ayisha's case it was only the connection with her mother's acute mental health problem which initiated the referral from the GP.

Assertive outreach

Tony is 25 and diagnosed with paranoid schizophrenia. He lives with his grandmother, Geraldine. In the past after admissions to the inpatient mental health unit Tony repeatedly stopped taking his antipsychotic medication, missed appointments with his CPN and became unwell, requiring readmission. However, in the last three years Tony has been being supported in the community by the assertive outreach team. The team visit Tony up to three times a week and check he is taking his medication and that he seems mentally stable. They also engage in activities with him, encourage him to lead an active life and develop his interests. At the same time when visiting the team support Geraldine in her role as Tony's carer. Sometimes the relationship between Tony and Geraldine is fraught. Occasionally Tony goes out in the evening and drinks alcohol and Geraldine rebukes him about this, which Tony interprets as her 'nagging'. The assertive outreach team provides the continued level of input Tony's mental health needs require.

With regard to the three areas of assertive outreach, crisis resolution and early intervention, in 2004 none of these were available in sufficient numbers and with enough staff to constitute a nationwide service, and most areas reported the service to be inadequate to meet local need (DoH 2004b). Among the explanations for the limited success in implementing these teams was a lack of supply of staff with the necessary skills, abilities and willingness to make such a radical transition in their working role. The remit of the new mental health teams also marked a radical departure from the previous community mental health nursing role with the emphasis on brief intervention, assessment and with a high level of responsibility for risk assessment and risk management.

Critics of the NSF point out that the standards are *minimum expectations* of mental health services as opposed to aiming for the highest possible care. It is also argued that trusts are not encouraged to develop services to their fullest capacity

(Morgan and Wetherell 2005). Furthermore, some of the NSF standards are vague – for example, Standard 5 states that where a service user requires inpatient care they should receive a bed in a unit as close as possible to their home, yet no specific distance is stipulated.

However, encouragingly the vision embodied within the NSF of a national service spanning primary and secondary care with specific standards and priorities has endured and been pursued as a consistent policy. Viewed in contrast to the lack of developed community services before 1999 the community-based mental health services can be seen as a 'work in progress' and a developing network which will continue to change and evolve.

Conclusion

In this chapter we have discussed the origins of care in the community and then identified the background and specific role and contribution of the NSF and the CPA. We then progressed to consider the range of community-based services which have been developed in the last 10 years and discussed examples of service users involved with these services.

These changes have represented an overhaul of the mental health services. However, in order to continue to improve services it is important that the existing form of mental health service provision is not accepted uncritically, but instead subjected to question. While the NSF represented the first ever national strategy for mental health care, this has also revealed the sharp divisions between primary and secondary mental health care and this in turn offers the opportunity for further changes in the future and the development of mental health services to more effectively provide access to people who require such assistance.

Creating new teams within the community required mental health nurses to develop skills which were not previously involved in their roles. The changing role of the mental health nurse in community care is often overlooked, yet forms a significant part of the identity of newly-qualified mental health practitioners who will be at the forefront of mental health nursing in the future.

References

Coppock, V. and Hopton, J. (2000) *Critical Perspectives on Mental Health.* London: Routledge.

DoH (Department of Health) (1990) *A Care Programme Approach for People with a Mental Illness Referred to Specialist Psychiatric Services*, DoH/Social Services Circular HC (90)23/LASSL (90)11. London: HMSO.

DoH (Department of Health) (1999) *National Service Framework for Mental Health: Modern Standards and Service Models.* London: DoH.

DoH (Department of Health) (2000) *The NHS Plan: A Plan for Investment, a Plan for Reform.* London: DoH.

DoH (Department of Health) (2004a) *The Ten Essential Shared Capabilities: A Framework for the Whole of the Mental Health Workforce.* London: DoH.

DoH (Department of Health) (2004b) *National Service Framework for Mental Health – Five Years On.* London: DoH.

DoH (Department of Health) (2006) *Mental Health Bill, 2006: Summary Guide.* London: DoH.

DoH (Department of Health) (2007a) *Commissioning a Brighter Future: Improving Access to Psychological Therapies.* London: DoH.

DoH (Department of Health) (2007b) *Improving Access to*

Psychological Therapies: Specification for the Commissioner-led Pathfinder Programme. London: DoH.

DoH (Department of Health) (2008) *Refocusing the Care Programme Approach: Policy and Positive Practice Guidance.* London: DoH.

Harkness, E. and Bower, P. (2006) National evaluation of the graduate worker initiative: current roles and future trends, paper presented at the Third National Graduate Worker conference, Nottingham, 17–18 January.

Jones, K. (1993) *Asylums and After: A Revised History of the Mental Health Services: From the Early 18th Century to the 1990s.* London: Athlone Press.

Layard, R. (2004) *Mental Health: Britain's Biggest Social Problem.* London: Cabinet Office.

Morgan, S. and Wetherell, A. (2005) Assessing and managing risk, in I. Norman and I. Ryrie (eds) *The Art and Science of Mental Health Nursing: A Textbook of Principles and Practice*, pp. 208–40. Maidenhead: Open University Press.

NICE (National Institute for Health and Clinical Excellence) (2003) *Depression: The Management of Depression in Primary and Secondary Care*, 2nd edn. London: NICE.

NIMHE (National Institute of Mental Health for England) (2003) *Primary Care Graduate Mental Health Workers: A Practical Guide.* London: NIMHE.

NIMHE (National Institute of Mental Health for England) (2004a) *Primary Care Graduate Mental Health Workers: A Practical Guide.* London: NIMHE.

NIMHE (National Institute of Mental Health for England) (2004b) *Enhanced Services for Depression Under the New GP Contract: A Commissioning Guidebook.* London: NIMHE.

Nolan, P. (1993) Guest editorial, *Journal of Psychiatric and Mental Health*, 10: 637–9.

Norman, I. and Ryrie, I. (2005) Mental health nursing: origins and orientations, in I. Norman and I. Ryrie (eds) *The Art and Science of Mental Health Nursing*, pp. 66–98. Maidenhead: Open University Press.

Pearson, A., Vaughan, B. and Fitzgerald, M. (1996) *Nursing Models for Practice*, 2nd edn. Oxford: Butterworth-Heinemann.

Rushforth, D. (2005) *Career Progression for Graduate Mental Health Workers in Primary Care: A Briefing Paper,* www.lincoln.ac.uk/ccawi/publications/ Career%20progression%20paper-Skills%20for%20all.April.05.doc, accessed 24 April 2006.

Salter, M. and Turner, T. (2008) *Community Mental Health Care: A Practical Guide to Outdoor Psychiatry.* London: Elsevier Churchill Livingstone.

Zengeni, M. (2008) The importance of being early, *Mental Health Practice*, 11(9): 38.

9

Secure inpatient and forensic mental health care for adults

Mark McGrath and Nick Wrycraft

Mark McGrath and Nick Wrycraft

Learning objectives

By the end of this chapter you will have gained:

- An understanding of the specialist role of secure inpatient and forensic mental health care services.
- An appreciation of the philosophy, goals and values of care and the whole person model of recovery within adult inpatient secure and forensic services.
- An understanding of the staff competencies required to work with people with these needs and how to engage effectively.
- An insight into risk assessment and management of offenders with mental health problems.

Introduction

In this chapter we will consider secure inpatient and forensic mental health services. While these apply to a relatively small number of people, they perform an important role within mental health care and have traditionally been regarded as a specialist service.

The chapter begins by providing a brief historical background before outlining the range of people with mental health problems who become involved in secure inpatient and forensic mental health services. We then consider the philosophy and values of care and look at the staff capabilities required to work with people in secure inpatient and forensic settings. Within this discussion we will consider a recovery and positive strengths-focused approach. Finally we will discuss risk assessment and management. A brief conclusion is provided summarizing the main issues covered.

Throughout the chapter there will be exercises and scenarios to provide you with opportunities to identify points for reflection and learning in the practice area.

Background

Historically mental illness within the UK has not been well understood. Often it was regarded as a homogenous term embracing a wide and varied range of human activities, behaviour and conditions. Often the mentally ill, socially disadvantaged and criminals were viewed as synonymous and a group of individuals was created whose only connection was their being perceived as a problem to society.

As noted in previous chapters, until the middle of the twentieth century services for the mentally ill comprised of large-scale inpatient institutions. Michel Foucault (2001) suggested that the impetus to create institutions or asylums arose from society's wish to remove these people from our communities. For Foucault the asylums and mental health institutions had no focus on mental health. Instead he believed that all institutions, whether hospitals, prisons or schools, exist to make people 'normal' within the values determined by society. Foucault thought that institutions were society's attempt to impose state power and imprint identity on the individual as opposed to facilitating the person to be aware of the ability to control their own life and choices. In support of his view Foucault pointed to the design of institutions in the nineteenth century, which were built specifically so that inmates could be permanently under surveillance.

Before the creation of the NHS, mental health services were in a confusing situation, aligned as they were with several areas of the state. Officially mental institutions were managed by local authorities and regarded as part of the social welfare services, yet there was also a connection to the criminal justice system through mental health legislation.

Only towards the end of the institutional era did mental health services come under the remit of health. This was hastened by the emergence of effective psychiatric medication, psychological therapies and the realization that with these tools care in the community might provide a more positive alternative to institutions. At the same time more liberal attitudes became popular within society.

The emergence of care in the community led to the establishment of a range of specialist mental health services within a network. The effect of this has been that secure inpatient and forensic services have become a discrete area within mental health provision for those who require secure care, those with mental health problems who commit crime and people in prison who acquire mental health problems.

Secure inpatient and forensic mental health services are at the intersection of mental health and the criminal justice system where so much misconception and confusion has occurred in previous history. Often due to their association with control and security these services are assumed to be similar to the old-style institutions. Yet there are crucial differences, including:

- the use of effective psychiatric medication and psychological therapies;
- multidisciplinary input into care from a range of mental health professionals;
- mental health nursing philosophy of recovery, social inclusion and the promotion of empowerment;
- being a part of an interconnected network of

mental health services which actively promote reintegration and social inclusion in the community.

> **A mental health student comments on their placement in a secure setting** ...
>
> My first ever placement was a low secure acute inpatient setting. I was incredibly nervous starting the course with my first ever placement being in an area caring for individuals who were acutely unwell. Initially the ward was very daunting and almost intimidating. However, after one shift I was at ease. My mentor was brilliant as she always ensured that I had a debriefing after any specific incidents. My ward manager played a huge part in me being accepted on the ward. He made me feel part of the team from day one, which boosted my confidence and resulted in me presenting as more professional to the clients.

Who receives secure inpatient and forensic mental health services?

It may surprise you that there are only around 5500 people in secure inpatient and forensic mental health services in the UK. The reason for this is that the prevailing philosophy among mental health professionals is to provide a level of care appropriate to the person's need in the least restrictive setting. Even people with severe mental health problems are often cared for within non-secure settings.

Deprivation of a person's liberty is only used where absolutely necessary and only to an extent to ensure that appropriate mental health treatment is made available and to protect the person or others due to their mental illness. These tenets are enshrined within the legislation pertaining to mental health and implemented strictly by all mental health professionals. The reasons for placing a person in a secure unit include several quite specific factors:

- the person's mental health need(s);

- either criminally offending or highly inappropriate behaviour;
- associated risk factors of either actual or the potential of harm to self and/or others.

There are three levels of secure inpatient and forensic care. These are low, medium and high with the level determined by the degree of risk and severity of need.

While much of the discussion in this chapter will focus on working with people in secure inpatient settings as a mental health student you may also receive placements with court liaison nurses who assess people who are going through the criminal justice system. Alternatively, substance misuse teams often engage in work with service users as part of the criminal justice system. Therefore the work of mental health nurses with this client group is varied and not limited only to inpatient areas.

In the panel below we have listed the numerous locations in which forensic/secure nurses provide care for mentally disordered offenders.

Nursing locations for working with mentally disordered offenders

- Prisons.
- Courts.
- Police cells.
- Social services establishments.
- Generic community mental health settings.
- Forensic community mental health settings.
- Intensive therapy units.
- Units for behaviourally disturbed people.
- Units for those who are difficult to place.
- Minimum (low) secure units.
- Forensic adolescent services.
- High Security services (special hospitals).
- Forensic independent sector provision.

People are referred to forensic services from a wide range of agencies and the previous panel also lists some of the various referral sources into secure/forensic mental health services, such as intensive therapy units. People treated in secure inpatient and forensic mental health services fall into three main categories as follows.

- People with schizophrenia and other severe and enduring mental health problems.
- People with dual diagnosis, in particular substance misuse that is a common feature of people who do not respond to treatment.
- People with personality disorders. The reviewed Mental Health Act 2007 widened the category of people eligible to be treated within mental health services. Previously people with personality disorders were often denied treatment due to the lack of proven interventions for such conditions. However, the new Act specifies that care should be provided based on need rather than diagnosis.

There are also other emerging groups, such as adults with autistic spectrum disorders and people who present challenging behaviours in the context of severe personality disorders or severe neurotic illnesses.

However, not all people in secure inpatient and forensic services also demonstrate criminal behaviour. Within low secure care the majority of people will be formally detained under Section 3 of the Mental Health Act 1983 for treatment of their mental health. Often the decision to impose the section is the person not consenting to necessary treatment to remedy an acute mental health problem and/or their presenting a risk to themselves and/or other people due to their mental ill health. Within medium and high secure care most people will have demonstrated criminal behaviour and be formally detained under Sections 37 and 37/41 of the Mental Health Act 1983.

Philosophy of care

It seems logical that people in a secure/forensic environment will share the same aspirations as us all for:

- independent living;
- recreation;
- employment;
- social and sexual relationships;

- material goods;
- being able to engage in practices relating to our preferred religion;
- having cultural needs met.

(Holloway 2005)

Yet for people within the secure and forensic mental health services these goals are sometimes compromised by the care environment. People are generally referred to specialist secure services after a very lengthy psychiatric career by which time a range of 'secondary impairments' can become apparent. These include the emotional, cognitive, social and functional effects of being a patient (Holloway 2005). Living within a hospital for a sustained period of time can negatively impact on the person's pre-existent sense of identity, values and priorities and the capacity for autonomy, decision-making and goal-setting. The person may also experience *conation* which is a lack of motivation to carry out activities and can lead to marked self-neglect.

People often come into secure inpatient and forensic mental health services having demonstrated criminally offending behaviour, multiple mental health needs and complex risk factors. These are sizeable issues with which to work, however, if the person is to make progress, their level of motivation will be pivotal. There are wide variations between people concerning their willingness to change but among the factors which determine their view are insight into their problems and the capability to sustain the work necessary to make positive change.

The recovery model

The role of the mental health nurse and other multidisciplinary health care professionals in secure and forensic services is extremely important in supporting the person to retain a sense of hope and identity in often challenging circumstances. The philosophy that provides a guide on how we can practice in accordance with this goal is the recovery model. *Recovery* can be defined as:

A whole system approach to recovery from mental ill health which maximizes an individual's quality of life and social inclusion whilst effectively managing risk by encouraging their skills, promoting independence and autonomy in order to give them hope for the future and which leads to successful community living through appropriate support.

(Adapted from Killaspy *et al.* 2005)

The idea of recovery can be summarized as optimism about the future and it is well described in the following three statements (Anthony 1993):

A person with mental illness can experience recovery in spite of their illness not being cured.

Recovery is a way of living and a person with a mental health problem can still have a satisfying and hopeful life, and contribute meaningfully to society, even with the limitations caused by illness.

Recovery involves the development of new meaning and purpose in a person's life which extends beyond the catastrophic effects of mental illness.

These statements represent a set of principles with a focus on:

- holistic assessment of the needs of the person experiencing severe mental illness;
- awareness of the person's strengths, social, spiritual and cultural environment;
- a determination to work with the individual to achieve the best possible clinical and social outcomes which are set by the person experiencing the illness.

Staff competencies

To move beyond words and implement this approach in practice as professionals we need to:

- work collaboratively in partnership with people and/or carers to identify realistic life goals and enable them to be reached;
- genuinely promote social inclusion in whatever way we can and however small these interventions might seem (Pratt *et al.* 1999);
- be optimistic about the possibility of positive individual change.

When working within secure settings nurses take the lead in most aspects of security, which creates a dilemma in striking a balance between 'care and containment'. A prime objective for nurses is to establish and sustain therapeutic relationships with people who have mental health problems. Yet within secure services people present with severe challenging behaviour and may have committed offences as serious as rape or murder. Nurses have to reconcile the obligation to provide a secure environment with the need to form therapeutic relationships with the person in order to effectively address issues of need and risk and produce positive change (Caplan 1993).

Six categories of nurse-patient interactions have been identified concerning verbal and social interaction in the nurse-patient relationship (Rask and Brunt 2007). These are:

1. building and sustaining relationships;
2. supportive/encouraging relationships;
3. social skills training;
4. reality orientation;
5. reflective interactions;
6. practical skills training.

Reflecting on the categories

- Read the above categories again.
- Now reflect on your own current practice experience and consider how each of these categories could be applied.
- Think of the implications and possible uses of each category.
- How could each category potentially enhance positive change for patients?
- Write some notes for each category.

When you have finished, place your notes in your professional portfolio.

Staff attitudes and values

Research into features of positive staff attitudes that enabled them to work with patients who have a personality disorder within a high secure setting gives some indication of the most important attributes for staff to possess when working in this environment (Bowers 2002):

- professionalism;
- individualized care;
- crime and harm prevention;
- focusing on the illness;
- able to accept abusive backgrounds of patients;
- universal humanity;
- can separate behaviour from the person;
- puts the person first;
- non-judgementalism;
- able to reason;
- expressing feelings to colleagues;
- understanding;
- perseverance;
- able to facilitate complaints.

However, it was reported that while staff had positive attitudes, this did not stop them receiving abuse from some of the people they were caring for. What seemed to keep the therapeutic relationship intact was the moral commitment of dedicated staff and an ability to endure behaviour that most cannot: in essence, 'tolerating the intolerable'. Therefore a willingness to work with people and attempt to understand behaviours that society finds unacceptable are prerequisites for working successfully within this environment (Bowers 2002).

Is this type of work for you?

Take a few minutes to answer the following three questions.

- Should I do this kind of work?
- Do I want to do this kind of work?
- Can I do this kind of work?

The first question is a values question and reflects your unique set of values and the principles to which you anchor your values.

The second question is a motivation question and deals with your innate passion and drive. What motivates you to do this kind of work? Why do you want to do this kind of work? Of course only you can answer these questions. If you are answering 'yes' to the first two questions and for the right reasons the third question is slightly easier.

The third question is a competency-based question: with positive values and motivation you are in the optimum position to train, develop and learn the knowledge and competencies needed to work with some of the most challenging and fascinating individuals within society.

However, before you get to the question 'Can I do this kind of work?' it is advisable to check you have answered the values and motivation questions honestly. Not to do so would be to do yourself and the individuals you subsequently come into contact with a disservice.

When you have finished, place your notes in your professional portfolio.

If a group of staff are not collectively 'signed up' to the core values and principles that underpin their work, then their ability to respond to people's needs is diminished. The question you must ask yourself is 'Are my values based upon principles?' Principles of respect, fairness, trust, kindness, integrity, honesty, service and contribution are essential for staff working within secure settings. These principles are aligned with moral authority that never changes and crosses all religious and cultural boundaries. In discussing the importance of principles and values to practice, Covey (2004) suggests that principles lead to consequences, and behaviour is determined by values: therefore, we should always value principles.

Engaging with people in a secure inpatient or forensic setting

Equipped with a sense of values and principles to underpin our practice we next consider how we might engage with people in the secure inpatient and forensic setting.

Often in such settings we are confronted by challenging behaviour which can be extreme, hostile or unpredictable. In these circumstances the following questions provide a useful guide to opportunities to understand the behaviour in a therapeutic context:

- What needs does this pattern of behaviour or emotion serve?
- What function does it have?
- How can it be replaced with a more empowering alternative?

This approach removes the pejorative aspects of dealing with people with significant challenging behaviour.

If we consider the people with mental health problems we are working with as on a continuum of care with the start point as their admission and the finish point being their discharge, we can create something akin to Figure 9.1 (Jeffcote and Watson 2004).

At the starting point the important factors are mainly containment, both in the physical and psychological sense, the safety of other people with mental health problems on the unit, the safety of the staff, and of course security. As the person progresses along the continuum, other factors become important such as specific programmes

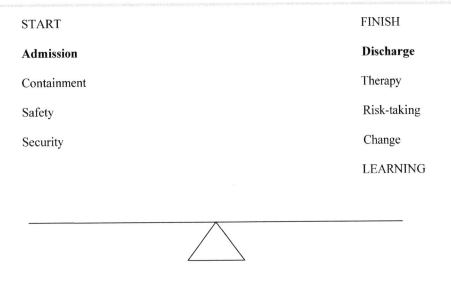

START   FINISH

Admission   **Discharge**

Containment   Therapy

Safety   Risk-taking

Security   Change

                                         LEARNING

Figure 9.1 A continuum of care

and therapy. Risk-taking is also an important concept where we look for positive change and progress in the person and for learning to have taken place which ultimately can lead to discharge.

A significant influence on the continuum is the person's individual ability to learn. If we know how the individual learns, we can understand what we are trying to achieve. In Figure 9.2 we have added the person's individual learning process by listing five factors that influence successful learning (Race 2004) and 'working through'.

Admission   **Discharge**

Containment   Therapy

Safety   Risk-taking

Security   Wanting to learn   Change

                          Needing to learn   LEARNING

                          Making sense (digestion)

                          Learning from feedback
                          Learning by doing

Figure 9.2 Learning through the continuum of care

The two factors that sit below the line of the continuum of care are 'learning from feedback' and 'learning by doing'. The initial work that we need to do must therefore focus on these two influential learning factors.

Within this model, recovery is promoted by encouraging the person to develop the skills, strategies, motivation, beliefs and hope to meet their own needs despite the presence of a mental disorder. This approach will also reduce aggression and challenging behaviour as these often stem from needs not being met or the behaviours fulfilling the need. For example, a person may carry out self-harm as a way of exerting some control.

Due to the complexities of people's individual mental health needs, risk factors and individual motivation and capabilities, not everyone will reach the finish point. Some people will require continued support or remain at various points on the continuum of care in receipt of varying levels of organizational and service input.

Scenario: Errol

Errol is 28 and has previous criminal convictions for violence and aggression, a history of drug and alcohol misuse and a tendency to become violent when under the influence of these substances. He was arrested by the police following a fight with a neighbour in the housing association-owned block of flats where he lives while under the influence of drugs.

Errol was referred to a low secure psychiatric unit following a risk assessment, and appeared to be experiencing acute delusional symptoms and presenting a risk of aggression to others. He was placed under Section 3 of the Mental Health Act and over the last two months has continued to be disorganized in his thinking and to display paranoid ideation and thoughts of aggression towards others.

Errol's memory is impaired at times. On the unit the staff encourage him to engage in groups and to make use of individual time with his allocated keyworker. Errol's mental health has gradually improved and he has developed therapeutic relationships with the staff, feeling able to share his thoughts and 'self-monitor' the fluctuations in his mood. Errol is still very disorganized in his thinking and experiences paranoia, but has engaged with the mental health services.

Risk assessment

In secure inpatient and forensic mental health services we routinely work with people who display high levels of risk and dangerousness and this forms a major part of our work. In this part of the chapter we will discuss risk assessment and risk management measures.

The last 10 years has seen an exponential increase in public and political interest in the assessment and management of risk and over this time the concept of risk has evolved considerably. A major theme throughout all recent mental health policy has been the high priority that mental health services need to give to issues relating to clinical risk assessment and risk management in mental health practice.

The Care Programme Approach (CPA) (DoH 1999) was introduced to ensure the effective coordination and delivery of mental health care. While risk assessment and risk management are central to the effective practice of mental health care (Paley 2003), the National Suicide Prevention Strategy (DoH 2002a) and the *National Confidential Inquiry into Suicides and Homicides by People with Mental Illness* (University of Manchester 2006) also emphasize the need for professionals to gain knowledge and skills in risk assessment and practice. While risk assessment has gained momentum among mental health professionals, strategies for managing risk are at times inconsistent (Milner and Myers 2007).

Although secure mental health units work with people who need to be detained in secure environments, they are NHS hospitals and not penal establishments. Their purpose is to provide care, treatment and recovery-focused services for people and it is necessary to achieve a balance between these requirements and the need for physical security.

The panel below identifies the range of general risk considerations which need to be taken into account in a secure inpatient unit environment (DoH 2002b).

Security needs

- *Environmental security:* perimeter security, the nature and height of perimeter fences and measures to prevent absconding.
- *Internal security:* the design and layout of the care environment, some of which will hinder escape. For example, entry systems, secure windows and alarms. Other design aspects will reduce the potential for injury such as safety glass, secure furniture, the absence of ligature points and materials that could be used for self-harm.
- *Procedural security:* organizational policies and processes that help maintain a safe and therapeutic environment. Examples include limiting the use of lighters and policies on cutlery use, kitchen use and possessions. Also the prevention of entry and possession of weapons, alcohol and drugs. These rules may be enforced by entry procedures for visitors and mail checks.
- *Relational security:* this is a function of the nature and the quality of the therapeutic relationships between patients and staff. Relevant influential factors include the staff/patient ratio, specific policies relating to staff/patient interactions (e.g. the way in which increased observation is managed) and the training of and interventions provided by the staff group.

There are 14 specific risk-related behaviours which can be applied to people with mental health problems in secure care. These are listed in the next panel.

Specific factors of risk assessment

1. Aggression.
2. Fire risk.
3. Physical health.
4. Security/absconding.
5. Self-harm.
6. Inappropriate behaviour.
7. Sexual offending.
8. Substance misuse.
9. Suicide.
10. Theft.
11. Vulnerability.
12. Risk to children.
13. Non-compliance with medical treatment.
14. Other.

Under each risk category there is a rating of probability in the current setting: low, medium or high.

- *Low* means that despite previous risk indicators the likelihood of this risk behaviour occurring within the current setting is low.
- *Medium* refers to a possibility of the risk occurring.
- *High* suggests the risk is active and ongoing and likely to occur within this setting.

Furthermore, in assessing risk we need to establish the type of risk we are dealing with. There are five dimensions to consider (Maden 2007):

- the nature of the risk or risks posed by the service user;
- the potential severity of that risk in terms of its impact to potential victims or the person;
- the probability that the risk will occur;
- whether the risk behaviour is a 'one-off' or a repeated event;
- when the risk behaviour is predicted to occur.

Based on the premise that previous behaviours are best predictors of future behaviours, the clinical risk assessment document provides up-to-date information regarding recent risk behaviours. This provides the best basis for the short-term assessment of risk. Other structured clinical risk assessment tools are useful in guiding risk assessment. The HCR-20 (Webster *et al.* 1997) is a validated and structured tool for the assessment of violence in both forensic and non-forensic areas. The Risk of Sexual Violence Protocol or RSVP (Hart *et al.* 2003) is a similarly structured tool that gives an estimate of future risk of sexual offending. Both these tools are better as medium- to long-term predictors of the risk of future violent behaviour and are integral components of risk management and discharge planning. These tools tend to involve a mixture of historical variables that are known to increase risk, current clinical variables and risk issues that may increase risk in the environment outside the secure setting. If the HCR-20 or an RSVP is completed, these are discussed at clinical meetings.

While government policy and guidance have placed significant emphasis on risk assessment, risk management and risk reduction, there are no guaranteed evidence-based measures which will eradicate risk from our clinical environments. Instead we rely on vigilance in clinical practice, good decision-making, astute observation and assessment, and the communication of perceived risk within the nursing and multidisciplinary team. The rest of this chapter focuses on clinical risk management.

Risk management

Risk management logically follows risk assessment and consists of the specific actions that are taken to minimize the severity, likelihood, imminence and frequency of risk behaviours. With effective therapeutic treatment the nature of the risk behaviours can also be reduced.

Accurate predication of all risk is not possible. Even the most comprehensive risk management procedures can never hope to reduce risk to zero. Risk management practices aimed at reducing risk have to be balanced against the concept of positive risk-taking that is an integral part of the process of recovery.

Guided by the principles of the CPA, clinical risk

is regularly reviewed by the multidisciplinary team and the person's clinical risk assessment together with the multidisciplinary care plan form the core documentation of the person's progress and treatment. They are an integral part in the discharge planning process and should always be discussed at every CPA meeting.

For many people the risk of absconding behaviour is high and this necessitates their detention in a secure environment. Reflecting this factor each person will have a missing patient management plan form completed. This will provide a brief clinical summary, a description of the person, any history of absconding behaviour, risks to self and/or the public, if absent without leave, as well as likely absconding destinations. This form can provide rapid access to vital information that is needed by services and/or the police in tracking an individual who has absconded.

Consistent with government initiatives to reduce the rates of suicide it is required that the clinical risk assessment document notes any risk of self-harm and suicidal behaviours as separate but interrelated entities. There are also further and more detailed assessment tools which can be used where there is a specific identified area of risk. These include risk assessments for parasuicide, suicide and homicide, and the Parasuicide, Suicide and Homicide Intent Scale.

Every risk management plan has four elements, as shown below.

The four elements of risk management
- *Monitoring:* how frequently is the person being monitored? What specifically is being monitored?
- *Supervision:* what restrictions are necessary to minimize the likelihood and impact of any given risk?
- *Treatment:* what treatment does the person require to reduce the likelihood and severity of risk behaviour?
- *Victim safety planning:* what specific actions need to be taken to reduce or minimize the impact on potential victims?

The four elements of the risk management process are usually considered at the level of the individual and at the level of the unit.

At the level of the individual

Monitoring

As standard practice each person's whereabouts is known at least every hour. Depending on the risk assessment the person may be placed on continuous observation which will either be at 'arm's length' or within eye sight, depending on the nature of the risk, or on higher frequency checks – for example, every 15 minutes. The individual circumstances would dictate what is being monitored but would tend to include assessment of mental state, assessment of expressed suicidal ideation, and the presence of delusional beliefs. The monitoring would be geared towards factors known to increase risk behaviour.

Where risk behaviours are a frequent occurrence, the nursing staff in conjunction with psychologists and other professionals may construct a behaviour checklist on which key risk behaviours as well as key positive behaviours are noted each shift and this data is used to guide the risk management plan.

It must be emphasized that any management plan based on a behaviour checklist is focused on risk and on a balanced view of both the negative and positive behaviours displayed by the person, and is *not* a punitive device. When used well, it can provide a clear structure and clarify expectations between the patient and the staff.

Supervision

Depending on the nature and perceived imminence of the risk, some restrictions may be placed on a person beyond standard ward practice – for example, they may be supervised when shaving, they may not have access to the main courtyard area or have certain items that are regarded as a source of risk removed from their room. In all the above cases there will be a clear rationale for these decisions based on the risk assessment.

Treatment

It is routine for there to be full multidisciplinary input and discussion about the best treatment options for somebody who is posing immediate and serious risk behaviours. This may involve options such as medication changes, additional psychology input, creative/innovative programmes and diversionary activity.

Victim safety planning

If the person is known to target certain individuals, then attention will be paid to where he or she is nursed in relation to other individuals with regards to their safety.

At the level of the unit

Monitoring

Audits linked to clinical risk are routinely carried out as part of the secure mental health unit's audit cycle. These include regular audits of the use and practice of seclusion facilities, regular reviews of potential ligature sites and quarterly figures reviewing trends in the numbers of accidents, incidents, self-harm episodes and absconding episodes. It is standard practice for there to be room searches where there is a sound supporting rationale for this action.

Supervision

All secure mental health units have a policy whereby drugs, alcohol and other contraband substances are not to be brought onto the unit by service users, staff or visitors. The list of contraband items which are prohibited changes with reference to wider legal restriction and evolving technical and electronic equipment which can detect the presence and usage of these substances. A list of items not to be held by people on the unit or brought in by visitors or staff is given in the next panel.

Contraband items

- Aerosols.
- Glass.
- Illicit substances.
- Alcohol.
- China.
- Broken or unsealed tobacco.
- Lighters.
- Cameras.
- Equipment with voice-recording facilities.
- Canned drinks.
- Lighter fuel.
- Mobile phones.
- Pagers.
- Weapons.
- Matches.
- Plastic bags.
- Sharp implements.
- Prescribed drugs.
- Items considered fragile or breakable.
- Mirrors.
- Solvents.
- Bank or debit cards (these are not to be held by the patient within the unit. The patient may be granted access to them when necessary on community leave as per individual risk assessment).

Each individual ward/unit will have its own specific items that are contraband in line with the perceived risks of their service user group. The purpose of the contraband policy is to ensure that staff and service users are working in a safe and secure environment conducive to the recovery of the service users. As part of a hospital policy all parcels will be opened in front of a member of staff to ensure the safety of their contents.

A mental health student comments on their placement on an acute adult ward

. . .

As my second placement I started on the ward with some knowledge, but very little knowledge of ward-based activities. The first day seemed so chaotic and unorganized. I just didn't know what I should be doing or when and who I should be working with. However, after a few days it became obvious and the ward actually ran like a well-oiled machine, where everyone knew their role and got on with the day without much instruction.

It did not take too long to find a place in the team and get on with my day in the same way as the others. It was a very enjoyable placement and a great learning experience.

Treatment

The long-term reduction in risk behaviours can only come about through the recovery of the person based on a holistic care plan whereby all of their human needs are met. Therapeutic programmes that specifically address the underlying factors behind risk behaviours are required to support recovery. Examples of these include anger management programmes, substance misuse groups and cognitive behaviour therapy programmes both at the individual and group level.

Victim safety planning

Every person who is admitted to an inpatient secure or forensic unit is assessed by both a doctor and a nurse and their care reviewed each week to ensure that any person who is admitted is appropriate for the level of security that the hospital/unit provides. Where a person poses a continuous and serious risk, the multidisciplinary team would seek second opinions and advice but also consider the appropriate level of security for the person.

Conclusion

In this chapter we have considered secure inpatient and forensic mental health services. The chapter began by providing a brief historical background to establish the context of the development of this area of the mental health services.

We then looked at the range of people with mental health problems who become involved in secure inpatient and forensic mental health services.

The discussion progressed to consider the philosophy and the values of care and discussed the capabilities nurses need to possess to work in this setting. We next considered a recovery and positive strengths-focused approach in working with people in secure inpatient and forensic settings. Finally, the chapter considered risk assessment and risk management in some detail.

While this area of work involves difficult challenges, the secure inpatient and forensic setting provides immense rewards and job satisfaction. Furthermore, as community care continues to develop it is likely that this specialism will continue to form an essential part of the network of mental health services.

References

Anthony, W. A. (1993) Recovery from mental illness: the guiding vision of the mental health services system in the 1990s, *Psychosocial Rehabilitation Journal*, 16(4): 11–23.

Bowers, L. (2002) *Dangerous and Severe Personality Disorder: Response and Role of the Psychiatric Team.* London: Routledge..

Caplan, C. (1993) Nursing staff and patient perceptions of the ward atmosphere in a maximum security forensic hospital, *Archives of Psychiatric Nursing*, 1: 23–9.

Covey, S. (2004) *The 8th Habit: From Effectiveness To Greatness.* London: Simon & Schuster.

DoH (Department of Health) (1999) *Effective Care Co-ordination in Mental Health Services: Modernising the Care Programme Approach.* London: DoH.

DoH (Department of Health) (2002a) *National Suicide Prevention Strategy for England.* London: DoH.

DoH (Department of Health) (2002b) *Women's Mental Health: Into the Mainstream.* London: DoH.

Foucault, M. (2001) *Madness and Civilization: A History of Insanity in the Age of Reason*, trans. R. Howard. London: Tavistock.

Hart, S.D., Kropp, R., Laws, D.R., *et al.* (2003) *The Risk of Sexual Violence Protocol (RSVP): Structured Professional Guidelines for Assessing Risk of Sexual Violence.* Burnaby, British Columbia: Mental Health Law and Policy Institute, Simon Fraser University.

Holloway, F. (2005) *The Forgotten Need for Rehabilitation in Contemporary Mental Health Services: A Position Statement from the Executive Committee of the Faculty of Rehabilitation and Social Psychiatry.* London: Royal College of Psychiatry.

Jeffcote, N. and Watson, T. (2004) *Working Therapeutically with Women in Secure Mental Health Settings.* London: Jessica Kingsley.

Killaspy, H., Harden, C., Holloway, F. and King, M. (2005) *What Do Mental Health Rehabilitation Services Do and What Are They For? A National Survey in England.* London: Department of Mental Health Sciences, Royal Free Campus, Royal Free and University College.

Maden, T. (2007) *Treating Violence: A Guide to Risk Management in Mental Health.* Oxford: Oxford University Press.

Milner, J. and Myers, S. (2007) *Working with Violence: Policies and Practices in Risk Assessment and Management.* London: Palgrave Macmillan.

Paley, G. (2003) Implementing a trust-wide strategy for clinical risk assessment in mental health, *Mental Health Practice*, 7(1).

Pratt, C.W., Gill, K.S., Barrett. N.M. and Roberts, M.M. (1999) *Psychiatric Rehabilitation.* New York: Academic Press.

Race, P. (2005) *Making Learning Happen: A Guide for Post-Compulsory Education.* London: Sage.

Rask, M. and Brunt, D. (2007) Verbal and social interactions in the nurse-patient relationship in forensic psychiatric nursing care: a model and its philosophical and theoretical foundation, *Nursing Inquiry*, 14(2): 169–76.

University of Manchester (2006) *Five Year Report of the National Confidential Inquiry into Suicide and Homicide by People with Mental Illness: Avoidable Deaths.* Manchester: University of Manchester.

Webster, C.D., Douglas, K.S., Eaves, D., and Hart, S.D., (1997) *HCR-20. Assessing Risk for Violence, Version 2.* Vancouver: Mental Health, Law and Policy Institute, Simon Fraser University.

The mental health of older adults

Alyson Buck, Amanda Blackhall and Steve Wood

10

Learning objectives

By the end of this chapter you will have:

- Gained an appreciation of the effects of ageing in a social, biological and psychological context.
- Developed an understanding of common mental health problems people experience in later life.
- Developed an understanding of the interventions which can be offered to older adults experiencing mental health problems.

Introduction

This chapter will focus on the mental health of people in later life. We begin by considering the effects of ageing from social, biological and psychological perspectives. These factors are often inter-related as older adults who have a mental health problem may also be experiencing coexisting physical ill health and long-term physical conditions. These can also impact on the person's mental well-being and therefore it is important that we understand how the problem specifically affects the person.

We then consider common mental health problems which can be experienced in older age before looking at the provision of mental health services for older adults and the national policy context. Finally, the chapter will discuss interventions which can be offered to older adults experiencing mental health problems. The chapter will end with a conclusion summarizing the points covered.

Throughout the chapter clinical examples will be used to illustrate the points made to encourage you to reflect on your experiences in practice. Answers to the scenarios are provided at the back of the book.

Ageing in context

In this section we will discuss the ageing process. Physical, psychological and social factors all con-

tribute in various ways to the process by which we 'grow into' old age. Such a viewpoint links with recent government policy which has changed the way we deliver mental health services for older adults. In particular the *National Service Framework for Older People* (DoH 2001) proposed multi-agency working and 'joined up' services for older adults and acknowledged that this group of people have specific needs, risks and concerns for which provision needs to be made.

Later life may be a time when increased mental and physical frailty means becoming reliant on others, including friends and family, to help with general and/or personal care. Informal caregivers have long been recognized as providing an invaluable service in supporting people which, if it did not exist, would place an unsustainable burden on the statutory health and social services. However, the emotional and physical impact of caring for a person with dementia, for example, cannot be underestimated. Non-statutory bodies which offer support to carers provide another invaluable service supplementing statutory health and social services. As older people with mental health problems may have an increased reliance on informal caregivers, mental health nurses are also called upon to be mindful of the needs and concerns of those carers and to actively foster partnership and collaboration.

Individuals have to cope with changes at all points across the lifespan and later life is no exception. Yet unlike other stages of life where there are definite milestones, ageing is characterized by being a gradual process. Yet how we age is not merely a biological phenomenon. If we are to understand how older people might experience mental health problems in later life, then we need to look at the multiple factors which influence ageing.

Social aspects of ageing

It is well understood that people in Britain are living longer. The increased demographic trend of the rising number of older adults is documented in the media and current statistics indicate that people over the age of 65 comprise 15 per cent of the population in England and Wales. In addition, there has been a significant rise in people over the age of 100 (ONS 2008). Evidence that we have successfully adapted to ageing does not just include physical health and lifespan but also our level of satisfaction and quality of life.

The increase in the number of older adults in our population is due to several factors which are listed below:

- public health improvements;
- institutional care;
- inception of the NHS;
- decreased birth rate.

People in the UK today can expect live to a 'good age' and in the vast majority of cases with an improved quality of life and independence, adding 'life to years', not just 'years to life'. It could be argued that the experience of later life is largely related to the person's previous socioeconomic status, emotional experiences and lifestyle. However, older people may well fall victim to discrimination on the grounds of age alone and face social exclusion (Biggs 1993).

Disengagement theory relates to the way in which older people may 'naturally' start to disengage from societal contacts and spend more time alone in pursuing solitary activities. However, it is worth considering whether older people make a *conscious choice* to disengage or whether instead modern society provides fewer opportunities for older people to meaningfully contribute to the community (Biggs 1993).

Society's perception of old age is constantly changing. The definition of *old age* as beginning at age 65 is a relatively recent phenomenon reflecting the creation of the old-age national insurance and pension schemes of various countries. The growing numbers of older adults, especially those aged 80 and older has resulted in the redefining of later adulthood into two distinct life stages or age groups (Suzman and White Riley 1985):

- the younger old from 65 to 75;
- the older old or oldest old of 76 and above.

In many countries the oldest old are now the fastest growing section of the total population. In the UK in 2005 it was estimated that there were 9,647,000 people aged 65 and over, 4,599,000 aged 75 and over and 1,175,000 aged 85 or over (Age Concern 2007). Yet in spite of the numerical size of this group of people, in reflecting on the recent development of the oldest old phenomenon Suzman and White Riley (1985: 177) observe that 'less is known about it than any other age group' and that there 'is little in historical experience that can help in interpreting it'.

For a small but significant number of older adults, retirement is not the end of working life. Many older people continue in paid employment in a self-employed capacity or in voluntary work. Many companies actively recruit older adults and value the knowledge, life experience and maturity these employees contribute to the workplace. In addition, informal carers are often retired from paid work and make an enormous contribution in providing child care, care for neighbours and friends and of course spouses, free of charge. As the media often reports, the economic impact of people living for longer will mean that the state retirement age will inevitably increase as we all live longer.

Biological theories of ageing

While ageing is an inevitable consequence of time passing and a universal experience, the rate at which our bodies age will occur at different levels and is caused by different factors (Bond *et al.*

1993). Many writers agree that ageing has a genetic cause and occurs at a cellular level (Kirkwood 2003). This theory suggests that all of the cells in our body are continually replicating at various rates. Eventually the body reaches an age where cell production begins to become inefficient and starts to deteriorate. This causes us to show the effects of ageing. It is not known whether our genes are pre-programmed to age at a certain point. However, it is believed that lifestyle, environment and family history all play a contributing part in how we age and so this process is unique to each individual.

The realization of ageing

- Think of an older person in your family. When did you first realize they were getting older and what led you to think this? For example, was it a particular physical change or problem which made you think they were no longer as young as they once were, or something else?
- Write down your thoughts.

When you have finished, place your notes in your professional portfolio.

A mental health student comments on their placement on an elderly mental health assessment ward ...

Even after six months on an acute ward setting I was not prepared for my first day on this ward. The chaotic noises and behaviour of the service users were hard to get accustomed too. Not only for me, but for many of the other service users. Every day was so very different, every service user could be so different on a daily basis, or even different times of the day, and my role within the team was different every day. It was a real working example of how order can be brought out of chaos, by a relatively small number of people.

The amount of physical illness of the client group was also a steep learning curve. The variety of the work was what made this placement so enjoyable.

The physical effects of ageing

Next we will discuss the changes we can expect to see with regard to each of the main areas of physical functioning.

The cardiovascular system

As we age the heart muscle becomes less efficient and has to work harder to pump blood through the body. Blood vessels become less elastic and hardened fatty deposits may form on the walls of arteries, narrowing the passageway through the vessels (arteriosclerosis). The natural loss of elasticity combined with arteriosclerosis makes arteries stiffer, requiring the heart to work harder to pump blood through them. This can lead to high blood pressure (hypertension).

The respiratory system

A number of changes occur with breathing as we get older. As with other muscles in the body the respiratory muscles become weaker and less effective, often resulting in the older person having to increase their efforts to breathe as the forces for inspiration and expiration are decreased (Farley *et al.* 2006). The respiratory rate is likely to increase with a range from 16–25 respirations per minute (Lueckenotte 2000).

Bones, muscles and joints

Bones reach their maximum density and mass between the age of 25 and 35 and as we age they shrink and lose density, with the result that a person may become shorter in stature (Jeukendrup and Gleeson, 2004). Gradual loss of density causes the bones to weaken and become more susceptible to fracture, and the healing process is less rapid and efficient. Muscles, tendons and joints also lose strength and flexibility.

Digestive system

Swallowing and the motions that move digested food through the intestines slow down with age. The amount of surface area within the intestines diminishes slightly and the flow of secretions from the stomach, liver, pancreas and small intestine may decrease. These changes generally cause little disruption to the digestive process but constipation sometimes increases (Farley *et al.* 2006).

Kidneys, bladder and urinary tract

With age the kidneys become less efficient in removing waste from the bloodstream and conditions such as diabetes or high blood pressure can occur. Some medications can damage the kidneys. A number of people aged 65 and older experience a loss of bladder control (urinary incontinence). This can be caused by a number of health problems such as obesity, frequent constipation and chronic cough. Women are more likely than men to have incontinence and those who have been through the menopause might experience stress incontinence as the muscles around the opening of the bladder or sphincter lose strength and bladder reflexes change. However, incontinence is not an *inevitable* consequence of ageing (Redfern and Ross 2001). As the production of a hormone called oestrogen declines, the tissue lining the urethra becomes thinner, pelvic muscles become weaker and so bladder support is reduced. In older men incontinence is sometimes caused by an enlarged prostate which can block the urethra. This makes it difficult to empty the bladder and can cause small amounts of urine to leak.

Eyes

With age, eyes are less able to produce tears, retinas become thinner and the lenses are gradually less clear. In our forties focusing on objects that are close up may become more difficult. In later life the irises stiffen and make the pupils less responsive which can make it more difficult to adapt to different levels of light. Other changes to the lenses can cause sensitivity to glare which presents a problem when driving at night. Cataracts, glaucoma and macular degeneration are the most common problems of ageing eyes (Farley *et al.* 2006).

Ears

Hearing loss is one of the most common conditions affecting adults who are middle-aged and older. It has been estimated that one in three people over 60 and half of all people older than 85 have significant hearing loss (Mayo Foundation for Medical Education and Research 2008). Over the years, sounds and noise can damage the hair cells of the inner ear, the walls of the auditory canals thin and the eardrums thicken. It can be difficult to hear high frequencies and/or to follow a conversation in a crowded room. Along with changes in the inner ear or in the nerves attached to it, earwax builds up and various diseases can affect hearing.

Teeth

Teeth and gums age according to how well they have been looked after. With age, the mouth often feels drier, gums recede and the teeth may also darken slightly and become more brittle and easier to break. Most adults can keep their natural teeth all of their lives but with less saliva to wash away bacteria the teeth and gums become slightly more vulnerable to decay and infection. If most or all of the natural teeth have been lost, then dentures or dental implants are common replacements. A dry mouth can lead to infections and can also make speaking, swallowing and tasting difficult. Oral cancer is more common among older adults. The number of taste buds can be reduced by up to two-thirds by the age of 80 resulting in preference for excess sugar and salt (Redfern and Ross 2001).

Skin, nails and hair

Skin thins and becomes less elastic and more fragile as we get older. Bruising happens more easily and decreased production of natural oils makes the skin drier and more wrinkled. Age spots can occur and skin tags are more common. Nails grow at about half the pace they once did. Hair may grey and thin. In addition most people perspire less, making it harder to stay cool in high temperatures and increasing the risk of heat exhaustion and heatstroke. Many factors affect how the skin ages, with the most significant being sun exposure over the years; however, smoking also adds to skin damage.

Sleep

Surprisingly, the need for sleep changes little throughout adulthood. However, sleep is usually less sound in old age, meaning more time in bed is needed to get the same amount of sleep. By the age of 75 most people find that they wake up several times at night.

Weight

With age, maintaining a healthy weight or losing weight can be more difficult. Metabolism slows down, meaning that the body burns fewer calories and the level of activity may decrease resulting in unwanted weight gain.

Sexuality

Sexual needs, patterns and performance usually change with age. A woman's vagina tends to shrink and narrow, and the walls become less elastic. Vaginal dryness is a problem and this can make sex painful. Impotence becomes more common in men as they age. By the age of 65 up to one in four men have difficulty getting or keeping an erection. For others it may take longer to get an erection and it may not be as firm as it used to be.

Brain and nervous system

The number of cells or neurons in the brain decreases with age and memory becomes less efficient. However, in some areas of the brain the number of connections between the cells *increases*, perhaps helping to compensate for the ageing neurons and to maintain brain function (Woodrow 2002). Reflexes tend to become slower and generally people become less coordinated.

Scenario: Martin

Martin is 79 years old and was admitted to hospital following a fall down the stairs at his home. He suffered a hip fracture but this has now been stabilized. He is recovering and is getting ready to go home where he lives on his own.

● What factors relating to his physical health should be taken into account for him to be able to do this?

Write down your thoughts and then place them in your professional portfolio.

The psychological effects of ageing

In this section we will explore the concept of old age from a life stage perspective and examine how psychology and physiology are interlinked in later life. Erikson's (1995) model of psychosocial development is an influential concept and helps us make sense of the issues we confront at various stages of the lifespan. The stages of Erikson's model are shown in Figure 10.1.

Psychosocial crisis stage	Life stage	Age range, other descriptions
1 Trust vs. mistrust	Infancy	0–1 years, baby, birth to walking
2 Autonomy vs. shame and doubt	Early childhood	1–3 years, toddler, toilet training
3 Initiative vs. guilt	Play age	3–6 years, preschool, nursery
4 Industry vs. inferiority	School age	5–12 years, early school
5 Identity vs. role confusion	Adolescence	9–18 years, puberty, teens
6 Intimacy vs. isolation	Young adult	18–40 years, courting, early parenthood
7 Generativity vs. stagnation	Adulthood	30–65 years, middle age, parenting
8 Integrity vs. despair	Mature age	65+ years, old age, grandparenting

Figure 10.1 Erikson's psychosocial model

Our attention in this chapter is focused on the last stage, which is maturity. There is a lot of debate concerning when maturity or old age begins. In Erikson's theory, reaching the last stage of life is a good thing as not getting there means the person did not successfully negotiate one of the earlier life stages.

Each of Erikson's life stages has a relevant challenge which must be overcome in order to proceed to the next. The challenge in the mature life stage requires that we develop 'integrity' rather than succumb to 'despair'. By reaching integrity we come to terms with our life and are able to look back and accept events and the choices we made as having been a necessary part of our life. Despair involves unresolved feelings about our past and involves emotions such as anger and resentment.

However, it is not necessary to have led a successful life to reach integrity. Erikson's theory retains a positive focus and we only need to accept ourselves as we really are. Even if we have led a less than good life and made many mistakes or experienced numerous failures, there is still the potential to achieve integrity and proceed to a peaceful death.

Boeree (2006) argues that the maturity life stage is the most difficult. As we have established, older adults often experience social exclusion. Together with this our bodies no longer function as well as they once did while often there is a noticeable deterioration in our physical health. Psychologically we become conscious of our fallibility and sometimes develop a fear of health conditions such as heart problems and cancer. Many older people also lose confidence and experience a general sense of physical vulnerability in terms of, for example, fear of falling over or have an excessive awareness of the threat of violence or abuse from younger people. This can cause them to avoid going out, leading to loneliness and limited opportunities for social contact and activity.

The increased awareness of our mortality in old age leads to concerns about death. A partner or spouse, friends and relatives and people of our generation die and there is the realization that death is near. It might seem natural to despair and some older people become preoccupied with the past. This is an understandable reaction because for many that was when they were at their busiest and most productive.

Scenario: Peter

Peter is an 80-year-old retired pharmacist who has been resident in a care home for the past two months. He moved there because his physical health had deteriorated to the extent that he became very frail and fell frequently, and he could no longer be cared for by carers in his own home.

Peter agreed to move to the residential home with considerable sadness at giving up the spacious seaside retirement flat he had shared with his late wife. He has become withdrawn, unhappy and tearful in the last few weeks and struggled to adapt to living with other people. He had always been a private and independent man who disliked having to rely on others to help him and had always felt embarrassed at carers having to carry out personal care. Peter started to spend longer periods alone in his room and stopped watching the television programmes which he had loved.

He showed no interest when his grandchildren came to visit having previously enjoyed helping them with homework. Care staff in the home and Peter's family became especially concerned when he started to refuse meals and looked considerably thinner as a result. Staff started to mutter to each other that they felt he was 'giving up' and that they did not know how best to help him. One morning Peter tells his carer to leave him alone and that he wants to die. He admits that he feels he has 'nothing left to live for'.

You are based within a community mental health team for older adults for one of your placements. An urgent referral is made by Peter's GP for a member of the team to assess Peter's mental state as soon as possible as he has deteriorated mentally and physically.

Your mentor, who is a community mental health nurse, asks you to accompany them for this visit. You observe the assessment process and reflect on the situation.

- Consider what Erikson says about the emotional 'tasks' and development relating to adults in the eighth life stage.
- Write down how the life stage theory can be applied to the difficulties Peter is currently experiencing under the headings of social, physical and psychological factors.

When you have finished, place your notes in your professional portfolio.

Common mental health problems in later life

While there are a range of mental health problems people can experience in later life this chapter will focus on the most common, in line with Standard 7 of the *National Service Framework for Older People* (DoH 2001) (NSF). This distinguishes three common mental health problems in later life: dementia, depression and delerium, and has provided a valuable spotlight on mental health problems in older adults that may often go undetected.

Depression

Depression is the most common mental health problem in later life. It can be easy to overlook and considered as a 'normal' part of ageing rather than a treatable condition. In older adults depression can be seen as a reaction to life events or severe and enduring ill health and pain. Alternatively it may be part of a lifelong pattern of low mood finally leading to contact with the mental health services.

In the same way as younger adults, an older person experiencing depression will report or demonstrate changes in their mood, thought processes, behaviour and physical state (Keady and Ashton 2005). It is important to listen to the individual and take into account their perceptions of the issue.

Table 10.1 Characteristics of depression in older adults

Symptom	Manifestations
Change in mood	Low mood for two weeks or more, apathy
Change in thought processes	Feelings of hopelessness or helplessness, worthlessness, guilt, reduced concentration and forgetfulness
Change in behaviour	Tearfulness, irritability, loss of interest in usual activities, withdrawal from contacts
Physical changes	Changes in appetite, weight loss/gain, sleep disturbance, low energy

It is important to remember that an individual may have characteristics of depression (see Table 10.1) together with other mental health problems. For example, a person may experience bipolar affective disorder with anxiety symptoms while people with dementia often become depressed.

Depression and suicide

Suicide is a significant risk factor to consider when the person is experiencing depression. Older men represent a particularly high risk group while studies have also shown that depression together with social isolation, living alone and alcohol misuse are all high risk factors for suicide.

Scenario: Dennis

Dennis is a 76-year-old widower who is brought in by ambulance to the A&E department of his local hospital. He was in a semi-conscious state after taking an overdose of prescription pain killers. Dennis's neighbours alerted the police after they noted his curtains had not been drawn and reported he had not been seen at the local social club for several weeks. Dennis was found collapsed on his bed with an empty packet of tablets beside him and had left a note addressed to his son who lives in Australia. Dennis appeared to have been neglecting himself and there were signs he had made superficial cuts to his wrists.

Dennis had a stroke in the last few months and is also being treated for a chronic and disabling lung condition which requires him to be on oxygen therapy for several hours a day.

Dennis appears to be very thin and is wearing soiled clothing which hangs loosely from his frame suggesting a large weight loss. His fingernails are overgrown and he is unshaven. He says very little and when he does it is in a barely audible whisper. He tells the nurse, 'It's all too late, I must face my punishment.'

A doctor has diagnosed Dennis as being severely depressed.

- From what you understand about depression, write down the ways that it has impacted on Dennis's life.
- Consider and write down what might have contributed towards Dennis becoming depressed.

When you have finished, place your notes in your professional portfolio.

What factors contribute towards depression in later life?

The NSF (DoH 2001) has identified factors which can contribute to a person experiencing depression and these are listed in the next panel.

Groups and life events predisposing to depression

- Those living in care homes.
- Those who have a long-term physical illness.
- Women.
- Exposure to traumatic life events.
- Bereavement.
- Loss of health, role, status, finances.
- Retirement.
- Alcohol misuse.
- Previous history of depression.

Dementia

While dementia is not an inevitable disease of old age, it is more likely to be seen in later life, although younger people can also develop this condition. Dementia is not just about 'being old and forgetful'. Instead it refers to an overall decline in mental, social and physical abilities. The term dementia refers to a deterioration in functioning, memory and cognition and includes a variety of conditions which all give rise to a *progressive* and *irreversible* condition (Lyttle 1986). It is important to identify a progressive dementia-type illness at the earliest stage so that the individual can have access to services and treatment and make informed decisions about their care.

The symptoms of dementia differ according to the type of disease. However, the experience of a dementia-type illness can be immensely devastating for the individual, their family and those who care for them. The NSF (DoH 2001) estimates that of the population aged over 65 years about 5 per cent have dementia and at any one time 10–15 per cent will have depression. The Alzheimer's Society (2009) identifies that as many as 700,000 people have dementia with the majority of 400,000 having Alzheimer's disease. Of those with mild to moderate Alzheimer's, 15,000 will be aged under 70 years, 75,000 between 70 and 80 years and

160,000 over 80 years. Around 80 per cent of people with dementia live at home while 23 per cent live alone and so it is clear that this is a particularly vulnerable group of older people.

In the next panel you will find a list of some of the types of dementia illness (Cayton *et al.* 2002).

Types of dementia illness

Alzheimer's disease

Accounts for about half of all cases. Deposits or plaques of an abnormal protein are found throughout the brain and tangles of twisted protein molecules appear in the brain's nerve cells. Scans can detect atrophy or shrinkage of the brain tissue and the widespread loss of brain cells.

Vascular (multi-infarct) dementia

Brain damage is caused by tiny strokes arising from an insufficient supply of blood to the brain.

Lewy body dementia

Regarded by some as a variant of Alzheimer's disease. Proteins build up in the nerve cells of the brain.

Frontotemporal dementia (Pick's disease)

There are similarities to Alzheimer's disease but many differences. Striking changes in behaviour precede memory problems and there is a marked loss of the person's ability to express themselves. Onset is typically when the person is in their forties or fifties.

Huntington's disease (Huntington's chorea)

A fairly rare inherited disorder which manifests itself in middle age. It is characterized by jerky movements in addition to progressive dementia.

HIV/AIDS-related dementia

Most people who are HIV-positive will not have dementia but many who progress to develop AIDS will experience severe dementia. The cause may be an HIV virus in the brain or as a result of tumours or infections resulting from reduced immunity.

Creutzfeldt-Jakob disease (CJD)

This rare type of dementia affects about one person in a million in the UK. 'Original' CJD usually occurs in middle age. 'New variant CJD' (vCJD) can be apparent in younger people and progresses rapidly, often leading to death within a year. There has been much publicity about the link between vCJD and eating beef from cattle infected with bovine spongiform encephalopathy (BSE).

Other

Dementia can also result from the excessive use of alcohol, brain tumours and Parkinson's disease (occurs in 10–20 per cent of cases). Some treatable causes of dementia include hormone and vitamin deficiencies, endocrine disturbances and infections, for example, neurosyphilis.

Dementia has a neurobiological origin. As the disease progresses and brain cells are lost, certain aspects of the behaviour of the brain are affected. While it is important to have some understanding of the action of the illness on the brain, the effects of dementia on the individual are not only physical. When working with people who are experiencing dementia it is necessary to maintain their sense of 'personhood' to prevent the despair which occurs through failing to negotiate the last stage of Erikson's model. As health care professionals we need to get to know the person and see the world through their eyes. It is important to view the person as having a wealth of life experiences which have value, and as someone who can still *feel* even if they are not always able to *remember*.

Scenario: Gita

Gita lives with Sanjay, her husband of 50 years. She was diagnosed with Alzheimer's disease two years ago.

Sanjay has not required any support from social services and manages to prompt Gita to attend to her personal care. Sanjay keeps in reasonable health despite his advanced years, and is visited once a week by a district nurse to dress a small leg ulcer.

Gita often fails to recognize Sanjay which causes him deep distress and he struggles not to lose his temper with her. Gita has at times left the house as she feels this 'stranger' should not be there and on one occasion she was picked up by the police in a highly agitated state, completely lost and bewildered. On another occasion Gita threw a heavy ornament at Sanjay in an attempt to defend herself against this perceived intruder. This previously devoted and gentle old couple appear to be living in a battleground with neither able to tolerate the other.

Sanjay feels he cannot take much more of Gita's accusations and admits he feels he is close to breaking point. Gita believes that Sanjay is doing wrong by allowing 'that funny old man' to come into their home.

You are on placement within a community mental health team and accompany one of the community mental health nurses following an urgent referral by the district nurse who has been attending to Sanjay. At first Gita seems very pleased to see you as she believes you can help to get Sanjay out of the house. She becomes hostile when you start to talk to him too and accuses you both of being 'his women'.

- Consider the above situation from both Gita and Sanjay's perspectives: how might Gita and Sanjay each be feeling at this time? Write down your thoughts.
- Can you think of any interventions that the nurse might use to help reach some degree of resolution here? Again write down the measures which might be taken.

When you have finished, place your notes in your professional portfolio.

For many years it was believed that nothing could be done to treat dementia and institutional care was the only option available. However, within, the last 10 years drugs have been developed which although not reversing the effects, act to slow down the progress of the disease. There has also been emphasis on diagnosing dementia much earlier and developing services to work therapeutically using a multidisciplinary approach with people with dementia and their families and carers. These new initiatives allow people to live for many more years with a higher quality of life following diagnosis.

Delirium
Delirium is a common mental health problem in later life and so we need to be aware of how this condition affects the individual. It also illustrates how physical problems can affect a person's mental functioning. Delirium is an acute

confusional state which is experienced at the extremes of life and people who have long-term physical conditions or are dependent on illicit drugs or alcohol are most at risk (Mayou *et al.* 2003).

Delirium produces a rapid onset of symptoms which have a physiological origin. The symptoms of delirium may lead us to believe that the person is experiencing an acute episode of mental rather than physical illness. Older adults who have dementia or long-term physical health problems are especially at risk. Delirium can affect the individual in several ways and be terrifying for the person who is affected, especially if they experience symptoms such as visual hallucinations and misinterpreting the actions of others as threatening. The scenario below is an example of a person experiencing delirium.

Scenario: Ola

Ola is a 78-year-old lady who lives alone. She has hypertension, angina and a history of alcohol abuse but over recent months has needed no care other than a repeat prescription for her medication (GTN spray, atenolol and temazepam). There is no previous psychiatric history. Her daughter, who lives nearby contacted the GP to say that on her recent visit her mother seemed confused, paranoid and aggressive. Ola has also been shouting at her neighbours, threatening them and accusing them of trying to poison her. She has been seen wandering outside at night in a state of undress and appears to have 'turned night into day', often being asleep when her daughter visits. Her daughter tells the GP that Ola's self-care seems to be deteriorating and that she is muddled, irritable and appears to be 'seeing things'.

When the GP visits Ola, she exhibits the following symptoms. Disorientation to time and place and talking about events from years ago. She appears paranoid, with rambling speech and fragmented thinking. There is poor concentration and fluctuating levels of consciousness. These problems apparently started about a week ago. Ola tells the doctor she decided to stop drinking about two weeks ago and, feeling tired, irritable and unable to sleep she had increased her dose of temazepam and so ran out of these tablets before her repeat prescription was due.

- Write down which of the characteristics that we have discussed concerning delirium you can identify as being present in Ola's behaviour.

When you have finished, add your notes to your professional portfolio.

Interventions for older adults with mental health problems

Psychiatric medication is often used throughout mental health services to alleviate distressing symptoms and in conjunction with 'talking therapies'. We suggest that you develop a thorough knowledge of the psychiatric medication prescribed to the people with mental health problem with whom you work.

Within this section of the chapter we will discuss psychosocial interventions or 'talking therapies'. You may find it useful to reflect on these techniques and to talk with your mentor and other health care professionals about how to positively use these methods.

The person who is depressed

Cognitive behavioural therapy (CBT) is often considered to be the most effective therapy for many of the mental health problems that occur in the adult age group. This includes treatment of depression, anxiety, eating disorders and behavioural problems. CBT can also have a long-term effect in preventing relapse and is often combined with drug therapy, although the benefits of this have not been extensively evaluated.

CBT is based on Beck's cognitive model and aims to develop client skills that modify the underlying inappropriate thoughts and beliefs that cause depression or anxiety. This is achieved by using techniques that identify and challenge the validity of such thoughts (Beck 1995). CBT is problem-focused and relies on an active collaboration between the person and therapist. A jointly agreed perspective of the problems is developed which relates the client's history to their current difficulties and then informs a range of suitable interventions. These may be, for example, behavioural approaches that challenge maladaptive beliefs or methods of modifying biased thinking by way of inter-session 'homework' tasks.

The success of CBT with younger people has now led to it being considered for use with older people. There are common cognitive problems associated with later life that can cause depression and may be amenable to being challenged successfully by CBT. These include difficulty in adapting to losses such as retirement, physical health problems, life review and self-morbidity. There may also be a tendency to hold unrealistic expectations of ageing and to attach self-blame to uncontrollable events. With anxiety-related problems, typical maladaptive beliefs are concerned with an overwhelming likelihood of threatening events, with a reduced capacity to withstand them. Thoughts may also be concerned with external threats such as harm to family members or the possibility of illness.

The person with dementia

The contemporary principles of caring for someone with dementia have been greatly influenced by the work of Tom Kitwood (1997). Within this person-centred framework, care is based on the assumption that all humans have five fundamental psychological needs:

1. *comfort:* receiving warmth and strength;
2. *attachment:* forming of specific bonds and relationships;
3. *inclusion:* belonging to a group;
4. *occupation:* being involved in the process of life;
5. *identity:* having a sense and feeling of who we are.

Based on these assumptions Tom Kitwood undertook research into *personhood* which refers to how biography and personality influence a person's experience of dementia. His research sought to provide a better understanding of how personhood was undermined for people who were living with dementia. He also sought to understand how 'good' dementia care could be implemented through the adoption of positive person work and dementia care mapping. He believed that to view dementia as an 'organic mental illness' ignored the important human issues and so attempted to change the perspective of dementia to one in which 'the person comes first'. Kitwood's work has provided the impetus for the development of individualized and holistic care approaches including personal biographies and the sharing of the lived experience of dementia.

In addition to these approaches the therapeutic interventions most commonly used for supporting someone with dementia are as follows.

- *Reality orientation* (RO) is a therapeutic approach that can be used by practitioners, care workers and carers who are supporting people with dementia. RO is concerned with taking regular opportunities to sensitively orientate the person. For example, to tactfully inform the person of the time of day and the location. There are a range of RO strategies that can be utilized on an individual or group basis including charts and orientation aids and prompts. While there is some evidence to suggest that RO can be effective in changing the behaviour and awareness of individuals with dementia, there have also been concerns over its inappropriate use. If applied without sufficient sensitivity it can cause the person considerable distress and so it is advisable to use it only where there are important orientation aims and as part of an individualized care plan.
- *Reminiscence therapy* is concerned with stimulating the recall of past memories or events using music, video, photographs and images. For example, recordings of popular musicals, viewing film clips, the use of cards displaying images from the past, books with pictures of past events and listening to music from the past. All of these techniques serve to stimulate recognition, discussion and interaction. Reminiscence therapy is based on the

premise that long-term memories tend to be retrievable even in advanced stages of dementia. Practitioners have become very skilled in utilizing a range of innovative approaches when delivering this therapy and so its use embodies the principles of a person-centred approach to care. Although the effects of reminiscence therapy have not been systematically studied there is no doubt that people with dementia find it stimulating and enjoyable.

- *Validation therapy* utilizes a number of specific approaches and was developed by Naomi Feil in 1963 when working in a nursing home in the USA (Feil 1992). This therapy is concerned with attempting to enter the inner emotional and personal world of the individual with dementia and involves seeking to develop an awareness of their feelings and the underlying meaning of verbal communication. In validation therapy the therapist attempts to understand the world from the perception of the older person rather than interpreting the situation from their own perspective. There is no attempt to impose a current reality in terms of dates and times; instead the practitioner explores the underlying meaning of the person's behaviour and speech. This therapy offers some very helpful communication techniques and often facilitates an understanding of what may appear to be confused and inappropriate behaviour. For example, a person with dementia who consistently wakes early and checks door locks might have previously taken his dogs for an early morning walk before going off to work. Or an older person who expresses anxiety about her daughter's whereabouts might believe she has to take her to school.

Conclusion

In this chapter we have considered the effects of ageing on people socially, biologically and psychologically. We then looked at the mental health problems people can experience in later life before discussing the services and policy pertaining to older adults. We ended the chapter by briefly outlining therapeutic interventions in older adults from a nursing perspective.

Working with adults in the latter years of their life provides unique opportunities and challenges for the student within practice settings. Working with older people often requires nurses to reflect on their attitudes and beliefs about older adults and their own ageing processes. We work with individuals whose mental health problems may leave them in a position of vulnerability as their usual levels of functioning and thinking decline towards the last period of life. For many, their first contact with mental health services will be in later life. Having a sound knowledge and understanding of how we age and the processes we go through on a physical, social and emotional level enables us to give the older person appropriate care and place that care in the context of their lives.

By working in collaboration with the older person, family, friends and the range of appropriate care professionals, we can promote and maintain positive mental health. Reaching old age should be viewed as an achievement of a life well lived and with thoughtful care and skilled nursing interactions we can help the older person face the end of life with integrity rather than the despair that affects so many.

References

Age Concern (2007) *Older People in the United Kingdom: Key Facts and Statistics 2007*. London: Age Concern.

Alzheimer's Society (2009) What is dementia? www.alzheimers.org.uk/factsheet/400, accessed 25 February 2009.

Beck, J.S. (1995) *Cognitive Therapy: Basics and Beyond*. New York: Guilford Press.

Biggs, S. (ed.) (1993) *Understanding Ageing: Images, Attitudes and Professional Practice*. Buckingham: Open University Press.

Boeree C.G. (2006) Erik Erikson 1902–1994, webspace.ship.edu/cgboer/erikson.html, accessed 25 February 2009.

Bond, J., Coleman, P. and Peace, S. (eds) (1993) *Ageing in Society: An Introduction to Social Gerontology*, 2nd edn. London: Sage.

Bond, J. and Corner, L. (2004) *Quality of Life and Older People*. Maidenhead: Open University Press.

Cayton, H., Graham, N. and Warner, J. (2002) *Dementia: Alzheimer's and Other Dementias*, 2nd edn. London: Class Publishing.

DoH (Department of Health) (2001) *National Service Framework for Older People*. London: DoH.

Erikson, E. (1995) *Childhood and Society.* London: Vintage.

Farley, A. *et al.* (2006) The physiological effects of ageing on the activities of living, *Nursing Standard,* 20(45): 46–52.

Feil, N. (1992) *Validation: The Feil Method. How to Help Disoriented Old-old.* London: Atlantic Books.

Jeukendrup, A.E. and Gleeson, M. (2004) *Sport Nutrition: An Introduction to Energy Production and Performance.* Champagne, IL: Human Kinetics.

Keady, J. and Ashton, P. (2005) The older person with dementia or other mental health problems, in I. Norman and I. Ryrie (eds) *The Art and Science of Mental Health Nursing: A Textbook of Principles and Practice*, pp. 552–93. Maidenhead: Open University Press.

Kirkwood, T.B. (2003) The most pressing problem of our age, *British Medical Journal,* 326(7402): 1297–9.

Kitwood, T. (1997) *Dementia Reconsidered: The Person Comes First.* Buckingham: Open University Press.

Lueckenotte, A.G. (2000) *Gerontologic Nursing,* 2nd edn. St Louis, MO: Mosby.

Lyttle, J. (1986) *Mental Disorder.* Eastbourne: Baillière Tindall.

Mayo Foundation for Medical Education and Research (2008) *Senior Health: Hearing Loss,* www.mayoclinic.com/health/hearing-loss/DS00172, acessed 25 February 2009.

Mayou, R., Sharpe, M. and Carson, A. (2003) *ABC of Psychological Medicine.* London: BMJ Books.

ONS (Office for National Statistics) (2008) *Population Trends,* www.statistics.gov.ik/downloads/theme_population-trends-134.pdf, accessed 23 February 2009.

Redfern, S.J. and Ross, F.M. (2001) *Nursing Older People,* 3rd edn. Edinburgh: Churchill Livingstone.

Suzman, R. and White Riley, M. (1985) Introducing the oldest old, *The Milbank Memorial Fund Quarterly, Health and Society,* 63(2), Special Issue, Spring: 175–86.

Woodrow, P. (2002) *Ageing: Issues for Physical, Psychological and Social Health.* London: Whurr.

Section 3
Therapeutic and theoretical perspectives

Physical health issues in mental health practice

11

Mary Northrop

Learning objectives

By the end of this chapter you will have:

- Gained an understanding of how physical baseline observations are measured.
- Developed an insight into some of the symptoms of physical health problems which can affect people.
- Acquired knowledge of the common physical health problems people can experience.

Introduction

This chapter focuses on the role of the nurse in assessing physical health care needs. In all practice settings we will encounter people who have physical health problems. These may be in relation to neglect of personal physical care, for example, nutrition or hygiene. Or the person may experience a physical illness such as diabetes, respiratory or cardiac disease. As mental health nurses our role is to assess the person's need and provide or access appropriate interventions to assist in addressing their health problem(s).

While this book focuses on mental health, physical health issues are a very prominent area of our work. People living with mental illness are more susceptible than other groups in society to acquiring a range of physical health conditions. Therefore it is likely that the mental health nurse will be involved with physical health care issues. People with a mental health problem also experience exclusion from society and difficulty accessing health care services. Therefore mental health nurses can and should perform a crucial role in advocating and negotiating on behalf of people with mental health problems in accessing health care.

The chapter will begin by considering the range of different baseline observations. These include pulse, blood pressure, respirations, temperature,

urinalysis and weight. We will then progress to look at some common physical health problems which are encountered in practice. These cover a wide variety of conditions that affect different systems in the body and include hypertension and acute myocardial infarction. We will then look at asthma, acute breathing problems, other respiratory conditions and chronic obstructive pulmonary disease (COPD). We then move on to look at obesity, diabetes, epilepsy and arthritis, and conclude with a brief overview of issues in relation to psychophramacology in order to highlight its importance in relation to the physical effects of taking medication.

Scenarios and examples of health problems will be presented throughout the chapter to help you make links with your practice experience and answers are provided at the back of the book.

Physical observations

When assessing a person's physical health we form impressions before we even speak to the person. These are made based on the evidence of our senses and in physical assessment we primarily use those of sight and smell. Yet it is important to provide an effective nursing assessment, so that we can trace the evidence to support our observations.

Initial impressions and observations

Think of a person you have recently met for the first time on placement. Now consider:

- What were your initial impressions?
- What observations did you make and why?
- How did these observations influence the physical assessment carried out?

Write down your reflections and when you have finished, place them in your professional portfolio.

Some of the first information we observe about people is their gender, age and ethnicity. Our sense of sight will alert us to self-care and whether, for example, the person's clothing and personal appearance are well maintained or unkempt and dishevelled. Using our sense of smell will corroborate our visual impressions. In some cases bodily odour can result from the neglect of personal hygiene but could also be due to a physical health problem. We can also observe whether the person's hair is washed and groomed or shows signs of neglect and if their fingernails are clean and well kept or in poor condition. The size and shape of the person will allow us to identify if they are overweight, within perceived normal limits, or underweight.

Mobility is a crucial part of physical functioning. Whether the person can walk unaided or, for example, experiences breathlessness or pain on mobilizing will provide important information. Often people with advanced arthritis experience acute pain when carrying out certain movements and in some instances joints will emit an audible cracking noise when being moved which will provide an indication of pain and difficulty in mobilizing for the person. Other information can be gained from whether the person requires aids such as a walking frame or wheelchair.

An important consideration is the environment in which the person lives. If the assessment is carried out in the person's own home we can observe whether this is well maintained or neglected. We can also assess whether the environment poses any risk to the person, for example, if a frail older person lives in a home without working heating during the winter. If family or friends are present, observing the interactions between them and the person we are assessing can provide an indication of whether relationships are cordial or strained and any problems or positive supporting factors.

A mental health student comments on their placement on an adult general medical ward

I had been warned that insight placements are often not happy experiences, but went with an open mind. On my first day I was told how lazy mental health nurses were and that they were not able to cope in the busy environment of an adult ward. I thought the best way to prove them wrong was to get on with it and not comment.

At the end of the placement I had used the experience to learn many aspects of physical care and worked as part of the team. I am still in contact with the ward and I am considering going back for my negotiated placement, to increase my knowledge of physical care before qualifying.

Baseline observations

When people come into a mental health inpatient area it is necessary to collect their baseline observations. The purpose of taking these is to enable comparison with any future changes and to assist with the detection of physical health problems of which the person is unaware. Often people have problems such as high blood pressure, heart disease or diabetes but are oblivious as they do not experience any symptoms of these potentially very harmful and even fatal illnesses.

A number of observations, particularly the pulse, respiration and blood pressure are affected by the 'fight or flight' mechanism of the central nervous system. Admission to hospital and the prospect of being examined by health professionals can be anxiety-provoking and lead to inaccurate observations. Instead, the effects of anxiety can be reduced by the staff introducing themselves, being friendly and explaining their roles and showing the person around the ward. Also allowing the person to acclimatize to their environment by permitting them time to unpack their belongings before carrying out the baseline observations will allow them to feel more relaxed in a new environment.

Carrying out the baseline observations in a private area or clinic room is advisable in order to respect the person's dignity and privacy. It is also advisable to take precautions to avoid interruptions including switching off mobile phones, putting polite signs on the door of the room and advising other staff that a consultation is being carried out. The observations can also be prepared for in advance by ensuring that the necessary equipment has been checked and prepared in readiness for use where possible. This will allow the nurse to concentrate on the person and the procedure and reduce the time the person has to spend waiting which might increase their anxiety.

Baseline observations

- Write down a list of baseline observations you would expect to be carried out.
- What are the normal ranges for these?

When you have finished, place your notes in your professional portfolio.

The most common baseline observations are pulse, blood pressure, respiration, temperature, urinalysis and weight.

Pulse

The pulse is the number of rhythmic expansions of arteries in response to the contractions of the heart over one minute. There are numerous areas in the body where the pulse can be taken but generally the *radial* pulse located in the person's wrist is used as it is easily accessible. A number of helpful observations can be made about the pulse. These include the rate, number of beats per minute, volume, strength, rhythm and whether the beat is regular or irregular.

To accurately assess the pulse the person needs to be resting and either lying down or sitting.

Physical activity, emotional upset and cigarette smoking all lead to a more rapid pulse rate and these factors need to be taken into account.

The pulse is best assessed by being taken manually as electronic measurement will not identify differences in strength or rhythm. The procedure is carried out by the person presenting their arm upturned. It may be more comfortable for them to rest the arm on a pillow or cushion while the pulse is being taken. The pulse is taken by placing the index and middle finger below the person's thumb on the wrist area and applying a very gentle pressure to *palpate* the pulse sufficiently to feel a beat by lightly pressing the person's artery against the bone. The person should not be in any discomfort during this procedure as detecting the pulse depends more on feeling in the right place rather than the amount of pressure applied. Therefore it is worth practicing on ourselves to ascertain where to locate the pulse.

The reading is taken over a full minute in order to fully assess the pattern of the pulse as changes in rhythm may not be regular and can be missed if measured over a shorter period. A fast pulse is referred to as *tachycardia* while a slow pulse is called *bradychardia*. The average pulse varies between 60 and 80 beats per minute for adults and is more rapid in children.

Taking the pulse

Take your own pulse and write down the reading after:

- resting for 30 minutes;
- doing exercise, whether this is going to the gym or a vigorous walk.

Write down the number of beats per minute and the strength of the pulse.

- What are the differences?
- Why are there differences?

When you have finished, place your notes in your professional portfolio.

In the exercise above you will probably find that the pulse rate is lowest after resting and fastest after exercise. Your level of fitness will affect the time it will take for the pulse to return to the resting state.

Blood pressure

Blood pressure is the cardiac output from the heart multiplied by the peripheral resistance of the vessels within which the blood is contained. Whereas observations concerning the pulse can tell us about the rate and strength of the heartbeat, the blood pressure gives an indication of the functioning of the heart and circulatory system. High blood pressure suggests the heart is under greater stress and can be an indication of a risk of stroke or heart attacks.

Blood pressure is measured using a *sphygmomanometer* and these can be either manual or electronic. It is important that whichever machine is used it is checked regularly to ensure accurate readings. If using a manual sphygmomanometer, a *stethoscope* is also required which allows the heartbeat or pulse to be heard.

When taking a person's blood pressure the procedure needs to be explained and the person to have provided verbal consent. They are then asked to present the inside of their arm which for comfort during the procedure can be rested on a pillow or cushion. Measuring blood pressure requires a situation to be created where blood is forced through the vessel and the circulation needs to be temporarily stopped. However it is important to ensure that the blood supply is not restricted for too long and no more pressure is applied than is necessary for the procedure to be carried out.

A cuff is then placed around the person's arm just above the elbow. There are different sizes of cuff and care needs to be taken to ensure the correct one is chosen for the person. Clothing may also need to be adjusted as if there are buttons or fasteners underneath the cuff the person's skin may be bruised or damaged.

If using a manual sphygmomanometer the *brachial* pulse needs to be located in the inside area of the person's elbow. By palpating or applying a very gentle pressure to the area and listening with the stethoscope the nurse can detect the person's pulse. The cuff is then inflated using a hand pump. A point is reached where the person's pulse can no longer be heard and this means the

blood supply has been stopped from the vessel due to the constriction of the inflated cuff. The pressure is then released at a steady rate. An electronic sphygmomanometer automatically inflates the cuff to a point where a reading can be taken and will also release the pressure.

The blood pressure reading consists of two measurements. If using a manual sphygmomanometer, the first is when we hear the person's heartbeat again on releasing the pressure on the cuff. This is the *systolic* reading which is the maximum pressure of the blood on the wall of the vessel following the contraction of the heart. The second measurement is the *diastolic* pressure which is when the sound of the heartbeat disappears (Marieb and Hoehn 2007). An electronic sphygmomanometer will automatically display the person's blood pressure reading.

Blood pressure will therefore be expressed as two readings. Normal blood pressure ranges from 100/60 to 140/90mm of mercury which was traditionally used in manual sphygmomanometers. Blood pressure changes with age and often increases as we grow older. This is due to the walls of the blood vessels losing elasticity or narrowing through a build-up of cholesterol deposits and the body being required to work harder to transport blood around the system.

Blood pressure can differ depending on posture because the sympathetic nervous system has to respond to postural changes. Often when being monitored on an ongoing basis measurements are taken of the person standing and then sitting to identify a contrast (Marieb and Hoehn 2007). Blood pressure can also be affected by a range of factors including age, sex, weight, mood, anxiety and stress, exercise, smoking, caffeine and having just eaten (Marieb and Hoehn 2007). Another factor is 'white coat hypertension' where a person's blood pressure is higher than normal when measured in the medical environment but is within normal parameters during everyday life (Celis and Fagard 2004).

Respiration

Respiration is an automatic act under the control of the nervous system and sensitive to the amount of carbon dioxide in the blood. The respiratory tract is made up of the nose, pharynx, larynx, trachea, bronchi and alveoli. Damage or infection to any of these areas can lead to breathing difficulties while trauma to the chest area will also affect respiration.

Respiration is a two-way process where we breathe in by inhaling oxygen from the air which then enters the bloodstream and is transferred from the blood to the tissues. We then exhale carbon dioxide which is a byproduct of energy production from the bloodstream through the lungs and out of the body into the air (Marieb and Hoehn 2007).

The rate of respiration is an indication of the amount of oxygen needed for the body to function. Measurement of respirations is achieved by observing the rise and fall of the chest and counting how often this occurs in one minute. The normal range for adults when at rest is 16 to 18 per minute.

Respiration

Count your own rate of respiration over one minute for the following:

- When resting.
- Immediately following exercise, for example, going to the gym or after a vigorous walk.

- What differences did you note?
- Why do you think there are differences?

Place your notes in your professional portfolio.

It is likely that you found your rate of respiration to be higher both in number and volume after exercise. This is in order to meet the increased requirement of oxygen to produce energy when exercising.

The rate of respiration is not the only observation that can be made. Others include:

- the *tidal volume* or depth of respiration or the amount of air the individual inhales and exhales;
- the *pattern of respiration* and whether the intervals between breaths are regular or irregular;

- *dyspnoea* is a condition where the person's breathing can sound laboured and they are gasping for breath;
- alternatively it is possible for people to have intervals when they stop breathing or *apnoea*;
- *cyanosis* can also occur where the person lacks oxygen and this is apparent where there is a blueness around the lips and fingernails.

A number of physical health conditions can affect respiration. These include asthma, chronic obstructive pulmonary disease, common colds and chest infections.

Temperature

Temperature measures the warmth of the body. Like the pulse there are a number of sites where this can be taken including the ear, beneath the armpit or rectally. While the most common method is in the mouth, people may have different preferences and if, for example, the person is unconscious another route may be necessary.

Electronic thermometers are now the most frequently used equipment in this procedure. Care ought to be taken to ensure that for hygiene purposes sheaths are changed after each use of the thermometer and that the thermometer is regularly cleaned in accordance with the manufacturer's recommendations. Health care staff should also change gloves after taking each person's temperature to avoid the risk of cross-infection.

The body's temperature is indicative of changes within the body and the environment. While the normal range is from 36 to 37.5°C, there is a variation between the sites where the temperature is taken with oral readings 0.2°C below those of rectal readings (Jamieson *et al.* 2008).

The regulation of temperature within the body is monitored by thermoreceptors and the hypothalamus in the brain. Changes in body temperature produce a range of responses. *Voluntary mechanisms* include the person taking action as a result of feeling hot or cold, for example, either by removing clothing or putting on additional layers. *Autonomic responses* are a physiological responses and *vasoconstriction* occurs when we are cold and, for example, the skin puckers up into 'goosepimples' and is a set of responses with the collective intention of retaining heat within the body. In contrast *vasodilation* occurs when we are hot and represents the body acting to release heat and cool the body down (Marieb and Hoehn 2007).

Nursing measures to reduce temperature include increasing air flow around the body if the person's temperature is too high by removing excess clothing or bedclothes and using a fan. Regular changes of clothing and bed linen and washing the person with tepid water will also reduce body temperature and make them feel comfortable.

Urinalysis

Urinalysis is a non-invasive method of assessment which can identify a range of factors. Urine is formed through the filtration of plasma in the kidneys by nephrons (Alexander *et al.* 2006). Urine contains 95 per cent water, and several other substances. The main ones are urea which is waste product from protein metabolism, creatinine and a range of electrolytes including potassium and sodium.

In hospital settings reagent strips are dipped into a sample pot of urine which has been collected and stored in a clean and dry container. Urinalysis is particularly important to identify levels of substances which are normally not secreted and might indicate the presence of an underlying physical health problem. Analysis has to be carried out while the sample is fresh as leaving any delay can result in false readings as the bacteria present in the urine will react with any glucose which is present.

Components of urine (Higgins 2008)

Urine is comprised of:

- blood/haemoglobin, the presence of which may indicate trauma;
- erythrocytes, the presence of which may indicate bleeding in the genital-urinary tract, kidney stones or infection;
- white blood cells, the presence of which may indicate infection;
- PH, the acidity or alkalinity of urine;

- glucose, which may indicate hyperglycaemia;
- ketones, which may indicate keto-acidotic states or starvation;
- protein, which may indicate hypertension, kidney or heart dysfunction, or infection.

If any of the above factors are found, then further investigations are necessary.

Other important observations which can be made are the colour and smell of the urine. Urine is normally straw coloured and becomes darker or lighter depending on concentration. Blood in the urine or *haematuria* will appear as a pink or red pigmentation although very small amounts will not be visible. The normal smell of urine is inoffensive and therefore a foul-smelling sample indicates the possibility of infection.

Weight

Observations of a person's weight should not only include the individual's physical measurement but factors which may indicate sudden weight loss or gain – for example, the wearing of very loose or oversize clothing or very tight clothing. Through asking the person it is possible to ascertain if the variation in weight was planned or due to other reasons such as change in eating habits, lifestyle or, for example, a period of immobility. As part of a physical assessment on admission to hospital a person will be weighed as a baseline measurement in case there is later concern regarding their weight change during their time in hospital.

Good practice related to recording of weight includes:

- ensuring the scales used are regularly checked and calibrated;
- using the same scales on each occasion;
- weighing the person at the same time of day;
- ensuring the person wears similar clothing on each occasion they are weighed.

Common physical conditions

A wide range of research has examined the links between physical health problems and mental

Physical illness and schizophrenia

Higher prevalence rates in the following:

- HIV infection
- Hepatitis
- Osteoporosis
- Obstetric complications
- Cardiovascular disease
- Overweight
- Diabetes
- Dental problems

Appear to have lower prevalence rates:

- Rheumatoid arthritis
- Cancer

illness (Colton and Manderscheid 2006). People with schizophrenia have a greater mortality rate for heart disease and respiratory disorders than other people in the community (Harris and Barraclough, 1998). Among the reasons for this are lifestyle factors such as smoking (McCreadie 2003), while the long-term use of some antipsychotic medication also increases the risk of cardiovascular disease (Tham *et al.* 2007; Daumit *et al.* 2008). Antipsychotic medication is also linked to an increased risk of diabetes and cardiovascular disease (Wirshing *et al.* 2002). Lifestyle and diet are also reasons why people with severe and enduring mental illness are at greater risk of obesity and diabetes (McCreadie 2003; Kreyenbuhl *et al.* 2008). It has also been found that there are higher rates of respiratory problems and weight gain in young people with behavioural and emotional problems (Aarons *et al.* 2008).

The Disability Rights Commission (DRC 2006, 2007) reported on the lack of equal treatment in relation to physical health needs for people with a mental health problem or learning disability. They highlight that individuals with schizophrenia are twice as likely to experience bowel cancer as the general population but less likely to receive screening. The DRC also discusses the interpretation by health professionals of symptoms as part of the mental illness or learning disability and not as a physical health problem leading to inadequate health screening and late diagnosis.

The next part of the chapter focuses on some of the more common physical conditions that people experience.

Hypertension

Hypertension is a specific disorder, but along with diabetes and obesity is also a major contributory factor to a range of other health problems. According to NHS Direct 40 per cent of adults in England have high blood pressure and there is an increased occurrence in people of African-Caribbean and South Asian origin (www.nhs direct.nhs.uk). Diagnosis of hypertension is defined as a sustained blood pressure of 140/90 mmHg or above. The symptoms of hypertension are summarized in the panel below, however, individuals very often do not experience any symptoms at all.

Symptoms of hypertension

- Headache that lasts for several days.
- Nausea.
- Dizziness.
- Drowsiness.
- Blurred or double vision.
- Nosebleeds.
- Irregular heartbeat (palpitations).
- Shortness of breath.

If hypertension is diagnosed there are a number of risk factors which cannot be modified including age, family history and previous experience of a heart attack or stroke. There are a number of measures which can reduce blood pressure. These include smoking cessation where relevant, change of diet to reduce cholesterol, salt intake and loss of weight. Engaging in regular exercise is also beneficial but needs to be related to the individual's fitness level and gradually increased.

Acute myocardial infarction

Acute myocardial infarction is commonly known as a heart attack and affects 275,000 people in the UK each year (DoH 2008). Heart attacks are the most common cause of sudden death in the UK. The condition occurs because of problems with the blood supply to the heart muscle and may follow intermittent chest pain for a few weeks before-hand. Risk factors include a family history of myocardial infarction, hypertension, diabetes and smoking. The person with a heart attack will be:

- in severe pain, often described as like a vice crushing the chest, and may feel as though it is located in the left arm, throat or jaw; normally this lasts for at least 30 minutes;
- pale or even grey and feel cold;
- sweating profusely;
- breathless and may feel nauseous;
- in an acute state of distress. (Al-Obaidi *et al.* 2004)

If you are on a placement and a patient suffers a heart attack, call the qualified members of staff for help immediately. On some placements there will be a designated emergency team, while at others it will be necessary to call the emergency services. If this is the case advise them of the person's symptoms and your location so that the emergency services can find you rapidly.

Medical emergencies

Often in emergency situations events happen quickly. Knowing important information in advance can save valuable time and help people who are severely ill.

- Either by asking the staff on your placement or checking the policies and procedures file, find out what to do in the event of an emergency. Make a note of any emergency numbers which need to be known.
- When beginning future placements make it a part of your orientation to become acquainted with the procedures to follow in the event of a medical emergency.

Cardiovascular accident/stroke

According to the Stroke Association (www.stroke.org.uk/information/index.html), around 150,000 people have a stroke every year and it is among the three top causes of death in the UK. Stroke also leads to severe disability with over 250,000 people

affected. Commonly stroke is more prevalent in people over 65 years but occurs in all age ranges.

Stroke is a disease of the blood vessels in the brain. The symptoms of stroke depend on the area of the brain which is affected and the severity of damage.

Common risk factors for cardiovascular accident/stroke (Hennerici *et al.* 2004)

- Hypertension.
- Diabetes mellitus.
- Smoking.
- Alcohol.
- Obesity.
- Myocardial disease.
- Transient ischaemic attacks.
- Atrial fibrillation.
- Chronic infection.

Initial diagnosis: the face-arm-speech test (FAST)

- *Facial weakness:* can the person smile? Has their mouth or an eye drooped?
- *Arm weakness:* can the person raise both arms?
- *Speech problems:* can the person speak clearly and understand what you say?

For more information consult www.stroke.org.uk/information/what_is_a_stroke/common_symptoms.html

---

A stroke can lead to a number of severe problems with the most common being *hemiplegia* or a weakness on one side of the body which is compounded by muscle spasms. *Dysphagia* or problems with swallowing occur in 50 per cent of cases and needs to be assessed to prevent complications such as choking and dehydration. Loss of continence of the bladder and bowel are also common. Other problems include difficulties speaking and understanding communication, the perception and recognition of common objects, short-term memory loss and difficulties with vision. Some problems improve over time as the brain recovers but some individuals will experience severe and permanent disability.

In the mental health setting stroke is one of the main problems that can occur. Living with the aftermath of a stroke can also lead to depression and isolation. The loss of physical functioning and changes to lifestyle can also cause a loss of self-esteem and change in body image. The impact on the family also needs to be considered.

Respiratory conditions

Asthma

According to Asthma UK, 5.2 million people in the UK currently receive treatment for asthma and there is one person with asthma in every five households. There are two forms of asthma. *Extrinsic* asthma is caused by allergens and occurs in children and young adults. *Intrinsic* asthma appears later in life and is associated with chronic respiratory conditions. Common triggers for extrinsic asthma include house dust mites, animal fur, pollen, tobacco smoke, cold air and chest infections. The symptoms of asthma which apply to both types are summarized in the panel below.

Symptoms of asthma

- Feeling breathless (you may gasp for breath).
- A tight chest (like a band tightening around your chest).
- Wheezing (a whistling sound when you breathe).
- Coughing, particularly at night (this is less common in adults than in children).

Typical symptoms of a severe asthma attack include:

- your symptoms will get worse quickly;
- breathing and talking will be difficult;
- your pulse may race;
- your lips and/or fingernails may turn blue;
- your skin may tighten around your chest and neck;
- your nostrils may flare as you try and breathe.

When the body detects an allergen it triggers defence mechanisms to fight the pathogens. In asthma the pathogens are inhaled and the body produces antibodies called immunoglobulin (IgE) (Marieb and Hoehn 2007). These antibodies bind to mast cells and basophiles which are located around the bronchial blood vessels. When the allergen is next encountered the antigen-antibody reaction releases histamines and bradykinin which leads to bronchial muscle spasms and swelling, and the excessive production of thick mucus.

In the case of intrinsic asthma, chronic inflammation of the bronchi and bronchioles is present along with oedema and mucus. Air becomes trapped in the alveoli making it difficult for the person to exhale. The progressive nature of the disease can even lead to deprivation of oxygen or *hypoxia*, hypertension and heart failure (Alexander *et al.* 2006).

Asthma can be controlled by the use of inhalers to reduce inflammation and swelling and make breathing easier. Information regarding the different types of inhaler can be found on the Asthma UK website (www.asthma.org.uk). More detailed information for health care professionals is available from The British Thorax Society guidelines (2008).

If you encounter a person experiencing an asthma attack it is necessary to sit the person down and summon help. Ask the person if they have an inhaler and let them administer this medication. Respiratory observations will also need to be made to check their rate of breathing has returned to normal.

Chronic obstructive pulmonary disease (COPD)

COPD is a collective term for a number of lung diseases including bronchitis, emphysema and chronic obstructive airways disease (COAD). COPD affects people over the age of 40 and causes 30,000 deaths a year. The main cause of damage to the lungs is attributed to smoking. As the condition develops, the person experiences problems breathing which increasingly impedes the capacity to perform normal daily activities and impairs quality of life. The disease may lead to heart failure as the heart has to work harder to pump oxygen round the body.

Symptoms of COPD

- Early morning smoker's' cough.
- Persistent cough.
- Production of mucus and phlegm.
- Wheezing.
- Tight chest.
- Difficulty breathing.
- Shortness of breath.
- Recurring lung and chest infections.

Initial treatment of the condition is through the use of bronchodilators and the input of specialist health care professionals including physiotherapists, occupational therapists and nurses. Interventions include exercise training, nutritional advice and education regarding the condition. Encouraging activity reduces the degree of breathlessness and anxiety (MacNee and Rennard 2004).

Scenario: George

George is 65 years old. He has been receiving support from the community mental health team (CMHT) for a number of years for management of his schizophrenia. He experiences auditory hallucinations which he calls Fred and Martha. Mostly Fred and Martha say positive things and do not affect his everyday life. Occasionally when he becomes stressed they are critical and he requires help in managing his anxiety and encouragement to continue taking his medication.

George has smoked since he was 12 and has a history of recurrent chest infections. He has recently become more breathless with a persistent cough which is affecting his sleep. He has been seen by the respiratory team and they have diagnosed COPD and prescribed inhalers.

George has been advised to give up smoking as he may need oxygen therapy in the future.

- How can you help George to come to terms with his diagnosis?
- What methods and support are available for George in relation to smoking cessation?
- What observations and assessments will be needed for both the COPD and the schizophrenia?

Diabetes

In Britain there are over 2.3 million people with diabetes and it is estimated another half a million do not know they have the condition (Primary Care Organization Progress Survey 2007). There are two types of diabetes. Type I is where our production of insulin is affected and needs to be replaced. This usually occurs in people under 40 and has a rapid onset with readily evident signs and symptoms. Type II diabetes is when the body still produces insulin but it is not sufficient or the insulin does not work effectively. Type II diabetes commonly occurs in adults over 40 years of age, however, childhood diabetes is increasing due to childhood obesity. The condition may be managed initially by dietary modification for three months, which is then reviewed.

Many people will need to commence oral hypoglycaemic medication and some will need insulin as the disorder progresses. For some individuals the signs and symptoms may not be obvious and diagnosis occurs when tests are carried out during routine health checks.

Symptoms of diabetes

- Feeling very thirsty.
- Producing excessive amounts of urine.
- Tiredness, weight loss and muscle wasting.
- Itchiness around the vagina or penis.
- Getting thrush regularly due to the excess sugar in urine.
- Blurred vision caused by the lens of the eye becoming very dry.

Epilepsy

At least 456,000 people have epilepsy in the UK and it is the most common neurological disorder in the world (The National Society for Epilepsy 2009). Epilepsy is a term which describes a range of disorders which are characterized by seizures or fits. The neurones in the brain work on electrical impulses and in epilepsy the electrical impulses are disrupted, causing the individual to have a seizure. This may appear as a momentary lapse in attention or a generalized seizure with tonic-clonic features.

Symptoms and types of epilepsy

Partial seizures

- *Simple partial seizure:* a seizure where the person remain conscious.
- *Complex partial seizure:* consciousness is affected, loss of sense of awareness, no memory of the event.

Generalized seizures

There are six main types of generalized seizure which are described below.

- *Absences:* this type of seizure mainly affects children. It causes the child to lose awareness of their surroundings for between 5 and 20 seconds.
- *Myoclonic jerks:* these cause the person's arms, legs or upper body to jerk or twitch in the same manner as if receiving an electric shock. They often only last for a fraction of a second and the person remains conscious during the episode.
- *Clonic seizures:* cause the same sort of twitching as myclonic jerks except the symptoms will last up to two minutes. Loss of consciousness may occur.
- *Atonic seizures:* these cause the muscles to suddenly relax and the person may fall to the ground.
- *Tonic seizures:* unlike an atonic seizure these cause all of the muscles to stiffen and the person loses their balance and falls over.
- *Tonic-clonic seizures:* this type of seizure has two stages. The person's body becomes stiff and their arms and legs will begin twitching. The person loses consciousness and will become incontinent of urine. The seizure lasts between one and three minutes. This is the most common type of seizure accounting for 60 per cent of all seizures experienced by people with epilepsy. Tonic-clonic seizures are typically what people are referring to when they use the term 'epileptic fit'.

People can experience any of the above types of seizure but usually the established pattern remains constant.

Auras

People who have epilepsy often get a distinctive feeling or warning sign that a seizure is on its way. These warning signs are known as auras. Auras differ from person to person. Some common auras include:

- a strange smell, or taste;
- a feeling of déjà vu;
- a feeling that the outside world has suddenly become unreal or dreamlike;
- experiencing a sense of fear or anxiety;
- the person's body suddenly feels strange.

Scenario: Hannah

Hannah has been admitted as an informal patient to an inpatient mental health unit with depression. She has a history of epilepsy characterized by generalized seizures which have been controlled with antiepileptic medication for the last five years.

Since she became depressed she has not always taken her medication and has experienced difficulty sleeping. She is at risk from a reoccurrence of tonic-clonic seizures.

- What further information do you need to minimize the risk of harm to Hannah?
- Find out about the first aid management for an individual experiencing a tonic-clonic seizure.
- How can you ensure Hannah's dignity is maintained during an epileptic seizure?

Arthritis

Arthritis is an umbrella term which covers a range of conditions characterized by painful joints and bones. The two most common forms are *osteoarthritis* and *rheumatoid arthritis*.

Osteoarthritis is the most common form of arthritis and is caused by the cartilage between the bones degenerating leading to the bones rubbing together at the joints. The cause is not known but it is thought that obesity, which imposes a strain on the joints, causes injuries to them and that jobs which involve repetitive movements of one particular joint are contributing factors (Hakim 2006).

Rheumatoid arthritis mainly affects the joints and tendons. It is caused by the auto-immune response which attacks the joints and leads to inflammation of the synovial membrane, tendon sheaths and bursae (Marieb and Hoehn 2007). It can occur at any age and in any part of the body but commonly starts in the wrist, hands or feet. The individual's experience will differ depending on the areas of the body affected and the pattern of the disease. It is characterized by active and inactive phases. During active phases the individual will feel generally unwell and tired and joints become inflamed leading to pain and loss of strength and movement. Joints become stiff, particularly after being immobile for periods of time. Treatment includes the use of disease-modifying anti-rheumatic drugs and non-steroidal anti-inflammatory drugs (Hakim 2006) and the assessment of the symptoms during the active phase, incorporating pain management. Provision of appropriate aids to enable independence as the disease progresses involves a range of health professionals.

Psychopharmacology

The role of psychopharmacology in managing the symptoms of mental illness needs to be taken into account when assessing the client. Some clients may be on long-term medication and experience side effects which can build up over time. For others new medication may produce initial side effects which they may not be prepared for or in some cases lead to syndromes such as neuroleptic malignant syndrome which occurs in 1 per cent of clients taking antipsychotic drugs, which if untreated can lead to renal failure and death (Anderson and Reid 2004).

Anxiolytics, antipsychotic and antidepressant medications can all lead to anticholinergic symptoms such as dry mouth, which can affect nutrition, cause gastrointestinal disturbances and may lead to falls due to dizziness. Some will result in postural-hypotension. Another factor in relation to medication is the possibility of withdrawal symptoms, particularly from benzodiazepines, which also needs to be monitored.

The use of monoamine oxidase inhibitors and lithium treatment also requires regular monitoring and blood tests to ensure they are within the effective therapeutic range.

Considering psychopharmacology

The majority of clients will be or have been prescribed medication to manage their symptoms. Look at the medication for two of your clients with different presenting problems and answer the following questions.

- What medication are they prescribed and why?
- What are the actions of the drugs and how do these contribute to symptom management?
- What are the side effects?
- How can you assess whether the client has side effects?
- What may be the consequences for the client of the side effects?
- Is the client on medication to address the side effects? If so, answer the same questions above.

Conclusion

The chapter has considered the range of different baseline observations that can be made. These include pulse, blood pressure, respiration, temperature and urinalysis. We then looked at the common physical health problems which are encountered in practice. We began with hypertension and acute myocardial infarction before looking at asthma, acute breathing problems including respiratory conditions and chronic obstructive pulmonary disease (COPD). We then moved on to look at obesity, diabetes, epilepsy and arthritis, concluding with a section on psychopharmacology.

Physical health issues are an important consideration in promoting the general well-being of people with a mental health problem. However, mental health nurses often feel ill-equipped to work with physical health issues. Developing your knowledge further in the areas covered in this chapter will provide you with the confidence and skills to give effective care in relation to the physical needs of people with mental health problems.

References

Aarons, A. *et al.* (2008) Association between mental and physical health problems in high-risk adolescents: a longitudinal study, *Journal of Adolescent Health*, 43: 260–7.

Alexander, M., Fawcett, J. and Runciman, P. (2006) *Nursing Practice, Hospital and Home: Adult*, 3rd edn. Edinburgh: Churchill Livingstone.

Al-Obaidi, M., Siva, A. and Noble, M. (2004) *Crash Course: Cardiology*, 2nd edn. Edinburgh: Mosby.

Anderson, I. and Reid, I. (eds) (2004) *Fundamentals of Clinical Psychopharmacology*, 2nd edn. London: Taylor & Francis.

British Thorax Society (2008) *British Guidelines on the Management of Asthma: Quick Reference Guide*, www.brit-thoracic.org.uk/Portals/0/Clinical%20Information/Asthma/Guidelines/asthma%20qrg%202008%20FINAL.pdf, accessed 10 November 2008.

Celis, H. and Fagard, R. (2004) White coat hypertension: a clinical review, *European Journal of Internal Medicine*, 15: 348–57.

Colton, C. and Manderscheid, R. (2006) Congruencies in increased mortality rates, years of potential life lost, and causes of death among public mental health clients in eight states, *Preventing Chronic Disease*, 3(2): 1–14.

Daumit, G. *et al.* (2008) Antipsychotic effects on estimated 10-year coronary heart disease risk in the CATIE schizophrenia study, *Schizophrenia Research*, 105: 175–87.

DoH (Department of Health) (2008) *Healthy Weight, Healthy Lives: A Cross-Government Strategy for England*. London: HM Government.

DRC (Disability Rights Commission) (2006) *Equal Treatment: Closing the Gap*, www.library.nhs.uk/mentalhealth/ViewResource.aspx?resID=187303, accessed 25 February 2009.

DRC (Disability Rights Commission) (2007) *Equal Treatment: Closing the Gap One Year On*, www.learningdisabilitiesuk.org.uk/docs/DRCrpt.pdf, accessed 9 November 2008.

Etter, M. *et al.* (2004) Stages of change in smokers with schizophrenia or schizoaffective disorder and in the general population, *Schizophrenia Bulletin*, 30: 459–68.

Hakim, A. (2006) *Oxford Handbook of Rheumatology*, 2nd edn. Oxford: Oxford University Press.

Harris, E.C. (1998) Barraclough B: Excess mortality of mental disorder, *British Journal of Psychiatry*, 173: 11–53.

Section 3 **Therapeutic and theoretical perspectives**

Hennerici, M., Bogousslavsky, J. and Sacco, R. (2004) *Stroke: Rapid Reference*. London: Elsevier.

Higgins, D. (2008) Client assessment, part 6 urinalysis, *Nursing Times*, 104(12).

Jamieson, E., McCall, J. and Whyte, L. (2008) *Clinical Nursing Practices*, 5th edn. Edinburgh: Churchill Livingstone.

Kreyenbuhl, J., Medoff, D., Seliger, S. and Dixon, L. (2008) Use of medication to reduce cardiovascular risk among individuals with psychotic disorders and type 2 diabetes, *Schizophrenia Research*, 101: 256–65.

MacNee, W. and Rennard, S. (2004) *Fast Facts: Chronic Obstructive Pulmonary Disease*. Oxford: Health Press Limited.

Marieb, E. and Hoehn, K. (2007) *Human Anatomy and Physiology*, 7th edn. San Francisco: Pearson International.

McCreadie, R. (2003) Diet, smoking and cardiovascular risk in people with schizophrenia, *British Journal of Psychiatry*, 183: 534–53.

Primary Care Organisation Progress Survey (2007) *Access to Healthcare Services at a Glance*, www.diabetes.org.uk/Documents/Reports/PCTandLHB2007AtaGlanceReport.pdf, accessed 23 February 2009.

Tham, M.S.P., Jones, S.G., Chamberlain, J.A. and Castle, D.J. (2007) The impact of psychotropic weight gain on people with psychosis – patient perspectives and attitudes, *Journal of Mental Health*, 16(6): 771–9.

The National Society for Epilepsy (2009) www.epilepsynse.org.uk, accessed 6 February.

Wirshing, D., Boyd, J., Meng, L., Ballon, J., Marder, S. and Wirshing, W. (2002) The effects of novel antipsychotics on glucose and lipid levels, *Journal of Clinical Psychiatry*, 63(10): 856–65.

12

Cognitive behaviour therapy

Henck van Bilsen and Lyn Parsons

Learning objectives

At the end of this chapter you will have:

- Gained an insight into how cognitive behaviour therapy (CBT) works.
- Developed an understanding of CBT theory.
- Developed an understanding of the development of CBT.

Introduction

CBT has emerged within the last 30 years as a widely used and popular treatment of choice. As a 'talking therapy' that is often only required for a brief number of sessions and has a practical focus there is an obvious appeal. Recent initiatives have also led to the development of more trained specialist therapists to increase its availability, making it possible to receive CBT from therapists working within GP surgeries for example.

This chapter will introduce you to the key principles of CBT. We begin by identifying the characteristics of CBT as a therapeutic approach. The discussion will then look at the theory underlying CBT before examining how it has developed. Finally, we will outline the evidence supporting CBT and consider the advantages and disadvantages. A brief conclusion will summarize the main points covered.

While we do not work as specialist therapists, mental health nurses spend more time with people with mental health problems than any other group of health care professionals. Developing an understanding of how CBT is applied will enhance our skills and effectiveness as student mental health nurses in the practice setting. Through appreciating how CBT theory perceives mental health problems we will gain an added insight into the process of mental health problems. Yet also by

understanding how CBT is carried out we will develop our skills and capabilities in working with people experiencing mental health problems.

Throughout the chapter there are reflective exercises and practice-based examples to help you to integrate the theories discussed within your understanding of the practice setting. An answer is provided to the scenario of Selina at the back of the book.

A mental health student's insight into CBT . . .

The good thing about CBT is that when you are talking to a person with a mental health problem on the unit, for example, in individual time, before I wasn't sure whether what I was saying was right. But CBT gives you questions you can ask. I can also see where other people are using this approach.

The principles of CBT

CBT is based on the notion that learning and thinking have an important influence in emotional and behavioural problems. These responses can be 'worked with' and modified to allow the person to develop positive adaptive ways of dealing with their problems.

Characteristics of CBT

- CBT is based on a cognitive and/or behavioural model of human thought in which mental illness results from maladaptive thinking.
- Therapy is brief and time-limited.
- A sound collaborative therapeutic relationship is essential.
- The interventions are structured and directive.
- The interventions are problem-orientated.
- The interventions are based on an educational model.
- Homework is an essential feature.
- They proceed according to the therapist's holistic conceptualization of the person's problem(s) and in collaboration with them.
- They use problem-solving techniques and break problems down into manageable units, identifying thoughts and beliefs which hinder problem-solving.

We will now discuss each of the features of CBT in more detail and where relevant make links to the case of Ann, whose details are provided below.

Scenario: Ann

Ann is a woman in her late thirties. She is referred by her GP to the therapist having been diagnosed as experiencing depression. Ann is very reluctant to accept that anything is wrong and would see an admission to hospital for depression as wrong and admitting complete defeat. She believes that everything in her life should be perfect and if things go wrong it is her fault. As a mother of two children with a part-time job as a sales assistant she is a busy woman for whom perfection is not easily achieved, which explains her negative outlook on life.

CBT is based on a cognitive and/or behavioural model

When a person becomes depressed, as in Ann's case, there is often a repetitious cycle of negative thoughts and expectations that reinforce each other and cause the person to become locked in a pattern of negative thinking which detrimentally affects their mental health. In Ann's case she has a belief that we are obliged to tolerate negative feelings. Also that it is weak to accept that these may impact in a damaging way on how she feels, which has eventually led her to experience depression.

An essential component of CBT is to understand and help the person appreciate that there is a link between what we believe and how we feel.

Interventions are brief and time-limited

CBT therapists work in a focused way that is time-limited and uses brief therapies. The purpose of this is to empower the person receiving therapy in two ways.

- To prevent them becoming dependent on the therapist or the process of therapy.
- CBT is focused on being active and helping the person to make changes to cope better with problems. After they have completed therapy the person becomes their own therapist as they will use the specific techniques developed in the sessions to deal with their problem(s). If they encounter other problems in the future they can apply the principles of CBT to develop new solutions.

In Ann's case the therapist will have discussed with her at the outset the length of time the therapy would last and the number of sessions. Later in the chapter, in discussing the evidence supporting CBT, we will see that there is even guidance to recommend the number of sessions.

A sound collaborative therapeutic relationship is essential

To be successful CBT requires the person receiving therapy to be willing to participate and to be prepared to contemplate change. In Ann's case she is reluctant to discuss her difficulties. Initially she did not agree with her family and GP that she needed help but does admit there is a problem.

The therapeutic relationship is the basis from which all therapeutic work flows as the person receiving therapy needs to have trust in the therapist and be confident that they can help. In Ann's case early on in therapy she was wondering how it could help and why she was there. The therapist used active listening and often summarized back to Ann the statements that she made. This gave her the space to arrive at her own understanding of how the sessions could help. Developing a therapeutic relationship relies on our skills as people to be able to relate to others and demonstrate understanding, compassion and interest in the problems the person is experiencing.

Interventions are structured and directive

CBT sessions begin with a discussion of the agenda: what the session will cover. Setting the agenda is not always a straightforward process but very important as it represents collaboration between the person and the therapist in establishing goals and priorities for the session. Often it is difficult for the person to identify specifically what it is they want to discuss and so some probing of the issues may be necessary.

In the extract of dialogue below the therapist uses a number of skills to clarify Ann's agenda items. Read through the dialogue and the comments on the skills being used.

Agenda-setting

T: Well, thank you, Ann, for coming back today. Our last session was a week ago and in that session if I can just briefly summarize, you decided that you might want to give CBT a go to see if it might be helpful for you to overcome some of the obstacles that you have in feeling happy within yourself. Is that still the case?

Therapist comments: opening statement, checking if client still wants to go ahead with CBT.

Ann: I don't know, as it's going to take a lot of time. Isn't it?

T: So you are wondering if it is going to take a lot of time? Well, that might be an issue that we might want to talk a bit about today. One of the ways that we try to work when we do CBT is that at the beginning of each meeting we make what we call an agenda, which is a list of things to talk about to make sure that all the things that you are worried and concerned about get discussed and all the issues that I would like to address are discussed. So this sounds like one of the things that we might want to put on the agenda. Is that OK?

Therapist comments: linking client's question with agenda-setting.

Ann: Yes. OK.

T: So you said, 'Is it going to take a lot of time?' Are there any other things that you would like to put on the agenda?

Therapist comments: agenda-setting.

Ann: Well, it does seem very odd, doesn't it, coming to talk to a stranger about things, you know? It's not exactly getting on with it, is it?

T: So, it is odd talking to a stranger.

Therapist comments: reflection.

Ann: Well, you just have to, you know, get your head down, stiff upper lip and I suppose that is what people will say – 'Just deal with it.' That is what life is like, isn't it?

T: 'Stiff upper lip. That is what life is like.' So we have got three things so far that we might want to put on the agenda:

1 Is it going to take up a lot of time?

2 It is odd talking to a stranger about these things?

3 Would it not be better to have a stiff upper lip and to get on with life and ignore the fact that you are unhappy?

Any other things?

Once the agenda is set, it is necessary for this to be followed and skill is often required to retain a focus on the agenda items and prevent the session from drifting.

Therapy sessions are problem-orientated

The therapist focuses on the problems the client wants to resolve. Complaints are translated into workable elements that can be changed in therapy. In Ann's case she did not feel that she was experiencing a mental health problem. However, she did admit she was experiencing difficulties. The therapist worked with Ann to identify what the problem was and understand the difference between her feelings and beliefs.

Sessions are based on an educational model

CBT uses learning to deal with our problems and is practical. The therapist educates the person so that they become knowledgeable about CBT and can make sense of their problem(s) from a CBT perspective. In the case of Ann, the therapist explained the principles of CBT and checked that she understood and could then apply this new information to her problems.

Homework is an essential feature of therapy

In CBT the therapy sessions are important but so are the tasks that the therapist and person receiving therapy negotiate to be undertaken between therapy sessions. These take different forms depending on the problem. Often behavioural experiments are used with the intention of giving the person the opportunity to try out and practice alternative or new behaviour to overcome problems. To have an impact, the person receiving therapy needs to work on therapeutic tasks between the sessions and be motivated. We will discuss CBT interventions in more detail below.

Therapy is based on a holistic conceptualization

The therapy and homework are structured based on the therapist's *conceptualization* or understanding of the person's problems. In some cases this may be as a result of a brief assessment. However, for people who have received CBT or other treatments before or for those with a severe and enduring problem the therapist will carry out an in-depth and detailed assessment.

In Ann's case the conceptualization was that her upbringing was very strict and that her parents had a 'stiff-upper-lip' attitude towards life. Ann adopted this belief herself and attempted to cope, however difficult life became, and she did not feel able to seek help and support. The problem was compounded as Ann did not communicate when she was experiencing difficulties. The combination of these factors led to her experiencing depression.

The therapy uses problem-solving techniques

CBT breaks down problems into manageable units by identifying the thoughts and beliefs that impede problem-solving and addressing these with a range of therapeutic interventions. All CBT interventions bring about change by influencing thinking and work on the premise that our thoughts are influenced by moods and the consequences of previous actions (Mahoney 1977; Bandura 1986). The techniques CBT uses are discussed in depth in the next section of the chapter.

In summary, CBT is a structured approach to working with people with mental health problems that has identifiable characteristics. However, a common misconception is that CBT works in a very mechanical and prescriptive way. The most important element of CBT is the therapeutic relationship and the success of therapy is determined by the extent to which the person engages with the therapy.

The development of CBT

CBT developed from two strands of psychological theory. These are *cognitive theory* and *learning theory*.

Cognitive theory

Cognitive theory functions on the premise that what we do and feel is influenced by our thinking. In situations where there is no right or wrong answer and limited factual or objective evidence to support a decision, the person is reliant on their personal opinion and/or preference. This offers the potential for irrational beliefs to become apparent and problems to emerge.

Within the cognitive model we can see the following group of attributes at work as depicted in Figure 12.1.

Feelings	Thoughts
Beliefs	Actions

Figure 12.1 Attributes of cognition

Our feelings, thoughts, beliefs and actions are all linked and mutually influential. Within CBT the therapeutic process assists the person in appreciating how these different attributes link together and can be made to provide more adaptive coping methods.

Learning theory

Learning theory considers how humans learn. The three most prominent learning theories are *operant learning*, *respondent learning* and *modelling*.

Operant learning works on the premise that we learn from the consequences of our actions. This could be an external event, for example, saying 'good morning' with a smile to our neighbour and their responding 'good morning' and smiling in return. However, it can also be an internal event. For example, if we are anxious about dogs and see a dog and then cross the street to avoid it this will put a distance between us and the dog. Behaviours that are followed by positive or enjoyable consequences are inclined to happen more often while behaviour followed by negative consequences tends to be avoided.

Respondent learning is when we make a

Scenario: Selina

Selina is 20 years old and believes she is overweight. Approximately a year ago she went on a radical diet and lost a lot of weight in a short space of time. However, she has still continued to strictly limit her food intake and to lose weight gradually. Selina will not eat any products with sugar in them as she is concerned this will cause her to gain weight. Her best friend Donna is worried about her and spoke with Selina suggesting that she return to a regular diet. However, Selina is concerned that she will put on weight if she deviates from her regime and insists on continuing to limit what she eats.

How would you place a cognitive interpretation on Selina's beliefs and behaviour?

connection between two events that originally were previously unconnected. A famous example is of Pavlov's experiments with his dogs. The dogs received food which caused them to salivate while at the same time a buzzer would ring. After a number of repetitions of this same exercise, setting the buzzer off would lead to saliva production in the dogs without food being provided. In humans this mechanism works in many anxiety situations where previous neutral events can trigger strong emotional reactions. An example is where a person has been in a car accident and the sound of a car engine makes them nervous.

Modelling works on the basis that people learn not only from their own actions but by seeing those of other people. An example is of parents who smoke. A child may see the parent frequently smoke and be influenced to participate in the same behaviour (Bandura 1977).

Learning theory suggests that our behaviour is linked to how we interact with our environment. Events that are seen as positive will make the behaviours preceding them more likely. Negative feelings can be triggered by previously neutral events and stimuli when they have been combined once – for instance, in a traumatic event – or many times – for example, being humiliated in a learning environment. Finally we also learn to feel and do from what we see others feel and do.

The cognitive and behavioural models are different as the behavioural approach focuses on the action in response to a stimulus while the cognitive approach relates to the emotions and feelings which underpin the response. However, CBT is taught as one model with an integrated approach (Gega 2005).

Within the CBT approach the cognitive and learning approaches are regarded as being complementary as changes in behaviour generally produce a change in thought, while a change in thinking usually causes changes in behaviour (Gega 2005). CBT therapists suggest that cognitions and behaviours are interrelated and not separate and therefore a good way of testing the CBT model is whether changes in behaviour and the re-evaluation of certain beliefs have occurred through receiving therapy.

An overview of CBT interventions

In this part of the chapter we will look at some of the therapeutic strategies used in CBT. These techniques function by helping people to understand how their negative thoughts and problems affect them. We will first of all consider **cognitive strategies** before progressing to look at **behavioural methods**.

The main cognitive strategy is *cognitive restructuring*. In this method the person learns to think differently in situations that previously led to negative feelings and/or negative behaviour. The main tool used for this is *thought records* where the person writes down the problem feeling and its strength and then focuses on the thinking involved that causes the feeling. Through this method the person learns to identify triggers for the problem feelings and behaviours.

Once the problem thinking has been identified, the person and therapist analyse it and try and identify *thinking errors* which are mistaken assumptions or biased thinking processes. Thought records are good homework tasks. By writing down the problem and the intensity with which it is experienced close to the time when it occurs the person is more likely to recall accurate and specific details. Particular patterns also become evident regarding when the person is more likely to experience the problem.

When the thought record has been completed, the original unhelpful thoughts are replaced with more rational alternatives. The final test is to develop new behaviours to support the new rational beliefs. The strategies we will explain next can all be used as part of working with thought records or as stand-alone techniques.

Identifying negative automatic thoughts

The person monitors their thoughts when they feel depressed, anxious or are experiencing other strong negative emotions. An example could be, 'When I noticed my breathing I thought I was going to have a heart attack'. There are a number of variations of irrational thinking strategies which can be identified through monitoring negative automatic thoughts.

Types of irrational thinking strategy

- *All-or-nothing thinking:* the person sees things in polarities. If their performance falls short of perfect then they are a total failure: 'If I don't do it perfectly, there's no point in doing it at all!'
- *Over-generalization:* single negative events represent a never-ending pattern of defeat. When expressing these beliefs the person uses words such as 'always' or 'never'. Examples include: 'I never get it right' and: 'Just my luck'.
- *Mental filter:* a tendency to pick out negative details and dwell on them exclusively so that the person's view of reality becomes negative. For example, where there are multiple queues at a petrol station or fast food outlet the person may believe they always choose the slowest queue and do not focus on how often they are in the queue to be fastest to be served.
- *Disqualifying the positive:* rejecting positive experiences by discrediting them. These beliefs are often prefaced by expressions such as, 'Anyone can do that it was easy'. In this way the person can maintain a negative belief that is contradicted by their everyday experience.

At various times we all use irrational thinking strategies. It does not necessarily mean we are mentally ill – just human. Read through the list of irrational thinking strategies above. Do any of them apply to your own beliefs? If so make a mental note of them and over the next week when you hear yourself using these irrational thinking strategies in conversation with other people or when they occur in your own thinking, reflect on why this is the case.

It is useful for the person experiencing the problem to develop an understanding of exactly how and to what extent their problem affects them. Once we have identified negative thoughts, the next stage is to work with them. The methods below provide strategies for investigating and understanding negative thoughts.

Rating negative thoughts

When the person has identified the negative emotion the therapist asks how strong this feeling is on a scale of 0–100 per cent. The person indicates which thoughts were associated with each of the negative feelings. Then all the thoughts are listed according to how much the person believed the thought at the time the feeling was present. For example: 'I felt 85 per cent depressed when I thought that I would never find someone who would love me. I believed this thought 100 per cent.'

Undertaking a cost-benefit analysis

The therapist asks the person to list all the advantages and disadvantages to themselves of continuing to hold the thoughts. They can follow this up by asking the person to divide 100 bonus points between these advantages and dis-

advantages. Seeing it clearly written down will help the person to make a decision about how helpful these thoughts are.

Investigating evidence

The person learns to look for 'real' evidence in support of their thoughts and beliefs. People learn to become 'personal scientists' and to evaluate the evidence. By seeking objective evidence and facts the person can check their beliefs and feelings in relation to the evidence and develop a balanced view. To feel that something is bad does not make it bad or to feel that people disapprove of you does not make it necessarily the case.

Placing events in perspective

This is an especially useful method where the person is *catastrophizing*, which is a tendency to think of the 'worst case scenario' and often a feature of anxiety-related problems. The person is asked to rate the event that triggered the catastrophizing thought, for example, 'He rejected me' or the thought, 'If he were to reject me that would be terrible' on a continuum from 0 to 100 with 100 being a catastrophe. The idea is then considered from the perspective of, 'How bad would it be if that happened?'

When the person has rated the thought or event, which is often in the 90s, the therapist asks them to rate an event that most people would rate as truly terrible. Examples include losing a limb in an accident or a loved one dying. The person is then asked to rate such an event on the same continuum. It is often a surprise for the person to see that they rate 'rejection' at the same level as a loved one dying. This allows them to reappraise how their beliefs can lead to irrational feelings and thoughts, and create a situation where they have unrealistic expectations in some life situations.

Investigating double standards

The person is invited to think about someone else in a similar position and asked whether they would apply the same standards to the other person as they believe are applicable to them. For example, if I believe that I have to succeed in everything I do in my work role, is it reasonable for me to apply this same rule to other colleagues with whom I work? Again, through realizing that our beliefs are not always correct, we can review whether our feelings and thoughts lead us to have realistic expectations.

Re-attribution of negative automatic thoughts and beliefs

After the person has disputed the negative automatic thoughts or irrational beliefs, another thought or belief needs to be formulated for the person. The goal of re-attribution is not to change the person's emotional state from depressed to happy but from feeling overwhelmed to a realistic appraisal. It is important not to demand too much

emotional change of the person. Certain situations are cause for apprehension, sadness or irritation but not for anxiety/panic, depression and anger.

The new thought should include and dispute all of the person's misinterpretations. For example, 'They are going to reject me and that is terrible. I will not be able to stand the embarrassment', could be changed to a more rational alternative. This may take the form of, 'There is no evidence so far that I will be rejected. That I expect to be rejected is a kind of automatic thinking I have taught myself. There is no evidence that it will happen. If I get rejected by him it does not mean that it is the end for me. It would feel unpleasant but would not be terrible. If he were to reject me that would mean he has different preferences than I have. It would not mean anything about me as a person.' People are assisted by the therapist in learning re-attribution and then are invited to try to do it by themselves.

Behavioural experiments

This is often mistakenly labelled as a behavioural strategy. It is used when a person is reluctant to engage in certain behaviours because they hypothesize certain things will happen as a result. Examples include, 'If I speak in the team meeting everyone will laugh at me', or 'If I disagree with my partner we will have a row that will never stop and it will be the end of our relationship'. The person and therapist work in the session to identify the beliefs and the therapist invites the person to collaborate on a thought record. The person therefore creates a set of rational thoughts to hold on to when they are actually in the challenging

---

Cognitive strategies

- Read through the above discussion of cognitive strategies. Think back on your experience on practice placements. Can you identify any situations where these strategies have been used in working with people receiving mental health services?
- Write down the circumstances. Remember to use pseudonyms for any names of staff or service users.
- What was the outcome? Was the intervention successful?
- From the list of techniques above, are there any you may prefer to use in your practice? Consider why you may prefer these interventions. Write down your reasons.

When you have finished, place your notes in your professional portfolio.

situation. The next step is to test things out in reality. In collaboration with the therapist the person may be given the homework task of speaking in the next team meeting and monitoring the reactions of colleagues. In the next CBT session the person and therapist will discuss whether the predictions made came true.

We will now consider behavioural strategies.

Setting behavioural targets

Specific behaviours that the person wants to change are highlighted. This is helpful as it specifically points in the direction of what needs to be done. Examples include statements such as: 'I hate feeling anxious all the time'.

Response/stimulus hierarchy

This involves constructing a list of the most to the least feared situations or responses. The list can be used in exposure and systematic desensitization which are both discussed below. Each of the situations/behaviours is rated for discomfort/ anxiety on a 0–100 rating scale with 100 being the most uncomfortable or anxiety-provoking. These ratings are called subjective units of discomfort or SUDS.

Exposure

This is a technique where the feared stimulus is confronted either gradually in *graded exposure* or by confronting the most feared stimulus in *flooding*. Often this means that people confront themselves with their feared situations one by one. The aim is to stay long enough in the feared situation to make the fear reduce or disappear altogether. Therapists should be aware of the level of fear oscillating or rising and falling repeatedly before finally going down. It is important for the therapist to provide reassurance that the person's fear will eventually reduce or disappear in order to promote the person's confidence in the therapy.

Modelling

Modelling involves the therapist demonstrating the desired response to the person. For example, in an exposure session with someone who has a compulsion to wash their hands out of fear of germs from door handles the therapist may demonstrate holding door handles firmly. Modelling can also be carried out by demonstrating assertive responses in other people. To provide the person with a wider range of models from which to choose, the therapist might ask them to observe others who demonstrate the target response appropriately and choose one to copy. Think of your own experiences on placement. If you have been working within a team of mental health nurses you will have noticed that there are a range of different styles of nursing. Was there one member of the team whose style influenced you and you wished to emulate and use as a model for your practice? What was it about their approach which you felt could add to your skills in mental health nursing?

Behavioural rehearsal

The person and therapist have identified a behaviour that the person wants to practice outside therapy. The person uses the therapy sessions as a forum in which to practice the desired behaviour while the role of the therapist is to shape the person's behaviour towards the target required.

Relaxation training

The person learns a specific strategy to relax. There are two techniques used to teach this method. The *progressive muscle relaxation technique* teaches the person to relax major muscle groups in the body and acquire the skill to bring the relaxation response under voluntary control. It is mainly focused on helping people to distinguish between tension and relaxation. With proper training people learn to relax within two to three minutes.

The second relaxation strategy is called *suggestive relaxation* and is based on undertaking guided imagery with the client and by doing so creating a state of relaxation.

Systematic desensitization (SD)

Relaxation training is a vital element of SD, which is used in the treatment of anxiety problems. The person first learns to relax. The second step is for the therapist to create a fear hierarchy. The person's fear is analysed and a list of stimuli created, ranging from being a little fearful to very anxiety-provoking. Then the person is asked to relax and the therapist asks them to imagine the situation that is lowest in the fear hierarchy. If the person can imagine the anxiety-provoking situation without losing the relaxation state then the next step in the fear hierarchy is taken. Often SD is combined with exposure. When the person has overcome certain feared situations in their own imagination, the therapist will suggest testing them out in reality.

Activity scheduling

In this intervention people learn to plan activities to restore a healthier balance in their lives. People with depression often have a general lack of activities and engage in few pleasurable and satisfying activities. For other people their balance of activities may involve too many demands on their time and not enough attention being given to activities they would prefer. By keeping a diary of activities and rating them on a 10-point scale for satisfaction and pleasure with 10 being the most pleasurable, we can ascertain a good picture of how the person's time is allocated and on what. The person and therapist can then set about correcting imbalances and planning a different activity schedule to achieve a better balance in the person's life.

Graded task assignments

Behaviours that are new to the person but they wish to incorporate in their behavioural repertoire are placed in a hierarchical order and then practiced from the least to the most difficult.

Assertiveness training

The person learns to assert their rights in a socially acceptable manner. Learning to say 'no', disagreeing with others, giving and receiving criticism, giving and receiving compliments and speaking out for their rights assertively, but not aggressively, are all elements of this strategy.

Communication training

This involves working with people to express positive and negative emotions and focuses on general communication techniques. It is beneficial in couple therapy or when helping people with interpersonal problems. Part of this is often active listening training and problem-solving skills training.

Training in self-reinforcement

People involved in learning how to bring about change in problematic behaviours also need to learn how to reinforce themselves for their efforts. Otherwise new behaviour patterns will not be maintained. This is especially important where the person demonstrates problems of excessive need such as addiction.

Behavioural strategies

- Read through the above discussion of behavioural strategies. Think back on your experience on practice placements. Can you identify any situations where these strategies have been used in working with people receiving mental health services?
- Write down the circumstances. Remember to use pseudonyms for any names of staff or service users.
- What was the outcome? Was the intervention successful?
- From the list of techniques above are there any you may prefer to use in your practice? Consider why you may prefer this intervention Write down your reasons.

When you have finished, place your notes in your professional portfolio.

The evidence base for CBT

Finally in this chapter we will look at the evidence base supporting CBT and consider the advantages and disadvantages of this approach.

There is significant research evidence on the positive effects of CBT and it is considered the treatment of choice for many mental health problems (Beck 1976; Beck *et al.* 1990; Roth and Fonagy 2004; NICE 2008).

CBT is effective in treating a range of mental health problems including depression and anxiety disorders with only a few exceptions – for example body dysmorphic disorder and hoarding. There is also evidence that CBT and family-based CBT are effective in assisting people with schizophrenia (Kingdon *et al.* 2006). It is also effective with people with a personality disorder although the results are not as impressive as for depression, anxiety and schizophrenia (Linehan 1993).

Most of the evidence relates to standard CBT interventions, for example, behavioural activation, cognitive restructuring and exposure and response prevention, and does not apply to more recent additions to the range of CBT interventions. The practical nature of CBT means that it is suited for use with service users in a community setting and it is also intended as a brief treatment. As few as six to eight sessions over 10 to 12 weeks have been recommended for the treatment of mild to moderate depression (NICE 2003). It has also been suggested that as few as four sessions in total can have a positive therapeutic effect (Parsons 1999). The optimal treatment input for major depression

Table 12.1 The advantages and disadvantages of CBT

Advantages	Disadvantages
CBT is a 'talking therapy' and does not have the stigma associated with drug treatments or with being 'on medication'.	Success largely depends on the motivation of the person receiving therapy. Many people do not engage successfully with CBT whereas receiving medication involves less personal commitment.
Offers practical solutions and is time limited.	There are no other therapies in competition so we cannot be sure how effective it is at what it does.
The CBT model is logical and can be taught to people receiving therapy to allow them to become their 'own therapist'.	Some people cannot comprehend the CBT model and may not succeed with the treatment.
Evidence has proven CBT to be effective in treating many mental health problems.	There are varying success rates between different conditions and caution should be exercised to avoid using it as a 'cure all' solution.
CBT has become extremely popular and is the treatment of choice.	There is a danger that mental health services recommend only CBT at the expense of developing other approaches such as brief solution focus therapy. It is well established that mental health issues are experienced differently between people and providing a range of therapeutic options seems preferable.
CBT focuses on the therapist developing an individualized relationship with the client, centred on their individual needs and problems.	CBT is often mistakenly perceived as a mechanical and robotic approach when in fact developing a therapeutic relationship and conceptualizing individual problems are different in each case.
CBT requires a good level of skill and knowledge of the model on the part of the practitioner. Commitment from the therapist and good supervision to support them are also required. Therefore CBT has a number of positive attributes as a high quality therapy.	Unfortunately expanding CBT into primary care and encouraging the use of CBT techniques by a wider range of mental health care professionals is often met with resistance by specialist therapists. This unnecessarily limits the development of mental health services.

is 16–20 hours although as few as 8–10 hours when supported by work outside sessions has proven effective. However, it has been recommended that sessions should be one to two hours each week for up to four months, supported by additional information and tasks (NIMHE 2004).

While the evidence for CBT is highly impressive, to lend a sense of balance to the debate we have provided a table summarizing the advantages and disadvantages of CBT (see Table 12.1).

Conclusion

In this chapter we have considered the key features and characteristics of CBT and how it developed. The discussion then looked at the theory underlying CBT before examining how various strategies are applied to problems from a cognitive and behavioural standpoint. Finally we outlined the evidence supporting CBT and considered the advantages and disadvantages of CBT as a therapeutic approach.

CBT offers a wide variety of different therapeutic strategies to adopt in working with people experiencing mental health problems and therefore is a rich source of interventions for mental health nurses. Often this therapeutic approach is kept within the bounds of professional practice of other disciplines. However, CBT techniques are highly suitable for use by mental health nurses and student nurses under appropriate supervision and can be applied safely within all clinical settings.

References

Bandura, A. (1977) *Social Learning Theory.* Englewood Cliffs, NJ: Prentice Hall.

Bandura, A. (1986) *Social Foundation of Thought and Action: A Social Cognitive Theory.* Englewood Cliffs, NJ: Prentice Hall.

Beck, A.T. (1976) *Cognitive Behaviour Therapy and the Emotional Disorders.* New York: International Universities Press.

Beck, A.T. *et al.* (1990) *Cognitive Therapy of Personality Disorders.* New York: Guilford Press.

Gega, L. (2005) Cognitive techniques, in I. Norman and I. Ryrie (eds) *The Art and Science of Mental Health Nursing: A Textbook of Principles and Practice*, pp. 704–18. Maidenhead: Open University Press.

Kingdon, D.G., Turkington, D. and Weiden, P. (2006) Cognitive behaviour therapy for schizophrenia, *American Journal of Psychiatry*, 163(3): 365–73.

Linehan, M.M. (1993) *Cognitive-Behavioural Treatment of Borderline Personality Disorder.* New York: Guilford Press.

Mahoney, M.J. (1977) Reflections on the cognitive learning trend in psychotherapy, *American Psychologist*, 32: 5–13.

NICE (National Institute for Health and Clinical Excellence) (2003) *Depression: The Management of Depression in Primary and Secondary Care*, second consultation. London: NICE.

NICE (National Institute for Health and Clinical Excellence) (2004) *Stepped Care Approach to Treating Depression*, www.nice.org.uk, accessed 10 May 2007.

NIMHE (National Institute of Mental Health for England) North West Development Centre (2004) *Enhanced Services Specification for Depression Under the New GP Contract.* London: The National Primary Care Research and Development Centre and The University of York in partnership with NIMHE.

Parsons, S. (1999) Working with depression, *Mental Health Practice*, 3(4): 32–6.

Roth, A. and Fonagy, P. (2004) *What Works for Whom? A Critical Review of Psychotherapy Research.* New York: Guildford.

Psychodynamic and psychoanalytic therapeutic interventions

Julie Teatheredge and Nick Wrycraft

13

Learning objectives

By the end of this chapter you will have:

- Gained an insight into how psychoanalytic therapy works.
- Developed an understanding of psychoanalytic theory.
- An appreciation of the development of psychoanalysis and psychodynamic theory.

Introduction

The aim of this chapter is to introduce you to the origins of psychoanalytic and psychodynamic theory and interventions. Psychoanalysts and psychodynamic therapists are trained specialists in their own particular area of mental health. However, mental health nurses can benefit from gaining an understanding of their view of mental illness in two ways. Firstly, through an appreciation of the psychoanalytic and psychodynamic perspective our understanding is enhanced of why and how people experience mental illness. Secondly, there are numerous therapeutic techniques used in this approach which can inform our skills in working with people experiencing mental health problems.

Psychoanalytic and psychodynamic approaches incorporate a wide range of various types of therapy and theories. The chapter intends to provide a brief overview of this complex area but there are many influential therapists you might want to read more about.

We begin by considering how psychoanalysis is carried out and what characterizes this particular therapeutic approach. The discussion then moves on to examine the theory underpinning psychoanalytic interventions and the origins of psychoanalytic thought. The chapter then considers a number of aspects of psychoanalysis including

defence mechanisms and metaphor, before moving on to look at free association and dreams. Within the psychotherapeutic relationship there are often difficulties. Key concepts which may exert an influence including resistance, transference and countertransference are then considered.

Finally, we very briefly look at the modern development of psychotherapeutic approaches and the evidence supporting psychoanalysis. In conclusion we will summarize the issues which have been discussed. Exercises and fact boxes will provide you with opportunities to reflect on practice experience and there is a detailed practice-based scenario to help you to appreciate the concepts and ideas discussed in a nursing-focused context. An answer to the scenario is provided at the back of the book.

A mental health student's insight into psychodynamic theory ...

Knowing the theory helped me understand the person a bit more. I could see how their background might have led to their problem and this helped me see the problem in a broader perspective.

An insight into psychoanalysis

Psychoanalytic therapy is a 'talking treatment' that aims to repair the mind (psyche). The goal of psychoanalysis can be defined as to 'alleviate the client's discomfort or pain, alter character structure and strengthen the client's ego, promote emotional and interpersonal maturation, and improve the client's ability to perform or act accordingly' (Shrives 2008:186).

Psychoanalysis is a long-term therapeutic relationship between a therapist and a client. The therapy is based on an interpersonal relationship and the same therapist works with the same person for the duration of that relationship. Usually sessions are once a week but can be up to three times a week depending on the therapist and the severity of the person's problems. Psychotherapy is available through the NHS, normally on a weekly basis, but can be as often as three to five times a week if paid for privately.

Boundaries are highly important in psychotherapy. Among the factors which need to be observed is confidentiality by the therapist, except where there are issues of a legal nature or child protection. The length of sessions is agreed at the beginning of therapy with appointments occurring at the same time of day, and on the same day each week. The rationale for this is to establish trust, reliability and consistency for the sessions (Bowlby 1953).

Once boundaries have been established, the process or the 'work' of therapy begins, and there are three distinct phases, as outlined in the following panel.

Phases of the psychotherapeutic process

1 Introduction.
2 Working.
3 Termination.

- *Introduction:* the introductory phrase involves setting and establishing the boundaries and assessing the person's problems and needs.
- *Working* involves 'working through' the person's issues, to arrive at a resolution to their problems and a sense of 'personal growth' (Maslow 1970), as well as developing adaptive defence mechanisms to enable the client to cope in the future. The 'working through' phrase can take many years and psychotherapy is not a magical cure for everyone. The therapist also receives monthly supervision sessions with a qualified psychotherapist to explore their own defence mechanisms.
- *Termination* refers to the ending of the therapeutic relationship which is negotiated after a successful 'working through' phrase and the achievement of 'personal growth'. Sometimes the person receiving therapy will terminate the relationship before they have been able to work through their issues due to their *defence mechanisms*. These can be experienced as very powerful feelings triggered in response to painful memories. Often the person is not aware of the connection of the defence mechanisms to the difficult memories and will interpret these feelings in different ways.

The basis of psychoanalytic therapy in theory

Psychoanalysis is a therapy which assists the person to develop an insight into the unconscious motivations and impulses by which they are driven (Carlson *et al.* 2004). Sigmund Freud (1896–1939) was the founder of psychoanalysis and originally practised as a medical doctor in Austria. However, he became fascinated by the complexities of the mind (psyche). Freud wrote prolifically and while his theories did not develop from research he drew heavily in his writing from wide clinical experience and case studies. Freud believed there was a structure to the psyche which comprised of differing levels of consciousness. These are the unconscious, pre-conscious and conscious which he developed into the topographical model (Freud, 1976).

Freud's topographical model – the conscious, pre-conscious and unconscious

- The **unconscious** can be understood as 'drives, feelings, ideas and urges outside of the person's awareness' (Shrives 2008: 405). In the *unconscious* pain, conflict and inappropriate social behaviour are driven by unconscious urges and are not part of the person's conscious awareness. Freud believed that through 'talking therapy' the therapist or the analyst could help the patient become conscious of these conflicts, and enhance their mental well-being by connecting the conscious and unconscious parts of the psyche.
- The **pre-conscious** is the second part of the mind 'Which contains experiences, feelings and thoughts from the past that can readily be brought into conscious awareness without a problem' (Rana and Upton 2009: 83). For example, a return trip to the dentist can result in a person remembering a previous anxiety-provoking visit.
- In contrast the **conscious** self in Freud's understanding of the psyche is 'The conscious level of the personality that is aware of the present and controls purposeful behaviour' (Shrives 2008: 405).

Freud compared his model of the mind to an iceberg (see Figure 13.1).

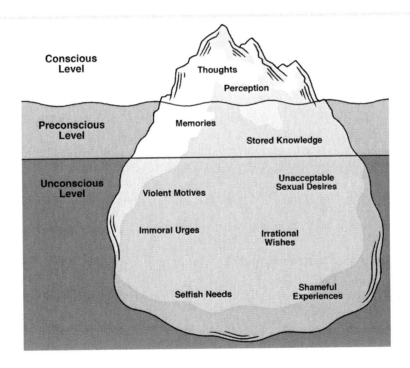

Figure 13.1 Freud's 'iceberg' metaphor for the mind

Only 10 per cent of the iceberg is visible and this is the conscious component of our psyche. The other 90% per cent is submerged under water and contains the pre-conscious and unconscious. Therefore the majority of our mental activity occurs at a level below that which is readily accessible to us in our day-to-day life. According to Freud, the pre-conscious is 10–15 per cent whereas the unconscious is 75-80 per cent of the psyche (Freud, 1976). While *material*, which Freud

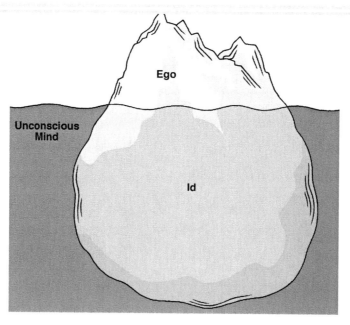

Figure 13.2 The id, ego and superego

defined as feelings, wishes, urges and desires passes between the conscious, pre-conscious and unconscious levels of the psyche, *unconscious* material cannot voluntarily be made available to the conscious. Freud believed that the only way in which unconscious material could be made accessible to the conscious level was through psychotherapy.

We have discussed how Freud saw the structure of the mind. Yet he also developed a model to understand how the mind worked, and in order to do this he developed three mechanisms called the *id*, the *ego* and the *superego*. These are not anatomical structures or physical parts of the brain but concepts to help explain how the psyche works. Within Freud's thinking the id, the ego and the superego all have specific roles to perform and relate to each other in particular ways to help us function in a manner which promotes our mental health, or leads us to be mentally ill.

Freud's model of the id, ego and superego

- *The id* 'is an unconscious reservoir of primitive drives and instincts dominated by the pleasure principle' (Shrives 2008 :405). The id is disorganized and at times very chaotic. It contains very primitive drives and instincts, including life and death, and the primitive drive for survival. Most of what the id contains would be morally and socially unacceptable in modern civilization.
- *The ego* 'meets and interacts with the outside world as an integrator or mediator and is the executive function of the personality that operates at all three levels of consciousness' (Shrives 2008: 406). The ego's role is to attempt to mediate between the id and the outside world, and form a balance between the id and the superego.
- *The superego* 'acts a censoring force or conscience of the personality, and composes of morals, values and ethics' (Shrives 2008: 406). The superego is shaped in our early development by our caregivers, for example, parents, guardians, carers and other influences, and the moral and judicial systems of the culture into which we are born. The superego operates at all levels of consciousness.

It is easy to see how conflict between the id, ego and superego can affect a person's mental well-being. A very critical superego can prevent the person seeking gratification of their drives – for example, the need for sexual pleasure and love. A very dominant id can lead people to exploit and abuse social conformity. The ego strains to balance the person's mental equilibrium. Yet when the ego is exhausted, it becomes depleted and the person can become depressed. The id's life instinct can then fail, leading the person to commit suicide, or turn to violence and crime. One of the aims of psychotherapy is to resolve the mainly unconscious conflicts that cause mental health problems.

Freud maintained that the source of these conflicts could usually be traced back to early childhood in the form of repressed material that is unacceptable and often of a sexual nature. Freud received much criticism for discussing sexuality in childhood and many people find these notions repugnant, although most theorists and experts on child development agree that sexuality is an element of a child's healthy development. Sexuality is also a term which has a different meaning in adult psychology than in children.

Freud's theory of mind suggests 'That unconscious conflicts based on the competing demands of the id (representing biological urges), the superego (representing the moral dictates of society), and the ego (representing reality) often lead to anxiety' (Carlson *et al.* 2004: 744). The reason for these conflicts is sexually based urges that are deemed unacceptable by the censoring influence of the superego. Repressed urges can cause mental health problems later in the conscious life of the individual and therefore one of the tasks of psychotherapy is to remove the forgetfulness of the painful memories which is imposed by deeper levels of the person's consciousness, by assisting them to revisit the earlier stages of their development, when these events occurred.

Defence mechanisms

Freud also believed that we protect ourselves from the damage of psychological trauma through the use of *defence mechanisms*. In spite of being a sophisticated tool, Freud believed that defence mechanisms develop from early childhood (and some later theorists believe they even develop from birth).

As the name suggests, defence mechanisms perform a protective function for the person as they help to avoid the need to confront the source of our problems because the feelings are too painful or distressing. While they work in the short term, over time defence mechanisms can be detrimental to our mental health and well-being as we experience powerful feelings, but are not able to identify why. In some cases the person uses defence mechanisms knowingly: 'As human beings we adopt various defensive mechanisms in order to avoid mental pain or conflict or to control unavoidable impulses. These defences vary from being almost wholly conscious to being completely unconscious. The end product for these defence mechanisms is often a maladaptive behavior or a neurotic symptom' (Malan 1979, cited in Barker 2003: 166).

Even if the person knowingly adopts a defence mechanism, the whole point of them is to avoid the person experiencing feelings directly related to the traumatic event and so there is a strong element of self-deception. A significant part of the work of psychotherapy is involved in understanding and overcoming defence mechanisms. There are numerous kinds and some are listed in the next panel.

Types of defence mechanism

- *Denial* is the 'refusal to acknowledge the existence of a real situation or the feelings associated with it' (Rana and Upton 2009: 92). It is also the refusal to perceive that painful facts exist. A person in denial is holding on to information they are not comfortable talking about. Often in the case of grief over bereavement we cannot accept the loss of someone close to us because acknowledgement they are gone is more than we can bear to accept at that time.
- *Repression* can be understood as pushing troubling thoughts into the subconscious so that the person retains no conscious memory of certain events. For example, a person who has difficulty forming intimate relationships as an adult may have experienced sexual abuse as a child but has no recollection of this.
- *Reaction formation* is responding to a fear with the opposite reaction. For instance, a person who misuses alcohol might often express strong views promoting abstinence.
- *Resistance* is 'the conscious or unconscious defence against bringing repressed thoughts into conscious awareness' (Shrives 2008: 185).
- *Projection* can be understood as applying the person's feelings which they find uncomfortable onto another person. This may take the form of a person who is being unfaithful to their partner believing their partner is having an affair.
- *Rationalization* involves the forming of an untrue but plausible justification for an action which is wrong. For instance, a person may avoid paying tax but state that the government sets taxes too high.
- *Regression* occurs where an adult adopts childlike behaviour. An example is where a student might start to carry around a teddy bear with them which they frequently hug.
- *Sublimation* is the redirection of uncomfortable urges into socially acceptable actions. An illustration of this is a person who experiences strong feelings of anger going to the gym on a regular basis and finding they experience less difficulty with anger management as a result.

Metaphor

Defence mechanisms function by distorting the person's perceptions of what has happened and so it is not unsurprising that sometimes people experience difficulty explaining what they are feeling. One therapeutic technique is to encourage the person to use a *metaphor* and identify an image or symbol which visually represents what they are feeling. This technique allows the feelings to be appreciated in the extent and specific way in which they affect the person.

An example of the use of metaphor is in relation to the defence mechanism of repression. A metaphor which is particularly helpful when a person is trying to explain repressed emotion is that of a bottle: the bottle inside the person's psyche becomes so full of repressed material that the cork or stopper pops out and a flood of emotions erupts.

As it is believed that people develop defence mechanisms from when they are very young, within the Freudian approach the psychotherapist will consider the whole of the person's life history as relevant and important in terms of how the person has coped at various stages, and how some unhelpful coping mechanisms may contribute to a crisis occurring at a later point in their life.

Scenario: Meera

Meera is 17 years old and has been referred to the community mental health team (CMHT) as part of her discharge plan and within the Care Programme Approach (CPA). Meera had been admitted to an acute adult inpatient mental health unit four weeks previously after severely cutting her wrists and consuming approximately 100 paracetomol tablets. She refused admission, but as she stated she still wanted to die she was compulsorily detained and admitted to the unit for an assessment of her mental health under Section 2 of the Mental Health Act 1983, 2007.

Meera has progressively improved over the last four weeks. She met with two community psychiatric nurses (CPNs) from the CMHT on the mental health unit. At first she was reluctant to talk and had a closed posture. Her shoulders were hunched with her arms tightly folded and she avoided eye contact. It was also evident that Meera was very underweight. The CPNs began to build a rapport with Meera and the information below was gathered during several meetings.

Meera's parents own a small hotel and wine bar in a well-known seaside resort. Meera is their only child but when she was 6 they adopted Karl who was 10 years old. Soon after Karl moved in, Meera's behaviour changed as she began to wet the bed at night and became very withdrawn.

The hotel and wine bar was very popular and Meera's parents were busy and had less time for either child beyond meeting their basic needs for food, shelter, warmth and clean clothes. Meera excelled at school and went to a girl's grammar school but continued to be socially withdrawn with no friends, and an apparent lack of interest in any social activity.

Her parents' relationship to both children continued to be distant though at the same time very strict. For example, Meera had to complete all her homework before she was allowed to have her tea. Karl left school when he was 18 and while studying to become a motor mechanic at a nearby college worked weekends in the local garage. When Meera was 15, one night Karl raped her. It was over in seconds but it felt like hours. Karl threatened that if she told anyone he would kill her. Meera did not tell anyone and the abuse continued repeatedly for approximately six months.

Meera became even more withdrawn and rarely spoke to her parents. She ate very little food and lost weight. Her parents attributed Meera's mood to adolescent behaviour. Her performance at school deteriorated and she lost more weight. Karl was now in trouble with the police for theft and on remand for drug dealing. When Meera was 16 she unexpectedly gave birth to a baby. Meera had no explanation for this and refused to acknowledge that she had given birth. With Meera's parents' agreement the baby was taken into foster care.

Meera returned home and carried on at school as though nothing had happened. She failed her GCSE exams. Meera's parents were both angry and disappointed with her and the baby was adopted after three months. One evening Meera's mother walked into the upstairs bathroom and found Meera unconscious in the bath: both wrists had been slashed and she had taken an overdose.

Following the lengthy assessment and gathering of information Meera was discharged home with the support of a CPN. She was referred for psychoanalytic psychotherapy because the causes of her depression were believed to be due to unresolved conflicts in relation to events in her life.

Linking theory to practice

- Write down a list of the issues that could have contributed to Meera's mental health problem.
- What do you think are the main causes of Meera's mental health problem?
- Which coping mechanisms has Meera used?
- Explain how you believe Meera understands the reasons for why she feels the way she does.

When you have finished, put your notes in your professional portfolio.

We will next look at other techniques which therapists use in psychoanalysis. As the purpose of psychoanalysis is to uncover unconscious forces, drives and impulses and make these accessible to the person, it is necessary for the recipient of therapy to be as relaxed as possible, so as to be able to impart this information. The techniques which can be used include free association and the interpretation of dreams.

Free association

Traditionally, during psychotherapy, the person receiving therapy lies on a couch, often with their eyes closed. The rationale for this is to bring feelings which are experienced as troublesome (the unconscious) into reality (the conscious) and through working with these difficult feelings the person's problem(s) are resolved by arriving at a new understanding.

Freud used a technique called *free association* which comprised of two stages. Firstly, the person is encouraged to speak about anything that comes into their conscious mind, without giving any thought to the meaning. Secondly, the therapist helps the person understand and make sense of these unconscious, unwanted feelings. The therapist's main role therefore is to interpret the clues that are revealed through the person's *free association.*

The importance of dreams

In psychoanalysis the therapist's goal is to pick up clues about the unconscious conflicts the person is experiencing. Often this occurs through the person talking about their dreams and memories. Freud subjected the dreams of the people with whom he carried out psychotherapy to rigorous examination. He believed dreams to be essential in highlighting the differences between the (primary) process of the unconscious and the (secondary) process of the conscious.

Freud believed that in contrast with our conscious experience, in the unconscious there is no organization or cohesion between different feelings and ideas, and physical laws are flexible and changeable (Freud, 1976). When we are dreaming, our unconscious influences thoughts and feelings. These may be represented by symbols and images which use our ideas, experiences and everyday events to make a patchwork narrative reflecting our concerns or emotional traumas. When we are asleep we are engaged in a mental life which is distinct from our everyday conscious experience. Yet often we can become confused between dreams and reality, because the content of our (unconscious) dreams involves elements of our (conscious) experience.

An example of the relationship between dreams and everyday reality, and the unconscious and conscious, is provided by the following example.

Dreams and the relation of the conscious and unconscious

Jane has just returned from a summer holiday abroad and is on a placement at a CMHT. She has a good tan but the cold weather is making her skin itch. It is a rainy day and a colleague used an umbrella to avoid getting wet. They have placed the umbrella in a plastic bin by a radiator next to the door. The fabric is red and white striped. Jane has a busy day and feels quite stressed at one point. She comes in and out of the office numerous times and sees the umbrella each time.

At night she dreams about being on holiday in a very hot climate where there are numerous red and white striped sun parasols. It suddenly rains and she can hear the raindrops beating on the fabric of the parasols. On waking Jane feels she has had a strange experience and cannot understand why she dreamt so vividly about striped parasols.

An explanation of the dream is that although Jane noticed the umbrella during the day she was preoccupied with other events. However, when she was dreaming her unconscious allowed her to exercise her interest in the umbrella, as shown by the rain beating on the fabric of the parasols in her dream.

Having recently returned from holiday the umbrella provided a metaphor for Jane's unconscious to reflect on the contrast of her recent experience of being in a warm climate and now being in a wet, colder climate, which has made her tan itch.

A connection may also be evident between Jane feeling stressed during the day and reflecting in her unconscious on the contrast with her holiday, when she might have felt more relaxed.

Dreams offer an excellent source of access to the unconscious. A basic assumption of Freudian theory is that unconscious conflicts involve instinctual impulses or drives that originate in childhood. The patient, through analysis, recognizes these unconscious conflicts and his or her adult mind can find solutions that were unattainable to the immature mind of the child.

There are ways in which the human responses and relationships involved in therapy can cause complications and problems. We will next consider the concepts of resistance, transference and countertransference.

Resistance, transference and counter-transference

Psychotherapy functions through the interpersonal relationship between the therapist and the client, acting as a useful medium for the development of a productive therapeutic rapport. However, sometimes people find it difficult to disclose very painful memories and this can produce powerful feelings which can be expressed in the relationship with the therapist. The therapist may also experience feelings or emotions towards the person they are working with which they cannot explain. Freud referred to these as resistance, transference and countertransference. The panel below provides brief definitions of the concepts.

Resistance, transference and counter-transference

- *Resistance:* the person receiving therapy can become defensive and display resistance which can be understood as 'unconsciously attempting to halt further insight by censoring their true feelings' (Carlson *et al.* 2004: 745). Often resistance will be evident in relation to feelings where the person feels particularly vulnerable or exposed.
- *Transference:* during psychotherapy the person can relive and revisit aspects of their past and childhood which can generate powerful feelings and lead to the person projecting these feelings onto the therapist: 'The client/patient's unconscious assignment to the therapist of feelings and attitudes originally associated with important figures in early life' (Shrives 2008: 185). Furthermore, Freud believed transference is evident in life, as from an early age we tend to form similar patterns, cycles or systems within relationships that can be effective or ineffective. Initially Freud thought transference interfered with therapy but later he identified it as a central component to the success of the analytic work: 'Whereas free association uncovers many of the relevant events and facts of the patient's life, transference provides the means for reliving early experiences. The therapist contributes to this experience by becoming a substitute for the real players in the patient's life and so becomes the tool for illuminating the conflicts of the unconscious' (Carlson *et al.* 2004: 745).
- *Countertransference:* Freud also considers the concept of countertransference, which refers to the effect of the person receiving therapy on the therapist, and can be defined as: 'the therapist's unconscious needs and conflicts in response to and during the therapeutic dialogue' (Shrives 2008: 405). The reason for countertransference may be patterns of past repetitive complicated relationships during the therapist's life. Often the therapist may be unaware of the effects of countertransference which is why clinical supervision is crucial. Through the objective perspective of the clinical supervisor the therapist will be able to identify where their response to the person is affected by their own emotions.

We have explored the foundations and basis of Freudian psychoanalytic thought and considered some of the techniques and methods used in the practice of this form of therapy. In the final section of this chapter we will discuss some of the modern developments in psychotherapy and how these contrast with Freud's earlier theory before considering the research and evidence base for psychotherapy.

The psychodynamic approach

Since Freud's era many other theorists have reviewed and expanded on his ideas, notably in the work of writers such as Anna Freud, Klein, Horney and Kohut, and the term *psychodynamic* is used to describe these newer approaches and developments in psychoanalytic theory.

A contrast of the psychodynamic and psychotherapeutic approaches

While modern psychodynamic therapy still focuses on conflicts in the unconscious there is less emphasis on the importance of sexual issues in child development and early childhood conflicts, and instead greater focus on interpersonal experience in social issues and the person's present life situation (Carlson *et al.* 2004). Although Freud believed the main role of the ego was to satisfy and mediate between the needs of the id and superego, modern psychodynamic theorists suggest that the ego has a more active role in influencing the person's actions, thoughts and psychological functioning and has much more control of the psyche.

While Freud believed that psychoanalysis was very complex and could often take years to complete, psychodynamic therapy can be achieved much more quickly, which has the advantage of reducing the dependence the client may develop towards the therapist.

While Freud mainly worked with people who were experiencing anxiety, modern psychodynamic therapies are used to treat many different forms of emotional disorder, ranging from depression and anxiety to behaviour disorders, severe emotional reactions, psychosis and addiction. Most psychodynamic theorists agree that the symptoms of mental illness have an integral component of chronic anxiety related to unresolved conflicts that in turn affect the person's quality of life.

Outcomes or evaluation of psychodynamic psychotherapy

Freud's work was highly controversial and has been much debated and discussed by many different writers. While there has been research into psychotherapy, the findings have proven inconclusive (Robinson 1993). Jeffrey Masson (1989) has written extensively in support of the view that psychotherapy is fundamentally wrong, and therapists exploit the people whom they treat to meet their own desires and needs which disempowers the person receiving therapy. Other writers also believe Freud's theories were doubtful on the basis that they have never been proved through rigorous research methods (Grunbaum 1984).

Among the reasons why it has been so difficult to obtain positive research outcomes for psychotherapy is that there are so many factors affecting the person's psyche *outside* of the therapy room. Also, psychotherapy takes a long time, often stretching into years, and so is not amenable to the brief trials used to test other therapies. Finally, success in psychotherapy is highly individual and depends on the level of commitment and motivation of the person receiving therapy (Carlson *et al.* 2004).

The National Institute for Health and Clinical Excellence (NICE 2004), which recommends treatment within the NHS based on the supporting evidence, has not advocated brief or long-term psychotherapy. However, while there is a lack of evidence supporting the effectiveness of psychotherapy, it has also been pointed out that research has not disproved psychotherapy as an effective treatment either, and the decision not to support the use of psychotherapy as a recommended treatment is controversial (Smith 2007).

Conclusion

In this chapter we have considered the origins of psychoanalytic thought and Freud's theory of how the human psyche is structured and functions. We then considered defence mechanisms and metaphor before looking at the techniques of free association and the interpretation of dreams. The chapter then moved on to discuss how the therapeutic relationship might be prone to negative feelings which can potentially affect both the person receiving therapy and the therapist, and considered the concepts of resistance, transference and countertransference. Finally, we looked at psychodynamic thought and the evidence base of psychotherapy.

While the research base supporting psychotherapy is very limited, nevertheless psychotherapy continues to influence health care practitioners and provide useful outcomes for many recipients of this form of therapy. The work of mental health nursing is very different from the intensive therapy in psychotherapy. Often in nursing we will be involved with people who are experiencing acute mental health problems on busy inpatient units. These are settings which are not conducive to the detailed examination of the person's feelings and emotions which are a part of psychotherapy. Furthermore, in the case study when Meera was experiencing her acute crisis, simply ensuring her safety and well-being would have been a priority, and psychotherapy would not have been appropriate. However, the theories and interventions we have considered offer highly illuminating perspectives which advance our understanding of these problems and can assist our work and interactions with people who experience mental health problems. Many mental health nurses incorporate psychodynamic thought in their work with people experiencing mental health problems and use this very effectively.

References

Barker, P. (ed.) (2003) *Psychiatric and Mental Health Nursing: The Craft of Caring*. London: Arnold.

Bowlby, J. (1953) *Child Care and the Growth of Love*. London: Pelican.

Carlson, N., Martin, G. and Buskist (2004) *Psychology*. Harlow: Pearson.

Freud, S. (1976) *The interpretation of dreams*. Harmondsworth: Penguin.

Grunbaum, A (1984) *The Foundations of Psychoanalysis*. New York: Berkeley.

Maslow, A. (1970) *Religions, Values and Peak Experiences*. New York: Viking.

Masson, J. (1989) *Against Therapy*. Glasgow: HarperCollins.

NICE (National Institute for Health and Clinical Exellence) (2004) *Depression: Management of Depression in Primary Care*. London: DoH.

Rana, D. and Upton, D. (2009) *Psychology for Nurses*. Harlow: Pearson.

Robinson. P. (1993) *Freud and his Critics*. Oxford, CA: California Open University Press.

Shrives, L.R. (2008) *Psychiatric-Mental Health Nursing* 7th edn. London: Lippincott.

Smith, J. (2007) From evidence base through to evidence base: a consideration of the NICE guidelines, *Psychoanalytic Psychotherapy*, 21(1): 40–60.

Recovery

David A. Hingley

Learning objectives

By the end of this chapter you will be able to:

- Appreciate the background to the emergence of the recovery-focused approach.
- Demonstrate an understanding of the concept of recovery.
- Identify the features of a model of recovery and how this can be used in practice.
- Appreciate the importance of promoting empowerment for people with mental health problems and their significant others and carers.

Introduction

In this chapter we will focus on the concept of recovery, which in recent years has become highly influential within mental health services. However, the importance of this term also reflects a dramatic change in the way mental health care is provided and the philosophy on which it is based.

We begin by considering the background which has led to the recovery model being adopted and replacing the paternalistic tradition. The discussion outlines the central principles of the recovery-focused approach, providing a model for practice. Next we consider a case study which allows us to contrast the paternalistic and recovery-focused approaches in practice and an answer is provided at the back of the book.

The chapter will then look at the concept of empowerment and how it is necessary for us to genuinely incorporate this within our practice if we are to facilitate the recovery of the people with whom we work. In conclusion the issues which have been covered in the chapter will be summarized.

The information panels and case study will illustrate the clinical and professional complexities involved and encourage your further reflections on practice.

Background

One of the most significant developments in the history of mental health care in the UK occurred in 1961. Enoch Powell, who was the then government Minister for Health, announced a policy to close down large-scale inpatient mental hospitals and relocate services in the community (Jones 1993; Coppock and Hopton 2000).

The transition took more than 30 years to implement due to resistance from within the services, yet more significant was the lack of a plan for new services in the community to replace mental hospitals.

During the 1980s and mid-1990s the last of the large long-stay mental hospitals were closed. However, there were repeated tragedies involving people with mental health problems returned to the community with inadequate support. The public response was to demand action. The measures introduced by the government, for example, supervision registers, appeared to regard people with mental health problems as offenders and not engender the trust and cooperation necessary to be a success (Coppock and Hopton 2000). Among the public a belief prevailed that through implementing care in the community the mentally ill had been abandoned to the streets and that this was not 'care in the community' but instead 'care by the community' (Powell 1999).

In 1997 a new government was elected after a long period out of office with a strong agenda for change and reforming zeal. One of their priorities was to improve mental health services and *Modernising Mental Health Services: Safe, Sound and Supportive* (DoH 1998) was published, which recognized that there was deep dissatisfaction with the way in which mental health care in the UK was organized. Yet this document also went further to suggest people with mental illness were unjustly disadvantaged in society as a result of stigma, discrimination and the negative perceptions of mental illness.

The document outlined a new strategy which sought to address public concern over the failures of the mental health services and spoke of the need to reduce the disadvantages experienced by people with mental health problems. However, also tucked away within its pages is a single idea that over the next 10 years became highly influential. It was suggested that people with mental health problems and their carers should be involved in their care and that services should communicate with them and seek to promote empowerment (DoH 1998). This simple idea is included because of the failure of existing services to meaningfully involve, inform and empower people with mental health problems in the care they receive.

Over the next decade the development of mental health policy is replete with the idea that services should be organized around the concept of helping people to recover from mental illness. In 2001 the Department of Health published *The Journey to Recovery: The Government's Vision for Mental Health Care* which made a commitment to involve service users at every stage of their care as equal partners. In 2006 and 2007, five mental health policy documents were published which all have recovery from mental illness as a core principle (DoH 2006a, 2006b, 2007a, 2007b, 2007c).

What is recovery?

At this point it is worth considering a definition of recovery. The Department of Health has produced numerous policy documents to provide a clear idea about what recovery is and guidance on how it should be implemented. *The Ten Essential Shared Capabilities for Mental Health Practice* (2004: 3) states that recovery is: 'Working in partnership to provide care and treatment that enables service users and carers to tackle mental health problems with hope and optimism and to work towards a valued lifestyle within and beyond the limits of any mental health problem.' While the Chief Nursing Officer's review of mental health nursing (DoH 2006b: 17) indicates that recovery means: 'working in partnership with service users (and/or carers) to identify realistic life goals and enabling them to achieve them; stressing the value of social inclusion (clear evidence exists which demonstrates that inclusion has a strong link with positive mental health outcomes) ... stressing the need for professionals to be optimistic about the possibility of positive individual change'.

However, it is a misconception to assume that recovery is an idea that has emerged from the Department of Health. Unlike all previous mental health policies which have been influenced by mental health professionals and experts, recovery came from people who really knew what they were talking about – people who had actually experienced mental health problems.

The traditional model of care for people with mental illness is *paternalistic*. People with mental health problems were seen as damaged, dangerous and disabled and therefore in need of professional care and guidance to live their lives. Within this approach the person's view of their needs was seen as irrelevant and unreliable because they were mentally unwell.

Today we are critical of the paternalistic approach, which was a product of the values inherent within society at the time and this philosophy of care matched the ordered and controlled environment of inpatient mental health institutions in which it was implemented. A problem with paternalism is that it disempowers the person receiving care, because rather than being engaged as an active partner in care, that person is not consulted or given information. For mental health services to be effective in the new environment of the community, a more collaborative approach was required.

The need to embrace a new philosophy of

mental health care has not only been influenced by the transition to care in the community. There have also been significant changes within society and the people who receive mental health care. Over the last 25 years the voice of service users has become increasingly prominent. Various groups of people who previously passively received treatment that was provided to them without question began to talk about the type of service that they wanted to receive. Perhaps this is unsurprising when we consider some of the changes that have happened nationally and globally within wider society. These include the following.

- The rise in popularity and easy accessibility of the internet, technology and information culture such as 24-hour news stations.
- Globalization has made travel much easier and many people are more inclined to regard themselves as citizens of the world rather than individual nation states.
- Human rights have become enshrined in law and governments are compelled to reject institutional practices and instead consider the real desires of the formally oppressed.
- Our relationship with authority has changed. Unquestioning obedience is no longer the norm and people expect accountability from our politicians, police authority, the legal system and most importantly for us, health services.

As a result, governments in democratically run countries have increasingly been required to respond to the changing nature of society and the wishes of various groups of people within it to retain their influence. Against this background, people with mental illness also began to search for a voice to speak out about the care that was being done *to* them, rather than *for* them. Mental health charity organizations such as Mind, The National Schizophrenic Fellowship (now called Rethink), Sane, and the Hearing Voices Network have become increasingly prominent. The predominant message from these groups asks for inclusion,

respect and collaboration rather than exclusion and oppression.

In summary, it is important to remember that recovery was originated by mental health service users and the adoption of the concept marks an important departure in government policy. Yet it is a concern that so many publications have been produced and so much work has been done on recovery by the government. A nagging concern remains that there is the potential for recovery to be usurped by mental health professionals and used to justify the continued monopolization of power over users of mental health services. Instead, for recovery to be applied meaningfully, it is necessary that we listen to the wishes of people with mental health problems, act collaboratively and actively empower the people with whom we work.

The concept of recovery

In this part of the chapter we will begin to build an understanding of a model of recovery to inform our approach to practice. It would be helpful if recovery could be encapsulated in a straightforward 'soundbite' but instead there are many different meanings because it is unique to each individual (Repper and Perkins 2003; Kelly and Gamble 2005). Patricia Deegan (1996) was one of the many voices that emerged in the 1990s to talk about her experience of recovery after receiving a diagnosis of schizophrenia, coupled with a poor prognosis of her future. She described recovery as referring: 'to the lived or real life experience of people as they accept and overcome the challenge of disability ... they experience themselves as recovering a new sense of self and purpose within and beyond the limits of the disability'. Within this understanding, mental illness does not mean that life is necessarily limited by it, or that rehabilitation is the best we can hope for, but that there is a possibility for growth because of its very presence in your life.

Postmodernism and recovery

Postmodernism is a concept that is being used to describe how ideas are being structured at the start of the twenty-first century. Postmodern thinkers, like Jean-François Lyotard and Jacques Derrida, suggested that rather than knowledge producing 'absolute' truths, it produces the possibility of many causes. This can be applied to mental health, in that rather than mental illness having a single cause and there being a correct way to treat it, there is instead the possibility of many causes. Included among the options are that mental illness is *not* a health problem but just a different way of being. Many of the characteristics of recovery reflect postmodern thinking. Mental illness may be just one explanation of understanding different or unusual experiences and some people on their recovery journey may choose that explanation to account for their experiences, while others may have a different explanation for similar experiences. Working in a recovery-focused way requires that we accept these different explanations, viewpoints and positions about the experience of mental illness to be able to work with people rather than challenging them. Or even worse, seeking to impose our own explanation and understanding on the person's experience.

Recovery is not specific to people with mental health problems but instead is applicable to anyone who feels that their life has been limited: through recovery those people can embark on a journey of growth (Repper and Perkins 2003). This idea is useful as it challenges the paternalistic tradition within mental health care of identifying and diagnosing mental illness and highlighting differences with a perceived norm. Through recognizing that we can all be engaged in growth, the desires of those who do not wish to be limited by their illness become closer to our own. We can therefore recognize people with mental health problems as similar to us as professionals rather than different. Service user research has helped to identify what people with mental illness want from services in order to be able to help them lead a normal life.

What people with mental health problems want from services (Faulkner and Layzell 2000)

- Acceptance.
- Emotional support .
- Finding a reason for living and purpose in life.
- Having choices.
- Feeling secure and safe.

- Shared experience – the company of others who have had similar experience (peers).
- Peace of mind.
- Relaxation.
- Finding pleasure in life.
- Taking control of life.

A happy and rewarding life

- Look at the panel above.
- Which of the factors do you feel are necessary for a happy and rewarding life?

From the above exercise it is highly likely that you identified many or even all of the things on the list as what you require for a happy and rewarding life. People with mental health problems are no different and recovery aims to achieve these things. Some of the central characteristics of recovery are listed and discussed below.

The characteristics of a recovery-focused approach (Repper and Perkins 2003)

- *Everyone's journey to recovery is different and deeply personal:* this places person-centred care at the heart of our work with people with mental illness. It means that if we are to help people recover there is no formula for success and no 'one size fits all' solutions. Medication may work for some people but not for others. Home treatment may help some people move through a crisis quickly and with minimal distress but for others a period of caring respite away from the home may be of more benefit. Mental health professionals need to stay open to the possibility that evidence-based interventions that 'should work' may not meet the needs of every person on the road to recovery.
- *Recovery is not a linear process:* relapse is not failure but a part of the journey.
- *Recovery is not a cure:* the idea here is that the problem of having a mental illness should interfere less with life. Deegan (1996) recounts how she was angry with the illness and this spurred her on towards growth. So the illness led her towards growth and recovery.
- *Recovery does not have an end point:* we gain experience through life and it is possible to adapt and evolve with each experience. Mental health practitioners working within a problem-orientated framework often focus on the successful outcomes of interventions and once the presenting problems are resolved, the work is done. However, for the person who has experienced the illness questions may remain about how they have been changed by the experience. As a consequence we may have to have a longer-term view of service users' lives and focus on the total experience rather than just immediate crisis resolution or risk management.
- *Recovery is a process that continues throughout life:* the experience of a mental health problem is not simply limited to the time for which the person can be described as being ill. Often people experience challenges to remain well and some therefore prefer the term 'recovering'. Also, rather than regarding the time when they were unwell as separate from the rest of their life many people find it useful to view their illness as a part of their life experience. This is a particularly helpful notion for people who experience prolonged or repeated episodes of illness.
- *Recovery can occur without professional intervention:* Wilson Besio as long ago as 1987 stated that service users were 'beginning to turn to each other rather than to professionals for emotional and instrumental support. They are finding that people with experiential knowledge (i.e. having learned through personal experience) are more able to understand their needs than are professionals who have learned through education and training. Moreover, they are finding the support and help they can give each other to be as valuable – or sometimes more valuable – than the interventions of trained professionals.'
- *Recovery is not limited to a particular theory about the causes of mental health problems:* this offers a significant challenge to mental health practitioners who may be more comfortable with the idea of being able to explain mental illness using a disease-based model. Working with medication and seeing the benefits as symptoms subside provides the reassuring knowledge that there is a biological basis to the illness. Faced with this evidence it is tempting to try to persuade 'the next patient' that they will experience the same benefit because the illness is 'obviously' biological in nature. However, the person receiving care may not share this theory and the danger is that rather than encouraging them to make discoveries that are helpful to them we become experts on the person's journey, preventing them from exploring their own resources.
- *Recovery is about taking control over one's own life:* this means that others including mental health professionals may have to give up some control. In some cases risk management may require mental health professionals to prevent people choosing actions or making decisions they might not when mentally well. However, there is a long history within the mental health services of the excessive and complacent use of control. Instead there is much to be gained from reflecting on how we can help people make choices and exercise control in their lives.

Recovery represents a real departure from the paternalistic past within mental health services. Yet it is important to retain a health-related focus in mental health care. We are still bound by our professional code of conduct (NMC 2008) to observe responsible and accountable practice and the policies and procedures of the organizations within which we work. For example, where a person is acutely distressed and we know that sedative medication has the potential to alleviate their trauma, it would be cruel and irresponsible not to act. However, rather than disregarding all that has gone before the recovery approach instead requires a better knowledge of mental health nursing and the principles of practice. Each new encounter offers the chance of an innovative or different solution which answers the problem. The scenario below will highlight the contrast of a paternalistic view with the use of a recovery-focused approach.

Scenario: Terry

The following is a case study during which various points are raised for you to consider. As you read think about how the beliefs held by different members of staff have influenced their practice and the way in which Terry has been able to live his life.

Terry is 40 years old, and since the death of his mother five years ago lives alone in a flat in the centre of town. Alison is a new member of the team and has just qualified as a community mental health nurse. She has been asked to take over Terry's care from another nurse, Peter, who has looked after Terry for 15 years and is retiring in six months' time. Over five visits Alison observes that Terry is a friendly man who only occasionally hears voices and sometimes says he is being harassed. Terry says his main problem is that he feels unable go out but is grateful that social services bring him shopping and help him with his bills, and so he does not really need to go outside his flat in order to meet his daily needs. The other main input that Peter had with Terry was to visit him fortnightly to monitor how he was feeling mentally and administer Risperdal Consta injections (a psychiatric medication) every fortnight.

- How have Terry's life chances been limited because he does not go out?
- Why do you think Terry has not been encouraged to get out more?

There's something else that Alison notices. Terry is fascinated with horses and he owns a large amount of objects related to horses including books, pictures on his walls and ornaments wherever she looks. Alison learns that he intended to be a jockey as a young man but when he became ill was discouraged from returning to work at the stables both by the consultant psychiatrist he had at the time and by the owner of the stable where he had once worked. Alison notices how animated he becomes when talking about horseracing and encourages him to share his knowledge with her. After a few visits where Alison makes sure they talk about Terry's interest, he even starts talking about wanting to go out and put a bet on a horse and Alison and Terry begin working out a plan to help him achieve this goal.

- Is it right for mental health professionals to discourage people from pursuing their interests and what are the possible long-term implications?
- Is it possible that the stable owner discouraged Terry because of negative attitudes towards mental illness?

At the office one day Alison mentions how well Terry is doing to a colleague. Peter overhears the conversation and interrupts, stating that when he was Terry's nurse he never asked about the horses and didn't think Alison should either. Peter explains that Terry's psychosis showed itself in a peculiar way in that when unwell he became childlike and would often act like a horse and canter down the corridors in the ward. Alison argues that there is a difference between behaving like a horse while psychotic and being interested in horses. Peter then makes the statement: 'We all thought he was responsible for those stabbings a few years back, when the horses in the fields were being attacked.'

Alison begins to worry that she has been colluding with Terry and his interest is in fact evidence that he is still ill and that she has been encouraging him to become unwell. She is also concerned that by encouraging him to start thinking about going out more he may be in a position where he is tempted to hurt horses. On her next visit to Terry's flat she feels tense and apprehensive and avoids any conversation about horses and instead focuses on his 'general well-being'. Terry notices the change and is concerned that Alison is not herself. He even rings the office the next day to see how she is. Alison continues to visit but feels unable to help Terry as much as she had been.

In the end Alison seeks a meeting with her clinical supervisor and described how difficult she is finding it working with Terry after she found about this risk. The supervisor suggests that she should ask to have another member of the team take over the case and focuses on the fact that she is inexperienced and this is an easy mistake to make.

Alison is unhappy with this solution and feels that she has failed. She is disappointed that all the good work that she believed she was doing has been wasted. After meeting with her supervisor she thinks once more about the principles of recovery and how Terry became more animated when talking about his interest. He became more trusting in his relationship with Alison and even started to work on his problems with her. Alison reads Terry's notes in detail but finds no record that Terry had ever been violent or aggressive. The reports of the time when he had psychosis suggest that he became irritated when he was stopped from 'trotting' down the ward but that he was more of an irritation to other people when he was ill than presenting any risk of violence.

Alison then speaks to Terry's consultant psychiatrist. He had not worked with Terry for the full length of time for which he had been in contact with mental health services but he did not know anything about Terry being a threat to horses or anyone else for that matter. Alison decides that Peter must have been mistaken about all this and asks him for more details about the risks that he mentioned. He is unable to elaborate but states that even if there was no evidence for the risk, nevertheless talking to Terry about his interest in horses was a risk he had not been willing to take and there was little point in talking to Terry about horses because he was 'a chronic schizophrenic and with a fixation about them'. Peter believes that when he worked with Terry he helped him stay well by ensuring he continued to receive his injection each fortnight and his mental health remained stable. He ensured that Terry had regular deliveries of food from social service support workers, and didn't want to tip Terry 'over the edge' by giving him any stress.

- Can you identify who between Alison and Peter was practising using a paternalistic approach?
- Write down which specific aspects of this approach to care were paternalistic.
- Write down what effects this had on the way Terry led his life.
- Can you identify who between Alison and Peter were using a recovery-focused approach?
- Write down which specific aspects of this approach were recovery-focused.
- Write down what effect this had on the way Terry led his life.

From the case study it is possible to see how difficult it is for professionals influenced by theories of mental illness that are often medical in orientation to find a way to behave that fosters rather than hinders recovery. Symptoms may interfere with the person's ability to achieve their own potential, but the way we provide services can also be damaging for the people with whom we work.

Empowerment in practice

The final section of this chapter considers the concept of *empowerment* and how this contributes to a recovery-focused approach to practice. We will discuss an understanding of empowerment before considering how we can shift the focus of our practice if we are to genuinely implement a recovery-focused approach.

In his excellent book, Peter Watkins (2007: 32) states of empowerment: 'personal power is that sense of autonomy and self-efficacy that enables us to become responsible and resourceful individuals, able to manage and influence the direction of our unfolding lives'. The process of empowerment involves the active facilitation of choice, freedom, autonomy and control through encouragement, nurturance and fostering. An empowerment culture (Watkins 2007) is where time is given freely by professionals with a view to talking, listening and engaging in joint activities. Relationships are founded on an equal basis rather than the professional being of a higher status or having greater influence than the person with a mental health problem. The person's rights to choose, take risks and make mistakes are acknowledged and respect is paid to the person's expertise, experience and any attempt to make things better for themselves. The exercise below will help you to reflect on whether your views promote or inhibit the empowerment of mental health service users.

Disempowering or empowering practice?

You may like to consider which type of nurse you are going to be. Rate yourself on the scales in terms of how strongly you side with the opposing statements.

People with mental illnesses don't get better	1 – 2 – 3 – 4 – 5 – 6 – 7 – 8 – 9 – 10	People with mental illness can, and do, get better
Medication is the best way to treat mental illness	1 – 2 – 3 – 4 – 5 – 6 – 7 – 8 – 9 – 10	There are many treatment options open to people with mental illness
I like to use medical terms	1 – 2 – 3 – 4 – 5 – 6 – 7 – 8 – 9 – 10	I like to use words that everyone understands
Mental illness is a brain disorder	1 – 2 – 3 – 4 – 5 – 6 – 7 – 8 – 9 – 10	I have some ideas about it, but I don't really know what causes it!
People with mental illnesses need to be looked after	1 – 2 – 3 – 4 – 5 – 6 – 7 – 8 – 9 – 10	People with mental illnesses are capable of looking after themselves

Low scores indicate that you have a very traditional way of thinking about people with mental illness. The statements on the left of the page represent ideas that are more paternalistic, while those on the right are the types of ideas that emerge from recovery. If you have rated yourself quite low on some of these scales, you may like to think about whether this view is really helpful to people who are already at risk of losing their own personal power.

Disempowering practice often stems from a belief that the person experiencing illness has 'lost their mind' and cannot make rational choices. The passing of laws permitting people to be detained against their will due to their mental ill health has made provision for the treatment and the protection of the person and general public. While sometimes it is necessary for these laws to be invoked, it is easy for a false and disempowering view to prevail where it is assumed the person was once unable to make 'good decisions' and this continues to be the case.

Empowering practice is based on the hope and possibility of change and the knowledge that compulsory detention, bad decisions and risky behaviours are a part of the person's overall journey but not the whole story. Therefore, we are required to continually reappraise our assessment of the individual's mental state and functioning and adapt our therapeutic response in the light of new information.

There tends to be an overemphasis on the influence and role of the mental health services and mental health workers. Often people with mental health problems recover regardless of the input of the mental health services. Promoting effective recovery requires us to facilitate the person to either re-engage in their social and family connections, former interests and lifestyle or support them to live the life that they would wish and become socially included.

Evidence supporting this notion is provided by Fisher (2005) who cites two studies by the World Health Organization (WHO) conducted in 1979 and 1992 which found that people in developing countries recovered more successfully from mental illness than those in industrialized counties. The reason for this was that in developing countries people with mental illness are supported by informal communities and remain integrated and involved in life. In contrast in the UK and much of the western world mental health systems involve expert teams, knowledge, diagnosis and legislation to manage the problem. Rather than being perceived as an aspect of the experience of some people in their lives, mental illness is regarded as separate from normality and extracted from society until it has dissipated. However, this view does not offer the means by which people can regain their former roles within society and it is assumed the person who has experienced a mental health problem can no longer take on a meaningful role in society.

Recent developments have also seen a growth in groups who either seek to represent the views of service users – for example, Mind and Rethink – and others that have been created *by* service users to help themselves, such as the Hearing Voices network. The work of Marius Romme and Sondra Escher (2000) has identified that more people experience hearing voices than the 1 per cent prevalence of schizophrenia would suggest and many people identify the voices as *useful* for them. While it is undeniable that many people do experience distress from hearing voices, this provides a contrast with the traditional view that voices are always a symptom of mental illness illness. The Hearing Voices movement have set up a network of independent self-support groups that endeavour to help each other by accepting and living with the voices they hear.

Conclusion

The chapter has discussed an understanding of the concept of recovery and the recovery model. Recovery focuses on the hopes and aspirations of the person and does not view mental illness as separate from other experiences in life. Instead many people incorporate their experience of mental illness within their growth and development.

We also considered the concept of paternalism and examined a practice-based case study illustrating the contrast of these approaches. In order to promote recovery it is necessary to give the person as much control as possible and we ended the chapter by defining the concept of empowerment and discussing how this can be incorporated in practice.

References

Coppock, V. and Hopton, J. (2000) *Critical Perspectives on Mental Health.* London: Routledge.

Deegan, P. (1996) Recovery as a journey of the heart, *Psychiatric Rehabilitation Journal,* 19(3): 91–7.

DoH (Department of Health) (1998) *Modernising Mental Health Services: Safe, Sound and Supportive.* London: DoH.

DoH (Department of Health) (2001) *The Journey to Recovery: The Government's Vision for Mental Health Care.* London: DoH.

DoH (Department of Health) (2004) *The Ten Essential Shared Capabilities: A Framework for the Whole of the Mental Health Workforce.* London: DoH.

DoH (Department of Health) (2006a) *Our Health, Our Care, Our Say.* London: DoH.

DoH (Department of Health) (2006b) *From Values to Action: The CNO's Review of Mental Health Nursing.* London: DoH.

DoH (Department of Health) (2007a) *Commissioning Framework for Health and Well-being.* London: DoH.

DoH (Department of Health) (2007b) *Mental Health: New Ways of Working for Everyone, Progress Report.* London: DoH.

DoH (Department of Health) (2007c) *Capabilities for Inclusive Practice.* London: DoH.

Faulkner, A. and Layzell, S. (2000) *Strategies for Living: A Report of User-Led Research into People's Strategies for Living with Mental Distress.* London: Mental Health Foundation.

Fisher, D.B. (2005) An empowerment model of recovery from severe mental illness: an expert interview with Daniel B. Fisher, MD, PhD, www.medscape.com/viewarticle/496394, accessed 20 October 2008.

Jones, K. (1993) *Asylums and After: A Revised History of the Mental Health Services from the Early 18th Century to the 1990s.* London: The Athlone Press.

Kelly, M. and Gamble, C. (2005) Exploring the concept of recovery in schizophrenia, *Journal of Psychiatric and Mental Health Nursing,* 12(4): 245–51.

NMC (Nursing and Midwifery Council) (2008) *Standards of Conduct, Performance and Ethics for Nurses and Midwives.* London: NMC.

Powell, M. (1999) *New Labour, New Welfare State?* Bristol: The Policy Press.

Repper, J. and Perkins, R. (2003) *Social Inclusion and Recovery: A Model for Mental Health Practice.* London: Ballière Tindall.

Romme, M. and Escher, S. (2000) *Making Sense of Voices: A Guide for Mental Health Professionals Working with Voice-hearers.* London: Mind Publications.

Watkins, P.N. (2007) *Recovery: A Guide for Mental Health Practitioners.* London: Elsevier-Churchill Livingstone.

Wilson Besio, S. (1987) *The Role of Ex-patients and Consumers in Human Resource Development for the Nineties.* Burlington, VT: Centre for Community Change Through Housing and Support.

15

Social inclusion

Allen Senivassen

Learning objectives

By the end of this chapter you will have:

- Gained an understanding of how social exclusion affects the lives of people with mental health problems.
- Developed an appreciation of factors which contribute to social exclusion including stigma, discrimination and popular misconceptions concerning mental illness.
- Gained an appreciation of how *The Ten Essential Shared Capabilities* (DoH 2004) are relevant to the promotion of social inclusion.
- Considered how mental health nurses play a positive role in promoting social inclusion and mental health through the application of the *Capabilities for Inclusive Practice* (DoH 2007).

Introduction

Mental illness is often experienced as deeply distressing. However, recently we have come to understand that the effects of social exclusion can also compound people's problems and lead to further disadvantage and hardship.

This chapter will assist you to appreciate the factors that are active in, and which cause, social exclusion, including stigma and discrimination. As mental health workers we are obliged to challenge negative attitudes towards mental illness and to promote the engagement of people with mental health problems in society so that they may access the full range of opportunities that their potential allows.

Therefore, it is necessary to develop a sense of positive values in our practice. These require an approach that regards people with mental health problems as individuals with strengths, abilities and talents together with the capacity to work innovatively in the context of community-based services. This is best begun from the very earliest stages of professional training.

The chapter next focuses in depth on two key documents: *The Ten Essential Shared Capabilities* (DoH 2004) and *Capabilities for Inclusive Practice*

(DoH 2007). We will consider each of the 10 capabilities, linking the discussion with practice and using these as a template to allow you to begin to develop your own understanding of how values and principles underpin practice. The chapter will end with a conclusion summarizing the main issues which have been discussed.

Scenarios and examples of mental health problems will be presented during the discussion to illustrate the clinical and professional complexities involved. Several exercises will help you identify areas for your professional development through reflection on practice experience.

The effects of social exclusion

Historically people experiencing mental health problems have been denied the social opportunities other groups within society take for granted, such as positive human relationships and access to community facilities. However, these are essential in maintaining a decent quality of life and mental well-being. 'Social exclusion' emerged as a new term in the late 1990s and is a concept which encompasses all of the social barriers and disadvantages faced by people who are marginalized in society, including mental health service users and their carers.

In an attempt to overcome the social barriers which marginalize people with mental health problems and their carers the UK government set up the Social Exclusion Unit (SEU) to promote measures to facilitate social inclusion (SEU 2004). The following quote graphically illustrates the social exclusion some people with mental health problems experience:

> For some of us, an episode of mental distress will disrupt our lives so that we are pushed out of the society in which we were fully participating. For others, the early onset of distress will mean social exclusion throughout our adult lives, with no prospect of training for a job or hope of a future in meaningful employment. Loneliness and loss of self-worth lead us to believe we are useless, and so we live with this sense of hopelessness, or far too often choose to end our lives. Repeatedly when we become ill we lose our homes, we lose our jobs and we lose our sense of identity ... so we are perceived as a social burden. Not only do we cost the government money directly in health, housing and welfare payments, we lose the ability to contribute our skills and economically through taxes.

(SEU 2004: 3)

Social exclusion and mental health problems

Mental illness is extremely common within our society. Research suggests that one in four people in the UK will be experiencing a mental health problem at any one time. Ninety per cent of people with a mental health problem are cared for by primary care services, such as their family and/or their GP and are not in contact with specialist mental health services (SCMH 2002). It is likely that all of us know someone who is experiencing a mental health problem and often such people live a perfectly normal life within the community.

Social exclusion can be understood as the combined and mutually compounding interaction of impairment and disability, together with the experience of discrimination, diminished role and a lack of meaningful economic and social oppor-

tunity. The effects of these factors are evident in a lack of status and unemployment, and also in the loss of the chance of having a family and limited or non-existent social networks, possibly exacerbated by racial or other forms of discrimination. Social exclusion is the experience of repeated rejection which leads to a restriction of the person's hope and aspirations.

Therefore, social exclusion is often experienced as a combination of interrelated factors. For many people it is more than economic disadvantage but rather the inability to engage in social life around them which most people take for granted (Repper and Perkins 2003). However, the relationship between mental health problems and social exclusion is complex with factors such as low income, unemployment and lack of a social network being both the cause of mental health problems and something people experience as a consequence.

Social exclusion is experienced differently between individuals with mental health problems (NIMHE 2004). While for one person it may begin with the experience of mental illness in the first place, for another it may be the absence of meaningful employment or rewarding relationships that gradually leads to social exclusion and a

Factors which interact with mental health problems and contribute to social exclusion

- Media stereotyping.
- Discrimination at work.
- Unemployment and lack of informal contacts.
- Lack of access to educational and training opportunities.
- Poverty and poor income.
- Homelessness and poor housing.
- Lack of social networks and disrupted family.
- Contact with the criminal justice system .
- Drug misuse and adverse effects of prescribed drug treatments.
- Physical health problems.
- Stigmatization health and social services.
- Rejection by the wider community.

detrimental impact on the person's long-term mental health and well-being. The factors which contribute to social exclusion will impact differently on people depending on their life circumstances, social situation and the nature of their mental health problem. On p. 208 is a list of factors that contribute to social exclusion (Repper and Perkins 2003).

Social exclusion can therefore be seen as having a number of different causes. However, many people experiencing mental health problems become caught up in a *cycle of exclusion* (SEU 2004) (see Figure 15.1).

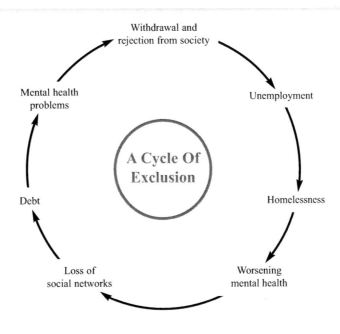

Figure 15.1 The cycle of social exclusion (NIMHE 2004)

People with mental health problems frequently have a low income. A lack of employment prospects and loss of hope of improving the person's circumstances can create a vicious circle which prolongs the experience of mental illness and predisposes their mental health to an increased risk of mental illness in the future (O'Brien *et al.* 2001; Singleton *et al.* 2001). As a result of social exclusion the cost of mental illness is increased in terms of the loss of quality of life to the individual, their families and carers, yet there is also a major social and economic cost to society (Layard 2006).

Scenario: Robert

Robert is 20 and lives with his parents. They feel he is extremely bright but he gets frustrated with the normal activities pursued by people of his age. At primary school he was quite outgoing and had many friends because of his sporting talent and academic ability. His ambition was to become an engineer like his father. In secondary school when he was 16, Robert's work began to deteriorate and he became involved with friends who frequently absconded from school. He left school at 16 with poor passes in most subjects.

Robert began taking illicit drugs and his friendly personality changed. He became distant to his parents and friends and aggressive at times. His mental state deteriorated and he frequently used cannabis and behaved suspiciously and strangely. At times he locked himself in his room for days with minimal contact with his family. Robert's parents were concerned about his safety and that of his younger siblings. Consequently he was admitted to the local mental health unit on two occasions under a Section of the Mental Health Act 1983; 2007.

Linking theory with practice

- Write down what type of social barriers is Robert likely to face as a result of his mental health problem?
- As time progresses how might his mental health lead to Robert experiencing social exclusion?
- When you have finished reading your notes consider how your own practice and that of other health care professionals might positively promote social inclusion.

The underlying causes of social exclusion

The SEU report (2004) identified five causes of social exclusion for adults with mental health problems.

1. Stigma, discrimination and the negative perceptions of society.

2. Mental health services are too medically oriented and professionals have low expectations of what individuals can achieve.

3. A lack of clear responsibility for improving vocational and social outcomes for individuals.

4. A lack of support for people to gain or return to work.

5. Barriers to engaging in the community.

While the causes of social exclusion are often inter-related, for the purposes of our discussion we will consider them separately.

Stigma, discrimination and negative perceptions of society

Stigma can be defined as evident where an individual is devalued, or possesses an attribute which is deeply discrediting (Goffman 1963; Repper and Perkins 2003). Often stigma is based on a misconception or exaggeration. The stigma attached to mental illness is extremely damaging and often society has intolerant views. For example, that

people with a mental health problem are regarded as malingerers who simply ought to 'pull themselves together'.

At the other extreme, people who are acutely mentally ill are feared and viewed as homicidal, crazed and unpredictable, and representing a danger to society (DoH 1998, 1999). These negative perceptions draw heavily on isolated high-profile cases, for instance the tragic death of Jonathon Zito who was killed by Christopher Clunis.

Many television, film and drama productions also contribute to detrimental perceptions of the mentally ill through negative portrayals as villains and bad people with malicious motives, prone to violence and aggressive behaviour, with few redeeming features (Sayce 2000). Yet while this may add to dramatic effect there is no evidence to suggest these distorted perceptions have any basis in reality (University of Manchester 2006). Within the general public perception there is a highly potent, media-fuelled fear of being murdered by a person with a mental health problem who was not known to the victim, otherwise known as 'stranger homicide' (BBC 2006). Yet care in the community has not increased the overall risk to the general public. 'Stranger homicide' and any other acts of violence are no more likely to be perpetrated by a person with a history of mental ill health than another person without a mental illness (SEU 2004; University of Manchester 2006). Instead, rather than violence towards others, people with mental health problems are more at risk of committing suicide, self-harming or of being a victim of violence, abuse or exploitation perpetrated by others (DoH 1998, 1999; University of Manchester 2006).

While generally opinion seems to suggest attitudes towards mental illness have improved, evidence of this is strikingly hard to find. The stigma around mental illness causes *discrimination* which can be defined as people being treated differently due to possessing particular characteristics. It is highly damaging where discriminating characteristics that are not relevant influence the making of decisions. An example is where a person who in all other respects is competent and equal to all of the other candidates does not receive a promotion at work because of their ethnic background, the colour of their skin or other physical characteristics. In this instance the decision has been made based on irrelevant information. Often people who experience discrimination feel ashamed, yet the responsibility for the social exclusion faced by people with mental health problems does not reside with the person who is stigmatized but instead with society, which discriminates against the person (Repper and Perkins 2003).

Reflecting on stigma and discrimination

- Reflect on who you are: consider your identity in relation to the following personal characteristics: male or female, rich or poor, the area where you live, education, ethnic background, age, height, weight, body shape, eye colour, choice of clothing, sexuality.
- Write down this description of your profile.
- Imagine someone did not like you because of one, or all, of these characteristics.
- Reflect on how you would feel.
- How might you react?
- We all have prejudices which might lead us to discriminate unfairly against others. Think of what yours might be.
- How might you change your views in future to be less discriminative, or promote anti-discriminative practice?

As evident from the above exercise, discrimination can be experienced in many areas of life and regarding numerous aspects of personal identity, for example, employment and education, race, culture, gender and age. However, it is possible that by placing an emphasis on tackling stigma we are only reinforcing the negative perceptions of this group of people. Within this view, people with mental health problems appear to be incapable of taking advantage of employment or social opportunities because of their problems, and society and employers have to make *special allowance* for their vulnerability (Sayce 1998). Furthermore, it has been argued that drawing attention to stigma leads to stigmatization as this encourages people to identify groups of individuals by a few crude characteristics which do not account for the subtle differences which makes us individuals (Repper and Perkins 2003).

Mental health services are too medically oriented and professionals have low expectations of what individuals can achieve

Traditionally, mental health services have focused on interventions, medical diagnosis of illness and treating psychological symptoms. There is often an assumption by mental health professionals that their role is primarily to deliver health interventions and treat symptoms to the point of restoring the person's normal functioning (Shepherd 2007). Yet the potential gain for the person's mental wellbeing through the promotion of social and vocational roles has often been neglected, even where the problem may be social in nature (SEU 2004).

It has also been suggested that mental health professionals often fall victim to the 'clinician's illusion' where, as a result of working for a sustained period of time with severely mentally ill individuals, it is assumed that there is very limited scope for recovery from mental illness and professionals often have low expectations of what people with mental health problems can achieve as a result (DoH 2004).

However, for many people with mental health problems recovering psychologically from an episode of acute mental ill health is only half the battle, and help is also needed to gain or regain a role and identity in wider society. The next step must be for mental health workers to also become involved with the vocational and social goals of service users to enable people with mental health problems to lead a more functional life in society with or without their mental distress.

Barriers to returning to work

The following is an extract from a personal account cited in the document: *Vocational Services for People with Severe Mental Health Problems: Commissioning Guidelines* (DoH 2006b).

> The stigma of mental health problems has certainly reduced the number of responses to my job applications and some diagnoses have more stigma than others. Another hindrance I have experienced is the attitude of some mental health professionals to discourage me from applying for paid work, and their insistence that claiming income support is a must. Also, it seems to me that there is no recognition that someone may be fit to work part time but not full time, in other words an all or nothing approach to medical certification.

A lack of responsibility for improving vocational and social outcomes for individuals

The severely mentally ill have the lowest employment rates of any of the main groups of disabled people (DoH 2006b). Therefore much work needs to be done to access the contribution people with mental health problems can make not only to the economy but to the voluntary and independent sectors (Allen 2008).

For people receiving mental health services it has been claimed that few mental health professionals put employment at the top of their priority list (Shepherd 2007). Fortunately, the tide has started to turn and mental health service providers have begun to see it as part of their responsibility to assist service users in vocational and leisure pursuits. The North East London Mental Health NHS Trust has launched 'Thinkarts' which is a

project providing arts-related events and vocational opportunities for service users and carers. The project links service users with commercial business and the community by bringing a collection of artists together to respond to the demands of the community (DoH 2007). Another service provider which has placed social inclusion and employment responsibility high on the agenda is South Essex Partnership Foundation Trust (SEPFT 2007). A service user research group works in partnership with Anglia Ruskin University and Professor Jenny Secker and has produced meaningful occupation and training through research projects for several service users (Secker and Gelling 2006).

A lack of support for people to work

Mental health is regarded as a taboo subject in the workplace. It has been suggested that in order to avoid attracting disapproval, people feel unable to phone in sick at work for mental health reasons and will instead offer an alternative physical reason which is more acceptable (Sayce 2000). Frequently people also avoid seeking help in the first instance for mental health issues as they fear for their job security or loss of promotion prospects and opportunities (DoH 2006a).

Many people with mental health problems who are not engaged in paid employment would like to work. Frequently, mental health professionals have not been sufficiently equipped with the belief and skills to support service users in gaining employment. However, in some areas where mental health services have recognized the importance of work as a valued social role for service users, greater effort is being placed on social inclusion activities. For example, individuals are being helped to develop vocational skills through meaningful activities that will eventually lead them to gain employment. There are a number of schemes to support service users including strong links with Jobcentre Plus and Pathways to Work, financial help with understanding disability benefits and paid employment, and individual placement and support (IPS). One mental health service user, who was helped to find a job after many years of being unemployed, commented: 'My new job has given me my life back, my sanity and some money to pay the bills.'

Barriers to engaging in the community

If we reflect on our own lives we frequently take for granted a wide variety of social and supportive networks in the community. These social contacts are gained and maintained through a diversity of means or activities such as the social networks listed below.

Social networks

- Family.
- Friends.
- Work colleagues, or people we meet if we work in a voluntary capacity.
- Acquaintances in the course of our daily life.
- People we meet while studying on courses.
- People we meet through sporting clubs and activities.
- Leisure interests and hobbies including evening classes.
- Involvement in religious or other groups.
- Social events and occasions, and festive celebrations throughout the year.

All these social networks help to preserve mental health and well-being, and instil a sense of personal identity, confidence, self-esteem, belonging and motivation. Yet imagine not being a part of these social activities. The absence of these meaningful aspects of our lives can crucially undermine a person's quality of life and sense of mental well-being. As innately social beings we acquire these social contacts without even being aware of it; however, many people with mental health problems experience isolation and do not have social companions to accompany them shopping or elsewhere in the community, have limited financial resources and may find public facilities intimidating or unwelcoming.

Education, sports, arts and leisure providers are often not aware of how they can make their services more accessible and beneficial to people with mental health problems. Some groups of people with mental health problems face particular barriers in accessing services and in getting their

mental health and social needs met (SEU 2004). People who are from ethnic minorities often feel alienated and not understood by those providing mental health services, and as a result they do not seek professional help. Their chances of securing decent education and employment are poor and they often find themselves involved with the criminal justice system. Another vulnerable group is young males with mental health problems who often become disengaged from education and employment and are at a high risk of social exclusion and suicide.

Promoting social inclusion and mental health

To allow individuals with mental health problems to feel socially included and able to contribute in society requires a multifaceted approach. In this section of the chapter we will focus first on how the government can intervene through legislation and policy initiatives to guide the priorities of mental health services. Then we consider how local communities are developing mental health services to involve local people and reduce stigma. Finally we will look at how mental health professionals can effectively engage with mental health service users, their families and the local community.

Government legislation

At a national level government legislation and policies can reduce discrimination against people with mental health problems and promote their well-being. For example, the Disability Discrimination Acts of 1995 and 2005 were passed to outlaw discrimination in employment and education, and permit access to public services and transport for people with disabilities including mental health problems. In 2000, the Disability Rights Commission was established to develop a code of conduct (Disability Rights Commission 2001) to provide practical guidance to employers on how to reduce discrimination and promote equality in the workplace and services for people with disabilities.

As a result of legislation, people who were being denied professional employment because of the stigma of mental illness are now able to engage in work. Within mental health nursing, students are joining the profession who have had mental health problems and they bring with them a valuable understanding of the experience of receiving mental health services which enriches discussion in the classroom and care planning in the practice setting. One student commented, 'I'm glad I'm able to share my experience of using the service with my fellow students. They are beginning to appreciate what it's like on the ward for service users who are in distress and wanting to talk, but staff are not available to talk because they're too busy with office work.'

There have been numerous other measures taken by the government to reduce discrimination and stigma and to promote social inclusion in society (DoH 1999; SEU 2004). A recent initiative from the National Social Inclusion Programme aims to coordinate an action plan to promote social inclusion (DoH 2006b). The National Social Inclusion Programme (NSIP) has engaged mental health service user representatives and professional mental health service organizations such as the Royal College of Nursing (RCN) and the mental health nurses associations to develop a set of capabilities for socially inclusive practice which will apply across all mental health professional disciplines engaged in care delivery.

In order to be effective, socially inclusive practice in clinical settings must be underpinned by a framework of professional values and attitudes. These have been provided through the *The Ten Essential Shared Capabilities* (DoH 2004) and more recently the *Capabilities for Inclusive Practice* (DoH 2007) which are discussed in greater detail later in this chapter and can be accessed online from www.socialinclusion.org.uk.

Local community action

Within local communities voluntary organizations have traditionally been more active than the statutory services such as NHS Trusts in leading the way, with strategies and actions to tackle stigma and discrimination. Local organizations are often involved in running campaigns to de-stigmatize mental illness and to recognize the contributions to the community of people with mental health

problems. Special events and exhibitions take place in local communities every year on 10 October to mark the celebration of World Mental Health Day. Mental health charities such as Mind, the Mental Health Foundation and Rethink, together with the local mental health statutory services, usually carry out events to raise public awareness of mental health issues on this day. Increasingly, celebrities are becoming involved in these events which gives them an opportunity to be more candid about their own mental health problems while also making communities more aware of how common mental health problems are within the population.

The development of mental health forums in most local communities is giving service users and carers the opportunity to express their concerns, learn about new mental health policies and interventions and gain increased influence and social inclusion for people with mental health problems. The forums are run by service users and carer organizations, and their meetings are also usually open to mental health workers and members of the public.

An example of a successful forum is North Essex Stronger Together (www.nest-network.co.uk) which is a mental health service user forum and holds monthly meetings in the local community. The items discussed range widely from incapacity benefits to employment, local initiatives to support social inclusion and research projects involving service users. The forum also provides a good opportunity to meet with service users in a different context where the power relationship between mental health professionals and service users is more equal.

Forums

The local mental health forum is usually an exciting place where people with mental health problems or interests discuss real concerns, current policies and interventions affecting the lives of sufferers and carers.

- Arrange to attend a forum meeting and find out for yourself about how service users and their carers address mental health issues.

The voluntary sector within mental health is predominantly composed of charities and actively promotes social inclusion as the workers or volunteers have a special interest in the welfare of people with mental health problems. Often people become involved who have experienced mental health problems in the past, or are or have been carers supporting someone with a mental health problem. People with personal experience of mental health problems are well situated to appreciate the perspective of service users and provide meaningful support. Voluntary services such as day centres are usually sited in the middle of the community and are seen as more accessible and less stigmatizing than statutory services in mental health trusts.

Statutory mental health services have tended to be reluctant to involve service users in the direct provision of mental health care which has led to divisions occurring between mental health service users and the providers of mental health services. However, it is increasingly being accepted that people with lived experience of mental health services are experts by experience (Perkins 2007). Many service providers are becoming less discriminatory and are offering employment to people with lived experience and their services are becoming more flexible to the needs of service users and carers.

Following the publication of Capabilities for Inclusive Practice (DoH 2007), it is now expected that mental health trusts will appoint social inclusion coordinators to create links with local community facilities, such as employment agencies, employers, education, leisure providers and religious centres, to ease access for people with mental distress. While in the past local mental health trusts provided mainly crisis treatment, the focus is now shifting towards social inclusion.

Engagement of mental health professionals

As mental health workers and students we owe it to all who use mental health services to prioritize social inclusion. Socially inclusive practice is based on principles and values but requires us to also be more creative in putting service users and their carers at the centre of care and not the organizations for which we work.

A useful guide in developing a principles-based approach to practice is provided by The Ten Essential Shared Capabilities (DoH 2004) which resulted from concerns that the mental health workforce were not meeting the needs of service users. Capabilities for Inclusive Practice (DoH 2007) adopted the framework of The Ten Essential Shared Capabilities but has placed greater emphasis on the social inclusion agenda.

Values-based practice

In this section we will focus on each of The Ten Essential Shared Capabilities (DoH 2004) and consider how we as mental health workers and students can develop the capabilities for inclusive practice, to enhance the way we work with individuals with mental health problems in the context of their local community.

To begin with it is important to define what we mean by capabilities. They are essentially the values, skills and knowledge that we require to develop as mental health workers. Values play a central role in our lives, guiding us in making decisions about issues in our personal lives and work, and our interactions with the outside world. They provide us with criteria for action and guide us in making judgements and choices (Woodbridge and Fulford 2004).

However, values differ from one person to another, from one health care profession to another and between mental health workers and users of the mental health services. Something one person prioritizes may be insignificant to another individual and in practice there is often discussion and difference in the perceived goals of care (Woodbridge and Fulford 2004). Developing a sense of values to underpin practice will provide a rational basis for practice.

The Ten Essential Shared Capabilities (DoH 2004)

- Working in partnership.
- Respecting diversity.
- Practising ethically.
- Challenging inequality.
- Promoting recovery.

- Identifying people's needs and strengths.
- Providing service user-centred care.
- Making a difference.
- Promoting safety and positive risk.
- Personal development and learning.

Working in partnership

This capability focuses on the development and maintenance of constructive working relationships between mental health workers and service users, their families, colleagues, lay people and the wider community. Building community networks includes establishing informal friendship networks and formal links with community organizations, such as Jobcentre Plus, colleges and the voluntary sector, to enable people with mental health problems to gain access to roles within the community.

Scenario: Victor

Victor is a 22-year-old student at a local university. He came to the UK two years ago as an asylum seeker from Zimbabwe, leaving behind his close-knit family. He is usually a rather quiet but dynamic person. His only close friend at the university, Joe, was expelled from the course four months ago. Gradually Victor became withdrawn and started missing classes. His landlady was concerned about his mental state as he stopped attending classes and spent much of his time in bed. He also seemed distant and low in mood and took a long time to respond to questions and lost a lot of weight. Finally Victor reluctantly agreed to be admitted to an acute mental health ward for his own safety.

- Imagine you are on placement and working with the mental health nurse who is admitting Victor onto the acute ward in the mental health unit (it is not necessary for you to have been on an acute ward to undertake this exercise).
- Think about and then write down how you would begin to develop an effective working relationship with Victor.
- Try to imagine what it might be like for Victor to be in a strange environment.

When you have finished, place your notes in your professional portfolio.

During assessment you may notice that Victor appears shy and evasive when answering questions. It is tempting to attribute his behaviour to his mental state, however, take time to consider other factors. An acute mental health ward is a strange setting for someone who may never have visited one before and the behaviour of some people who are acutely ill may be distressing. Victor may also be aware of, and frightened by, his own changing mental state which he may be going through for the first time. In addition to this, he is in an unfamiliar setting with people he does not know which may also be a source of distress and so it is not surprising that he may appear frightened and mistrustful of staff on the ward.

To build an effective working relationship you will need to communicate to Victor an empathetic understanding of his experiences. He will begin to develop trust in you if you act as a good host, welcoming him, explaining your role clearly and demonstrating how different members of the team will help him in his recovery. It is important that

Victor is helped early on to discuss his expectations of his recovery. In relation to working in partnership, your ability to be a resource for him will depend on how you value him as a person and also on how well you communicate with him about your role and that of other professional disciplines in the team. The student nurse who builds a good rapport with and works alongside other staff from different disciplines will quickly become aware of how the whole team can be helpful in the recovery of individuals. Assisting Victor to contact his relatives and access other facilities in the community at an early stage of his admission is a positive intervention unless there are specific risk issues involved. As part of the working relationship it is crucial that individuals are considered as equal partners and they are offered choice in the care they receive. The relationship is one of mutual respect between all disciplines, agencies, the individual and the family involved in the care.

Working effectively with other people requires us to be aware of and manage our emotions to produce healthy relationships. There may be occasions during interaction with others where our own unhealthy emotions – such as anger, irritation and fear – may interfere with building trusting relationships. Equally the emotional state of others may adversely affect their interactions. In these situations we must take steps not only to contain our own unhealthy emotions but also those of others, to recognize barriers in communication and accept others as they are. We also need to take steps to minimize the unhealthy emotions of other people and work positively with them to develop a good working relationship.

The working relationship must extend beyond the clinical setting. The inclusive nurse will enable Victor to maintain contact with his existing social networks and build new connections which will help to develop his self-esteem and recovery. Victor's confidence in developing relationships will grow as you enable him through your knowledge of the facilities in the neighbourhood to take advantage of the appropriate community resources.

Respecting diversity

As mental health nursing students we are required to work in ways that respect and value diversity. Diversity may be in terms of age, race, culture, disability, gender, spirituality or sexuality. In the first part of the chapter we discussed how discrimination and prejudice often impact on the mental health of the individual and on the delivery of mental health services. In providing care and treatment we need to be sensitive to individuals' own values, and respond to their needs as they perceive them.

Respecting diversity: Victor

In the scenario above, Victor comes from an ethnic minority. His culture is very different from mainstream British culture, and may also be different from that of Zimbabweans who have lived in this country for some time.

- How could you work positively with Victor so that he does not become a victim of discrimination and prejudice within the mental health system?
- How would you ensure that his cultural needs are realized?

Write down your notes and when you have finished, put them in your professional portfolio.

It appears that Victor became lonely when his friend Joe left the university. Victor was close to him and felt understood and accepted in Joe's company. They shared a similar culture and interests, and these were very important to Victor. As a student mental health nurse, awareness of the cultural, political and economic situation in Zimbabwe would enable you to communicate with him in a sensitive, respectful and meaningful way. It may be that his religious and spiritual needs are important to him and have previously sustained him through traumatic situations. Through making contact with people both inside and outside the care setting you may discover that there are facilities in the local community which would meet some of Victor's cultural and spiritual needs and rekindle his sense of belonging, which he lost when Joe left the university.

Providing culturally sensitive care is not always easy unless we are aware of our own cultural biases and prejudices. Sometimes these are so ingrained that we are oblivious to how they might adversely affect our relationships with others from diverse backgrounds. We sometimes discriminate against certain groups of people who are culturally different to our own. Our fear of some people may also stem from ignorance of their cultural values and lead us to discriminate and socially exclude them. It is for this reason that some people do not receive an equitable service from the mental health system. It is important for us to recognize and contain our prejudices and biases and treat everyone equally irrespective of their diverse cultural backgrounds.

Victor and diversity

Developing an appreciation of the different cultural beliefs and values of individuals and minority groups within the community is the first step in respecting diversity.

- How can you develop an appreciation of Victor's culture and that of other minority groups in order to help them to address their needs?

Write down your notes and when you have finished, put them in your professional portfolio.

We do not have to go far to gain insights into different cultures. The health service, the university and the local community all contain people from diverse backgrounds. Your own student group at the university may be a rich resource in providing opportunities to interact effectively with people different to you. You may start off by establishing a genuine interest in them and find out about their way of life and how their culture, education and economic situation have shaped that life.

Becoming an inclusive practitioner will require you to undertake specific searches for community resources which are targeted at minority and under-served groups within the community. In the case of Victor he may value joining a local community group where he feels his cultural needs or interests can be met. He may also need help securing appropriate housing, employment, occupational opportunities and welfare benefits, and with developing social networks to build his life.

Practising ethically

Recognizing and respecting the rights of service users and carers and responding to our legal and professional obligations in practice is a central part of responsible practice.

Victor and ethics

In the scenario, Victor was initially admitted as an informal patient. However, later on he was detained under Section 2 of the Mental Health Act for his own safety (1983, 2007).

- Write down what you think is the difference between Victor's legal rights as an informal patient and his legal rights as a detained patient.
- Now write down what your professional and legal obligations towards Victor are based on the Mental Health Act 1983, 2007, and our professional code of ethics.

When you have finished, place your notes in your professional portfolio.

For information about the legal rights of patients under different sections of the Mental Health Act, consult the Department of Health website at www.dh.gov.uk/publications for the 2008 code of practice.

When Victor was an informal patient he had the same rights as a patient admitted to a general hospital for a physical illness and could decide whether or not to accept treatment or care. If he was unhappy with the care he received he could have discharged himself against the wishes of the mental health professionals.

However, as a patient detained due to his mental health under a Section of the Mental Health Acts 1983 and 2007 some of these rights are suspended and he cannot leave the hospital without the authority of his responsible clinician (DoH 2008). There is an increased obligation on the ward staff and hospital management to ensure Victor's safety and to explain and safeguard his legal rights under Section 2 of the Mental Health Act (1983, 2007). Victor can apply for a Mental Health Review Tribunal (MHRT) hearing which is independent of the mental health services and if they find the detention criteria do not apply, the Section can be overturned. The mental health services encourage people compulsorily detained under a Section of the Mental Health Act to apply for a tribunal hearing. The reasons for this are to ensure decisions are subjected to maximum scrutiny and are therefore fair. It also means that people like Victor, who do not have the benefit of the support, advice and help of their relatives or carers, can have their circumstances considered and legal rights respected.

Even though he may be detained under the Mental Health Act, Victor should still be regarded as an equal partner in decisions about his personal recovery and in accordance with good practice, he ought to be advised at all stages of matters concerning his care. Inclusive practice recognizes that service users are also expert in a different way through their experience of living with mental health problems and this forms the basis for collaborative and equal therapeutic relationships.

Challenging inequality

Scenario: Robert

Robert is 35-year-old man who lives in a home with five other residents with mental health problems. He was an only child and his parents were very caring. As a child Robert made good progress at school and particularly enjoyed music and art. However, he got bored very easily and by the age of 16 had become increasingly isolated and failed to obtain any formal qualifications. He did various casual jobs from manual work to working as a shop assistant but these jobs never lasted long because of a gradual deterioration in his mental health.

When he was 22 Robert's parents became very concerned when they heard him shouting and swearing to himself for no apparent reason. It seemed that voices in his head were tormenting him. Eventually he was admitted to a mental hospital and over the next 10 years had numerous inpatient admissions. The voices no longer bother Robert as he has learned to tolerate them with the help of medication. Contact with his parents has been reduced as they find it difficult to travel to see him due to their old age. Like other residents, Robert spends much of his time idle or watching television in the home. Mental illness and social exclusion have reduced the quality of Robert's life.

- Think of, and write down, the ways in which Robert has become socially excluded from his community.
- How could you help Robert?

When you have finished, place your notes in your professional portfolio.

Unfortunately the gradual deterioration in Robert's mental state was not noticed by his parents, at school, by primary care services or by any of his employers. Although he received treatment at the hospital most of it was in the form of medication and unfortunately Robert did not receive psychological talking therapy to help him cope with the voices. As a result of his frequent hospital admissions he lost many things we take for granted including friends, other close relationships, social and vocational skills and any contact with his local community. His life of social exclusion was exacerbated by the lack of stimulation in the home. Robert will continue to be socially excluded as long as health and social care workers do not recognize his potential for social roles.

Promoting recovery

Recovery has a different meaning for each individual. While one person may wish to regain their former lifestyle prior to becoming mentally unwell, another person may choose to adopt a different way of life altogether. The key issue is that recovery must be meaningful and valued and the individual with the mental health problem be at the centre of all decision-making. Recovery is something that the person experiences as they become empowered to lead a valued social role in society. For many service users, however, recovery depends on the sense of hope and optimism of the mental health professionals working with them.

Promoting recovery for Robert

- How would you promote recovery which is meaningful and valued by Robert?

Write down your notes and when you have finished, place them in your professional portfolio.

Robert is a relatively young man, and if he wishes he could take advantage of further education or vocational training, develop a new circle of friends and engage in leisure activities. It would be helpful to find out what hobbies or work Robert used to enjoy and whether he would like to rediscover them or develop new ones to suit his current health situation. At one time Robert used to love music and art. He could be helped to renew his interest in these hobbies if he wishes. There are examples of projects where people with mental health problems have developed their creative talent even to the point of earning a living (Secker *et al.* 2007).

Through enabling Robert to search on the internet about local art networks, community centres and voluntary or paid job opportunities he may develop an interest in using the internet to extend his horizons. Over time Robert may develop new interests such as the wish to undertake further education and skill development which you could help him to arrange with the local college. Having a good knowledge of the local neighbourhood will be invaluable in assisting Robert to make choices.

The potential for Robert to develop socially and vocationally is huge. However, in the early stages of his recovery he may need extra help to overcome barriers such as the negative attitudes of some mental health staff and discrimination within the local community.

Identifying people's needs and strengths

Working with individuals with mental health problems in a positive way involves a whole-system approach and viewing the individual in the context of their environment. We are required to take into account personal, physical, social, cultural, emotional and spiritual needs and strengths. Working closely with individuals and their support network including relatives and friends will enhance the individual's ability to live the life they would like to choose and achieve their aspirations.

Nirali's situation presented an interesting

Scenario: Nirali

Nirali is a 40-year-old woman who came to settle in this country two years ago from India following an arranged marriage with her husband, Rajiv, a British citizen but of similar cultural background. Nirali was an independent and career-minded person before she arrived in this country and in India she had been working part-time as a typist while undertaking further studies in computing. On arrival in this country it took a long time before she found similar work and then the work did not last for long. She has become increasingly dependent on her husband who works in the catering sector and spends long unsocial hours at work. Their social network is somewhat limited because of Rajiv's work and the couple do not have any children.

Rajiv has become concerned that Nirali is spending most of her time in bed and often looks tearful and miserable. The GP has diagnosed Nirali with depression and has referred her to the community mental health team.

● Write down a list of the factors you would take into consideration in the assessment of Nirali's needs and strengths.

Place your notes in your professional portfolio.

challenge to the community mental health team (CMHT). John was the community psychiatric nurse (CPN) assigned to work with Nirali and Rajiv. He found them polite but not forthcoming during conversation.

The breakthrough came on John's fourth visit to their home when he was accompanied by Daniela, who is a first year student mental health nurse. Daniela recognized that Nirali found it uncomfortable talking to a man in the presence of her husband. While John was conversing with Rajiv, Daniela took the opportunity to chat with Nirali about her past in India. She learned that Nirali comes from a large family and misses her siblings, and although well educated she has found it difficult to find suitable employment in this country. Both Rajiv and she are unaware of the neighbourhood facilities. They have relatives in different parts of this country but seldom meet with them because of financial hardship and Rajiv's unsocial working hours. The one-hour interaction between Nirali and Daniela was most beneficial and it became apparent that she is not as shy and withdrawn as she previously appeared.

Focusing on the needs and strengths of an individual requires a shift in our thinking from the habit of seeing people as having problems. We need to develop a whole-system approach to working in partnership with the individual's family or other significant people in their life and the relevant support networks.

Providing service user-centred care

When working with a service user it is necessary to develop an approach which actively involves them in planning their care and develops realistic goals which the person genuinely values. In subsequent visits to Nirali and Rajiv's home, the interaction between Nirali and Daniela and between Rajiv and John became much more relaxed. However, when

discussing their work with Nirali and Rajiv in clinical supervision John and Daniela recognized they had to work at a pace which assisted Nirali but did not make Rajiv feel challenged or disempowered. Encouraging them to engage in joint activities would help Nirali while also supporting her married relationship with Rajiv.

Daniela and John discovered a local cultural centre which offered music classes and advised Nirali and Rajiv, who both began to attend. Nirali also enrolled on a part-time course at the local college to develop her typing skills. While Rajiv previously had responsibility for their food shopping, this become a joint activity which empowered Nirali in the relationship and enabled them to spend more time together.

From the example provided by Nirali's case we can see that when sensitively and creatively carried out in the family context, a user-centred approach to care can produce real benefits and should be widely encouraged.

Making a difference

The measures that we use must be *evidence-based interventions* which can be understood as having been systematically studied by researchers and proven to be effective in certain situations or with specific client groups. The National Institute for Health and Clinical Excellence (NICE) issues advice on the most effective treatments and interventions in all areas of health care and their website is www.nice.org.uk.

For people such as Nirali, who is experiencing depression, NICE (2007) recommend treatment ranging from drugs to psychosocial interventions and support depending on the severity to which the person is affected. While evidence-based approaches are effective, several points need to be made regarding how this is interpreted within values-based practice. We are all individuals and two people can experience the same illness very differently. Therefore, while an intervention may be recommended by evidence and appropriate for one person, it may not be suitable in another case, even if there are similarities in how the problem is experienced. Furthermore, mental health care involves interpersonal interactions with people and in order to be effective it is necessary for us to demonstrate a genuine interest in the issues which concern the specific individuals with whom we work. Finally, users and carers as well as colleagues will have more faith in our practice if we are able to integrate individually-orientated values promoting social inclusion with evidence-based interventions.

For many mental health service users and carers, what makes a real difference in their recovery is the ability of the practitioner to carefully select interventions which are not only evidence-based but sensitive to their needs and aspirations.

Promoting safety and positive risk

All of us engage in a certain amount of positive risk-taking. Empowering service users to decide the level of risk they are willing to take to achieve the goals they set for their own well-being is an important role of the mental health worker. Yet in a professional capacity there is a tension between promoting safety and positive risk-taking (NIMHE 2004).

Safety vs. risk

Often we engage in positive risk-taking in order to attain a certain level of well-being.

- Discuss with your fellow students some positive risks that you have undertaken which enhanced your quality of life.
- Write down the circumstances.
- Consider and then write down what steps you took to avoid compromising your personal safety.

When you have finished, place your notes in your professional portfolio.

Examples of the positive risks which you might have chosen include one-off events such as parachute jumps, water skiing or paragliding. For others it might be a life event such as moving to a new town, applying for a job or even this course. In undertaking the above exercise you will have recognized that positive risk-taking is sometimes necessary to boost our self-esteem, confidence and skills and in some cases it is essential for us to take risks if we are to progress and move forward.

People with mental health problems face different types of harmful risks. Some may be directly due to their mental health problems while others are the consequence of using mental health services. Some individuals may be at risk of self-harm and suicide because they do not know alternative ways of coping. Less frequently, the risk of harm is to other people, including carers or members of the public. There may also be a risk of self-harm or suicide as a result of negligence by mental health workers or ineffective treatment and care. Finally, we must not forget that the stigma attached to mental illness and to using mental health services has a major debilitating and discriminatory effect on service users in accessing community facilities and securing meaningful employment (Hammersley *et al.* 2008).

In the past, mental health workers managed risk on behalf of people with mental health problems which resulted in disempowerment. Instead, it is preferable to enable individuals to assess potential risks for themselves and to decide how to overcome them. Not everyone will be in a position to assess their own risks and in such situations mental health workers will work with them to promote their safety but without compromising their trust and dignity.

Personal development and learning

At all levels of practice, as health care professionals there is an obligation on us to continue to commit to learning and developing our skills. The best way of continuing to learn is to monitor our own performance in practice.

While there are many different ways of developing values and skills, why not start by reflecting on your practice experience and assessing to what extent you are displaying each of the essential shared capabilities (DoH 2004)?

Working alongside mentors and other qualified mental health nurses and staff from other health care disciplines will give you the opportunity to observe and reflect on positive practice. The use of a reflective diary to document your observations and impressions is an effective way of developing personally and professionally but also of remembering small but important details which might otherwise be overlooked. Seeking constructive feedback on your practice in supervision and from those receiving care will help in transforming the way you work in the future.

Conclusion

People with mental health problems frequently face social exclusion in a number of areas of their lives. While the nature of a person's mental health problem may contribute to their experiencing social exclusion, more often stigma, discrimination and difficulties accessing social opportunities play a major role.

Mental health nursing and working with people who experience mental health problems have changed significantly in recent years. There has been the realization that providing care during the acute phase of a person's illness is not sufficient and it is necessary to go further and work with people to regain roles in the community which will benefit the person and wider society.

As student mental health nurses we can help and support people to make a real difference to their quality of life through developing not only evidence-based practice but also values-based practice.

In this chapter we have used the frameworks of *The Ten Essential Shared Capabilities* (DoH 2004) and the *Capabilities for Inclusive Practice* (DoH 2007) as a template to show how we can promote social inclusion in our practice. As a result of mental health workers working in an inclusive manner, many service users and carers are being supported to engage in the social life around them in a meaningful way and to develop a sense of well-being.

References

Allen, D. (2008) Volunteering works, *Mental Health Practice*, 11(9): 6–7.

BBC (2006) Mental health peril 'not spotted', *BBC News*, 4 December, available from http://news.bbc.co.uk/1/hi/health/620356.stm, accessed 16 February, 2007.

Disability Rights Commission (2001) *Strategic Plan*. London: Disability Rights Commission.

DoH (Department of Health) (1998) *Modernising Mental Health Services: Safe, Sound and Supportive*, Mental Health Service circular (HSC) 1998/233: LAC (98) 25. London: DoH.

DoH (Department of Health) (1999) *National Service Framework for Mental Health: Modern Standards and Service Models*. London: DoH.

DoH (Department of Health) (2004) *The Ten Essential Shared Capabilities: A Framework for the Whole of the Mental Health Workforce*. London: DoH.

DoH (Department of Health) (2006a) Written ministerial statement on the government's policy in response to the judgement of the European Court of Human Rights in the case of HL v UK (the Bournewood judgement), 29 June, www.dh.gov.uk/en/Consultations/Responsestoconsultations/DH_4136795.

DoH (Department of Health) (2006b) *Vocational Services for People with Severe Mental Health Problems: Commissioning Guidelines*. London: DoH.

DoH (Department of Health) (2007) *Capabilities for Inclusive Practice*. London: DoH.

DoH (Department of Health) (2008) *Code of Practice: Mental Health Act 1983*, www.dh.gov.uk/publications, acessed 7 May 2008.

Goffman, E .(1963) *Stigma: Notes on the Management of Spoiled Identity*. Harmondsworth: Penguin.

Hammersley, P., Langshaw, B., Bullimore, P., Dillon, J., Romme, M. and Escher, S. (2008) Schizophrenia at the tipping point, *Mental Health Practice*, 12(1): 15–19.

Layard, R. (2006) The case for psychological therapies, http://cep.lse.ac.uk/textonly/research/mentalhealth/RL447_version2.pdf, accessed 22 October 2008.

NICE (National Institute for Health and Clinical Excellence) (2007) Clinical guidance on depression,www.nice.org.uk/Guidance/CG23/Guidance/pdf/, accessed 19 October 2008.

NIMHE (2004) *The Ten Essential Shared Capabilities*. London: NIMHE National Workforce Programme.

O'Brien, M., Singleton, N., Sparks, J., Meltzer, H. and Brugha, T. (2001) *Adults with a Psychotic Disorder Living in Private Households*. London: The Stationery Office.

Perkins, R. (2007) Promoting recovery and facilitating social inclusion: a strategy for practice and implementation plan, www.southwest.csip.org.uk/

silo/files/promoting-recovery-and-facilitating-social-inclusion.pdf, accessed 25 February 2009.

Repper, J. and Perkins, R. (2003) *Social Inclusion and Recovery*. London: Baillière Tindall.

Sayce, L. (1998) Stigma, discrimination and social exclusion: what's in a word? *Journal of Mental Health*, 7: 331–43.

SCMH (Sainsbury Centre for Mental Health) (2002) *Primary Solutions: An Independent Policy Review on the Development of Primary Care Mental Health Services*, briefing 19. London: SCMH.

Secker, J. and Gelling, L. (2006) Still dreaming: service users' employment, education and training goals, *Journal of Mental Health*, 15(1): 103–11.

Secker, J., Hacking, S., Spandler, H., Kent, L. and Shenton, J. (2007) *Mental Health, Social Inclusion and Arts: Developing the Evidence Base*, final report, www.socialinclusion.org.uk/publications/MHSIArts.pdf, accessed 25 February 2009.

SEPFT (South Essex Partnership NHS Foundation Trust) (2007) *Annual Report and Accounts*, www.nhsft-regulator.gov.uk/register/annual_report_2007_se.pdf, accessed 22 October 2008.

SEU (Social Exclusion Unit) (2004) *Mental Health and Social Exclusion*. London: ODPM.

Shepherd, G. (2007) Work – whose business is it anyway? *Mental Health Review Journal*, 12: 15–17.

Singleton, N., Bumpstead, R., O'Brien, M., Lee, A. and Meltzer, H. (2001) *Psychiatric Morbidity Among Adults Living in Private Households, 2000*. London: The Stationery Office.

University of Manchester (2006) *Five Year Report of the National Confidential Inquiry into Suicide and Homicide by People with Mental Illness: Avoidable Deaths*. Manchester: University of Manchester.

Woodbridge, K. and Fulford, K.W.M. (2004) *Whose Values? A Workbook for Values-based Practice in Mental Health Care*. London: The Sainsbury Centre for Mental Health.

Conclusion

This book has provided a 'students' eye' view of mental health nursing and an introduction to pre-registration training, which we hope you have enjoyed.

Over the last few years the growth of new multidisciplinary teams based in the community has transformed mental health nursing, requiring the development of new skills and proficiencies. These range from knowledge of the Care Programme Approach (CPA) and working as a CPA coordinator to skills in risk assessment and risk management. It is now also necessary for mental health nurses to have knowledge of opportunities for training, employment and education. This role also extends to recreational activities and local facilities – for example, advising people with mental health problems of exercise programmes and encouraging participation in social activities or events in which the person may be interested which will develop confidence and mental well-being.

The promotion of mental health is also crucial and includes liaison with family, carers, independent agencies and other stakeholders crucial in the care of people with mental health problems. Yet we also need to involve the wider context of local services, independent and voluntary agencies and facilities in supporting people with mental health needs to engage meaningfully in their communities.

The Ten Essential Shared Capabilities

Underlying these practice-based skills are positive values as stated within *The Ten Essential Shared Capabilities* (DoH 2004). These link principles with practice, applied to specific situations and clinical settings. Reflecting on how our work demonstrates these principles is important in developing in confidence and competence in our practice. The development of multidisciplinary teams within the community in recent years has sometimes been thought of as challenging the identity of mental health nursing. Yet nursing as a profession has traditionally involved a wide and diverse workload. Instead of identifying a range of tasks within this role it might be preferable to clarify how our work demonstrates practical application of the principles and values of the profession.

This book has sought to collect together the new themes and concepts which have emerged within mental health nursing in recent years, contributing to the training of mental health nurses. These range from Barker's tidal model of nursing to *The Ten Essential Shared Capabilities*, recovery and social inclusion. In addition, other long-established aspects of nursing continue to be relevant. The professional code of conduct for nursing continues to provide a clear framework for the pre-registration mental health nurse training (NMC 2008). Physical assessment skills are long established as being vitally important in nursing, which we highlighted in Chapter 11. At the same time, the therapeutic approaches of cognitive behaviour therapy (CBT) (Chapter 12) and the psychodynamic and psychoanalytic approaches (Chapter 13) are core components in the way in which nurses interact with people with mental health problems.

The future of mental health nursing

The prospects for mental health nursing in the future are very exciting. The existing provision of teams in the community is a 'work in progress' and is likely to evolve still further. Among the areas where improvements need to be made are continuing to widen access to mental health services. Unfortunately it is still the case that many decisions concerning access to specialist mental health services is severely limited, with only the most acute receiving attention. Many people with mild to moderate problems are required to wait, or do not receive care at the time it is needed. Many people in the UK are prescribed antidepressants and the vast majority of people with a mental health problem are never seen by the mental health services. Improving mental health services for this group of people is essential if we are to improve mental health within the wider population. Student mental health nurses are well situated to work in these services and identify ways in which we can better engage meaningfully in the lives of people with mental health problems.

Sadly, it also continues to be the case that society has negative perceptions of people with mental health problems, and often people report the effects of discrimination to be more disabling than their mental illness. It is ironic that as a society we are more aware of the importance of mental health and well-being than ever before. Often employers provide confidential counselling services and other measures to promote the mental well-being of employees. Equally it is not unusual for people to receive complementary therapies, read self-help books and literature, engage the services of a life coach, or practise yoga and meditation to relieve stress or uncomfortable feelings. In this context student mental health nurses can act as advocates and challenge discrimination while promoting positive perceptions of mental health.

We wish you luck on your journey!

References

DoH (Department of Health) (2004) *The Ten Essential Shared Capabilities: A Framework for the Whole of the Mental Health Workforce.* London: DoH.

NMC (Nursing and Midwifery Council) (2008) *Standards of Conduct, Performance and Ethics for Nurses and Midwives.* London: NMC.

Answers

Here we provide some guided answers to a selection of scenarios.

Chapter 3

Scenario: Dave

- Dave's state of mind will be predisposing him to feel negatively and not see anything positive in his life and then continue to feel as bad, or worse. Perhaps Dave has never experienced a major health problem before, and suddenly feels vulnerable and unsure of what he previously took for granted. His view of the world has changed and Dave has been forced to adapt and make changes in his life which he might not have otherwise chosen. Changing long-established patterns of lifestyle can be challenging, even when we know it is for our long-term benefit.

- Dave may speak in a quiet tone and use a monotonous voice. His manner and behaviour will lack animation and energy, and responding to questions could appear to require effort, or there may be a delay between you speaking and Dave responding, suggesting slowed-down thinking and low motivation. The words he uses might be the same as those in the questions he has been asked, and his replies may be brief and offer little information, or he may not answer the question. These factors could suggest a lack of concentration and difficulty thinking, or an absence (poverty) of thought. Dave might appear as though he is not interested in the conversation, reluctant to engage and avoid direct eye contact. The content of Dave's speech is likely to be negative and pessimistic. He may also be unaware of current events and issues in the news. Dave's body posture could appear to be hunched, suggesting he is tense and anxious, due to feelings of low self-esteem and confidence, or alternatively he may appear lethargic and bored as a result of his low mood. Dave's physical appearance will possibly be unkempt with his hair unwashed or untidy, and personal care neglected. He may appear tired and look pale and his clothing may be loose and baggy, due to his recent weight loss and low mood. It is necessary to assess and document risk in terms of Dave's potential for self-neglect, suicide and harm, both to himself and others.

Scenario: Sophie

- Speaking to Sophie in a non-threatening, friendly manner and drawing her attention to the bloodstains on her sleeve may be a discreet way of beginning a conversation. It might be helpful to mention to Sophie that open wounds can become infected, and the risk is increased if the wound is covered with an item of clothing on which there may be germs. It could be argued that shame and secrecy often characterize self-harming behaviour and this could lead to Sophie, if she is engaging in self-harm, taking further steps to conceal her actions. However, the fact other people notice evidence of a person self-harming can reinforce to them that they have a problem, and provide the impetus to review their behaviour or to access help and support. It is important to be aware of boundaries and to discuss the encounter with the practice mentor.

- Yes, the code of professional guidance states that the role of the nurse is to promote the health and well-being of service users in our care and their families and significant others.

Scenario: Asifa

- Not necessarily, as it is difficult to know from

the information we have whether Asifa's weight loss is due directly to an eating, disorder, as while it appears to be the case that she has lost weight over time through not eating, we cannot be certain. However, Asifa has undergone significant changes in her life since beginning the course. It is advisable in the first instance before notifying the university to speak with her directly about your concerns, yet in a supportive way, even if this is difficult.

- Even as students we are obliged to act in accordance with the code of professional conduct to promote the health and the well-being of others. The course of action suggested above might help. However, if it does not, and we continue to have concerns, we might need to think carefully about exactly what these are. If you are in the same tutor group as Asifa, the personal tutor at your university can offer help and support. This dilemma highlights the complex role we have as students at a university as well as future health care professionals.

Scenario: George

- Offer reassurance to Sarah and demonstrate understanding of the difficulties she is experiencing. Through learning about Sarah's perspective of the situation the wider picture of George's difficulty will become evident. It will also become clear what support she has provided for George, what he is like and his background. Ask her about details of George's memory problem in order to elicit specific information about the problem(s), and to support her to see the situation clearly.

Chapter 4

Scenario 1

- The person may be at risk of danger through trying to escape and not paying attention to their wider environment.
- Talking calmly and in a quiet tone to the person will avoid further increasing their fear and anxiety. Showing respect for them, using their name and communicating in a friendly manner

will also assist in developing a therapeutic relationship. Explaining who you are and your role, and what has happened and how the person came to be on the unit demonstrates honesty and openness. It is important to listen to the person's statements and beliefs but not to collude with them.

Scenario 2

- The person is at risk of eating very hot food and inadvertently burning their mouth; of choking through not cutting up their food sufficiently; or of injury through misusing cutlery. The person may also forget to eat and experience weight loss if this occurs over successive meals and for a period of time.
- The nurse can encourage the person to eat, tactfully suggesting what tasks they need to perform, drawing their attention to the food. During this process the nurse will assess the person's responsiveness and use of skills. In some cases where the person wishes to eat but cannot perform the mechanical task the nurse might cut up the food and assist. However, this step ought to be taken with caution, and balance the person's need for nutrition with the possible loss of independence through de-skilling. Consideration of the person's dignity and interacting with them psychosocially can be demonstrated through checking their dietary preferences if possible, mixing the foodstuffs in manageable amounts, selecting food from their plate in accordance with the order and combination in which they wish to eat, while providing the food at the person's pace of eating, interspersed with fluid to lubricate the person's mouth. While performing this task the nurse ought to explain what they are doing and engage the person in communication, although verbal interaction may be limited while the person is eating.

Scenario: Paul

- Paul discussed with his mentor that it was unusual for John to ask for individual time.
- He advised the other staff on the unit where he was.

- In the interview room Paul sat opposite a window from which he was visible to another member of staff.
- He had a personal alarm.
- The alarm had been tested and so he was aware it would work.

Scenario: James

- James has paranoid ideas and feels persecuted and threatened. As a young male, James is in a high risk category of possible physical aggression. He also has previous training in martial arts; while this is not a definite indicator of risk, it may suggest a potential for possible aggression.
- James has tended to isolate himself and displays paranoid ideas and mistrust of others. It is advisable for the staff to begin by attempting to develop a rapport and build trust with James. James lacks significant interpersonal relationships and making clear the role and function of the nurse will establish useful boundaries. A place to begin may be for the staff to introduce themselves, treat him with respect and courtesy, and orientate him to the unit, explaining the location of the facilities and showing him his room and where to put his belongings, to normalizse the ward environment and reduce any apprehension he may be feeling.

Chapter 10

Scenario: Martin

- As we grow older, our bone density decreases and so the extent to which Martin's fracture has repaired will be an important factor together with muscles, tendons and ligaments which may have also been damaged in the accident. It is likely that Martin will have received intensive input from a physiotherapist to regain the movement in his hip and to be confident walking again. However, before he returns home we need to assess his mobility to be sure there are no problems. This measure is lent added significance as there are stairs in his home and it may be necessary for him to have regained a high degree of mobility to be able to

manage. Other faculties such as eyesight, which may predispose him to a risk of falls, should also be assessed. Martin will also require an activities of daily living (ADL) assessment with an occupational therapist at his home. This is a comprehensive assessment to ascertain how he will meet his daily needs such as washing, dressing, cooking and shopping and arrangements will need to be made where there are deficits. Finally, we need to assess how Martin is overall, and how he appears in his general physical health. As we grow older we require more time to recover from setbacks and traumas.

Scenario: Peter

- Peter is in Erikson's life stage of maturity and the task is to achieve integrity against despair. Socially Peter is experiencing a loss of the independence he has valued and out of necessity has been required to adapt to a lifestyle he would not choose. As a pharmacist in his working life he no longer has the same empowered role in life and has a more limited role within the community.
- Physically, Peter's health has led to his requiring assistance which it seems he has never adapted to as he has always been very independent and private. Psychologically, it is highly possible that loss of confidence and an awareness of his vulnerability have led Peter to experience an increased risk of the repeated falls he had at home. Losing his wife will also have led to Peter becoming more aware that he is closer to death but also deprived him of his life partner. It is possible that within Erikson's theory, Peter's depression is despair. Often older people achieve a sense of integrity through connections with their family. Peter's grandchildren, whose company he used to enjoy, may have served as a positive factor but at the moment he is dwelling on a sense of despair at his current situation.

Scenario: Dennis

- Depression has impacted on Dennis's life in the following ways. He has neglected his former interest by not going to the social club. He has not been engaging in his usual pattern of other activities as neighbours reported his not opening his curtains aroused their initial concerns. It appears that Dennis has not been eating or looking after his personal care. His depression appears to have dominated his life as he appears low in mood, withdrawn and to have lost hope in life. From what he has said he appears to feel guilty and that he has no future. His apparently having taken an overdose of tablets and made superficial cuts to his wrists indicates serious intent to end his life.

- Dennis has experienced two acute physical health problems in recent months, a stroke and lung condition which requires intensive treatment. Physical pain and discomfort and physical limitations may have impacted on his mood. His neighbours called the ambulance and his note is to his son in Australia. It is possible that he has a limited social support network and may feel vulnerable, which can add to low mood. Loneliness can also exacerbate low mood and depression.

Scenario: Gita

- Gita is likely to be feeling frightened, confused and unsure of herself. It is very possible she is aware that something is deeply wrong but not sure exactly what. Gita's behaviour may seem strange at times and her motives unclear. Sanjay may feel resentful that the person he has lived with for so long has changed so much. He may feel betrayed and resentful towards her, or even angry at her hostility and suspicion towards him. He may feel embarrassed that they need help and that this is a sign of weakness or not coping. On the other hand he may feel very protective of Gita and that it is his duty to look after her.

- It is necessary for the nurse to develop a rapport with Gita and Sanjay and understand their relationship. This will allow the nurse to appreciate their human experience but also encourage to understand their history and view current challenges from that perspective. It would be useful to ask how they met and to see

photos of their wedding, and to encourage them to reminisce on key moments of their married life. This strategy will help the nurse understand Gita and Sanjay and remove any threat Gita may feel while reacquainting them both with the relationship they once had.

Chapter 11

Scenario: George

- The support George requires will depend on his level of understanding of the condition and what he feels are the main issues. Information will have been provided in the form of leaflets regarding the condition. George may require help to read this or want to discuss his understanding of the condition with a health care professional. Referral back to the nurse specialist for COPD will be necessary if he is struggling. The community mental health nurses can help George by encouraging him to attend appointments, maintaining regular contact with him and monitoring the effects of knowing that he has COPD on his mental health. NHS Direct provide a range of information on smoking cessation and the different methods involved. However, it will depend on whether George wishes to stop smoking as this requires significant motivation.

Scenario: Hannah

- Hannah's assessment will include whether she experiences any auras which may give prior warning of a seizure. More information regarding her medication and when she has taken it will also be helpful. Even though she is on an inpatient mental health unit as an informal patient Hannah can refuse to take her medication. As Hannah is at risk of a tonic-clonic seizure through omitting to take her medication the main dangers are of injury to herself during a seizure and obstruction of her airway.

- When Hannah experiences a seizure it is important to ensure she is given privacy and her dignity is respected. First Aid measures include the initial assessment of the environment by ensuring any furniture or objects that may lead to injury are moved or cushioned if safe to do so. During the tonic-clonic stage the main role is observation as attempts to control Hannah's movements may lead to injury. When the seizure ends, she should be placed in the recovery position in order to maintain her airway until she is fully conscious.

Chapter 12
Scenario: Selina

- We can see that what began as a concern has now became a rigidly held belief. Selina wanted to lose weight and went on a diet. As she lost a lot of weight she can understand the effect of the amount of food eaten on weight gain or weight loss but this has developed into an exaggerated belief. Evidence contradicts her view and to maintain health it is necessary to have a balanced diet of different foods and in sufficient amounts to support our bodily needs. We may be able to help Selina by supporting her to challenge her beliefs.

Chapter 13
Scenario: Meera

- The adoption of Karl. Meera's not having other siblings and feeling ignored and emotionally neglected by her parents. Her parents being strict and driving her educationally. A lack of friends and socially meaningful opportunities. Experiencing rape and sexual abuse. The trauma of giving birth, possibly to a child born as the result of her being raped.
- Denial regarding the birth of the baby. Repression by responding to her unloving home life by withdrawing. Sublimation by investing all of her energies in her schoolwork to the detriment of her social development and engaging in relationships. Rationalization may also be evident, as clearly Meera intended to end her life and still wished to die afterwards, and viewed this radical act as rational.

- A lack of rewarding relationships, emotional neglect and abandonment but also high expectation from her parents, and sexual abuse by her adopted brother.
- Meera may believe she is never good enough and cannot ever please her parents and is a failure and to blame for having the baby. She may know in her unconscious mind that she has been neglected and is a victim but is unable to express her anger as these feelings are too difficult to confront. As a result her actions have been to withdraw, control her eating and attempt to end her life.

Chapter 14
Scenario: Terry

- In the scenario Peter's views are representative of a paternalistic model of care. Terry was seen to be a vulnerable person and Peter believed he was not able to recover beyond a certain point of functioning. Decisions were made that meant Terry was discouraged from engaging in any activity in the community. Mental health and social services staff had become Terry's main contact with the outside world and his opportunities to develop as a person are limited by the type of conversations that people are willing to have with him. Despite this Terry has continued to be interested in horses even though he was discouraged from engaging with them. Alison on the other hand is practising a recovery-focused approach regarding Terry as a whole person and not just someone defined by his illness who cannot recover and to be regarded with suspicion. She sees Terry's interest as an opportunity to encourage his personal identity and autonomy to emerge. By looking at the two different approaches to Terry, we can see some of the differences between them.

Peter	Alison
Focused on minimizing risk	Focused on maximizing opportunities
Focused on preventing relapse	Interested in encouraging change
Does not talk about interests that were present during psychosis.	Talks about interests
Assumes risks to be 'self-evident'	Explores risks in detail
Considers diagnosis and symptoms as indicators of outcome	Considers engagement and relationship as indicators of progress
Satisfied with ensuring basic needs are met	Interested in encouraging clients to fulfil themselves

Glossary

Activist learners: seek out new experiences, are keen to volunteer, meet new people and engage in different activities. Activists prefer to learn by doing, and will get on with the job before receiving all of the instructions. While activists are adventurous learners, they are prone to spontaneity, tending not to complete one task before starting the next.

Activity scheduling: in this intervention people learn to plan activities to restore a healthier balance in their lives. By keeping a diary of activities and rating them on a 10-point scale for satisfaction and pleasure with 10 being the most pleasurable we can ascertain a good picture of how the person's time is allocated and on what. The person can then set about correcting imbalances and planning a different activity schedule to achieve a better balance in their life.

Acute myocardial infarction: is commonly known as a heart attack and is the most common cause of sudden death in the UK. The condition occurs because of problems with the blood supply to the heart muscle and may follow intermittent chest pain for a few weeks beforehand. Risk factors include a family history of myocardial infarction, hypertension, diabetes and smoking.

Advance decision: a person's decision concerning future treatment. It does not have to be written down but if expressed verbally, nursing notes documenting the decision can become the written record. These decisions are generally legally binding if certain criteria apply: the individual was 18 years or older when they made their decision and had the necessary mental capacity.

Advance statements: express a general treatment preference. These are not legally binding but subject to the 'best interests test' where if the health care team feel it is to the benefit of the person to have what they are requesting they may comply. However, they are not obliged to and could provide an alternative which they believe better meets the person's best interests.

Affective learning: concerns emotions and feelings. All such techniques serve to stimulate recognition, discussion and interaction. Reminiscence therapy is based on the premise that long-term memories tend to be retrievable even in advanced stages of dementia.

Alzheimer's disease: accounts for about half of all dementia cases. Deposits or plaques of an abnormal protein are found throughout the brain and tangles of twisted protein molecules occur in the brain's nerve cells. Scans can detect atrophy or shrinkage of the brain tissue and the widespread loss of brain cells.

Anxiety: is a functional mental health problem where a person is preoccupied and displays heightened or exaggerated concern and attention to specific issues. It exerts a detrimental effect on the person's functioning and quality of life. There are physical and psychological characteristics associated with anxiety. Physical characteristics are increased heart rate, increased rate of passing urine – micturition – and dry mouth. Psychological characteristics are agitation, feelings of fear or terror over a sustained period of time and an inability to concentrate. More extreme anxiety can manifest itself as panic attacks, where physical symptoms are experienced due to the body being highly responsive. These include palpitations, chills, hyperventilation, dizziness, chest pain, choking, nausea and stomach churning. Other forms of anxiety include phobias, for example, agoraphobia is anxiety pertaining to places or situations from which it may be difficult to escape or receive help if the person were to experience a panic attack.

Apprenticeship: traditional nurse training where students spent most of their time in the clinical setting. This model focused on gaining practical skills and technical competences.

Arthritis: an umbrella term which covers a range of conditions characterized by painful joints and bones. The two most common forms are osteoarthritis and rheumatoid arthritis. Osteoarthritis is the most common form and is caused by the cartilage between the bones degenerating, leading to the bones rubbing together at the joints. Rheumatoid arthritis mainly affects the joints and tendons. It is caused by the auto-immune response which attacks the joints and leads to inflammation of the synovial membrane, tendon sheaths and bursae.

Assertive outreach: was created to work with service users with severe and enduring mental health problems who are in need of continuing support and contact with the mental health services but are at risk of disengaging.

Assertiveness training: the person learns to assert their rights in a socially acceptable manner. Learning to say 'no', disagreeing with others, giving and receiving criticism, giving and receiving compliments and speaking out for their rights assertively, but not aggressively, are all elements of this strategy.

Asthma: there are two forms of asthma. Extrinsic asthma is caused by allergens and occurs in children and young adults. Intrinsic asthma appears later in life and is associated with chronic respiratory conditions. Common triggers for extrinsic asthma include house dust mites, animal fur, pollen, tobacco smoke, cold air and chest infections. The symptoms of asthma, which apply to both types are feeling breathless, a tight chest, wheezing and coughing.

Behavioural experiments: often mistakenly labelled as a 'behavioural strategy'. These are used when a person is reluctant to engage in certain behaviours because they hypothesize that certain things will happen as a result. The person and therapist work in the session to identify the beliefs and the therapist invites the person to collaborate

on a thought record. The person therefore creates a set of rational thoughts to hold on to when they are in the challenging situation. The next step is to test things out in reality. In collaboration with the therapist the person may be given the homework task of, for example, speaking in the next team meeting and monitoring the reactions of colleagues.

Behavioural rehearsal: the person and therapist have identified a behaviour that the person wants to practise outside therapy. The person uses the therapy session as a forum in which to practice the desired behaviour while the role of the therapist is to shape the person's behaviour towards the target required.

Biological theories of ageing: suggest ageing is an inevitable consequence of time passing and is a universal experience. The rate at which our bodies age differs and is caused by different factors such as genetics predisposition, lifestyle, family history and environment.

Bipolar mood disorder: a functional mental health problem which affects mood, thinking and behaviour and is characterized by mood swings. When in a high phase the person can display grandiose behaviour and express delusions, but when low they become deeply depressed.

Blood pressure: the cardiac output from the heart multiplied by the peripheral resistance of the vessels within which the blood is contained. Blood pressure gives an indication of the functioning of the heart and circulatory system. High blood pressure (hypertension) suggests the heart is under greater stress and can be an indication of a risk of stroke or heart attack. Hypertension is a sustained blood pressure of 140/90 mmHg, or above. The systolic reading is the maximum pressure of the blood on the wall of the vessel following the contraction of the heart. The diastolic pressure is when the sound of the heartbeat disappears.

Boundaries: highly important in psychotherapy. Among the factors which need to be observed are confidentiality, and the length of sessions, which should be agreed at the beginning of therapy with appointments occurring at the same time of day, and on the same day each week. The rationale for this is to establish trust, reliability and consistency for the sessions. Boundaries are a key concept for effective mental health nursing and managing our relationships with people with mental health problems in order to work therapeutically and in the person's best interests.

Bournewood safeguards: legislative measures to protect certain individuals and allow mental health services to provide the necessary level of care within the law. The safeguards protect those over 18 in a hospital or a care home, those experiencing a disorder or disability of the mind, individuals lacking the capacity to give consent to the arrangements made for their care and those whose care amounts to a deprivation of liberty but is considered after an independent assessment.

Capabilities: essentially the values, skills and knowledge that we require to develop as mental health workers.

Capabilities for Inclusive Practice: a document published by the Department of Health in 2007 which builds on the 2004 document, *The Ten Essential Shared Capabilities*. This document states that mental health trusts will appoint social inclusion coordinators to create links with local community facilities, such as local employment agencies, employers, education, leisure providers and religious centres, to ease access for people with mental distress to promote social inclusion.

Cardiovascular accident/stroke: a disease of the blood vessels in the brain. The symptoms of stroke depend on the area of the brain which is affected and the severity of damage. Commonly, stroke is more prevalent in people over 65 but occurs in all age ranges. A stroke can lead to a number of severe problems with the most common being hemiplegia, or a weakness on one side of the body, which is compounded by muscle spasms, and dysphagia, or problems with swallowing.

Care Programme Approach (CPA): introduced in 1990, the CPA provides a unified system of documentation for users of mental health services and links together the aspects of care in the community by health care professionals, allowing the development of care plans based on assessed needs. Every person whose mental health needs are assessed under the CPA has a named CPA care coordinator and receives regular reviews of care. Services are responsible for ensuring service users, their carers and significant others receive adequate care.

Chronic obstructive pulmonary disease (COPD): is a collective term for a number of lung diseases including bronchitis, emphysema and chronic obstructive airways disease (COAD). The main cause of COPD damage to the lungs is attributed to smoking.

Cognitive behavioural practice: is based on the key concept that all behaviour is learned and is therefore amenable to be unlearned or changed. The cognitive behavioural approach offers a framework for assessing the pattern of behaviour and a method for altering thinking, feeling and behaviour. The model aims to help the person become aware of how their thoughts and emotions are linked and enable them to acquire new life skills.

Cognitive behaviour therapy (CBT): a 'talking therapy' based on the notion that learning and thinking have an important influence in emotional and behavioural problems. CBT proceeds from the assumption that these responses can be 'worked with' and provides a problem-focused approach. First an active collaboration is entered into between the user and therapist. During therapy various techniques are used which identify and challenge the validity of unhelpful and negative thoughts and allow the person to develop positive adaptive ways of dealing with their problems. It is effective in treating a range of mental health problems including depression, anxiety disorders and behavioural problems.

Cognitive learning: refers to factual and empirical knowledge.

Cognitive restructuring: the person learns to think differently in situations that previously led to negative feelings and/or negative behaviour. The main tool used for this is 'thought records' where the person writes down the problem feeling and its strength and then focuses on the thinking involved that causes the feeling. Through this method the person learns to identify triggers for the problem feelings and behaviours. Once the problem thinking has been identified, the person and therapist analyse it and try and identify thinking errors which are mistaken assumptions or biased thinking processes.

Cognitive theory: functions on the premise that what we do and feel is influenced by our thinking. In situations where there is no right or wrong answer and limited factual or objective evidence to support a decision, the person is reliant on their personal opinion and/or preference. This offers the potential for irrational beliefs to become apparent and problems to emerge. Our feelings, thoughts, beliefs and actions are all linked and mutually influential. Within CBT (see above) the therapeutic process assists the person in appreciating how these different attributes link together and can be made to provide more adaptive coping methods.

Common Assessment Framework (CAF): provides a shared approach to an initial needs assessment for use by statutory or voluntary sector staff in education, early years, health, police, youth justice or social work. This will reduce the number of assessments experienced by young people and their families, prevent their being asked the same questions multiple times and promote better communication between health care professionals from different agencies.

Communication training: working with people to express positive and negative emotions and general communication techniques is beneficial in couple therapy or when helping people with interpersonal problems. Often this takes the form of active listening training and problem-solving skills training.

Community mental health teams (CMHTs): multidisciplinary CMHTs continue to be the focal point of adult mental health services. They support people with complex mental health problems and their families in the community when their needs cannot be met by their GP, primary care or generic social services.

Community psychiatric nurses (CPNs): are mental health nurses who work with people who experience mental health problems in the community.

Cost-benefit analysis: the therapist asks the person to list all the advantages and disadvantages to themselves of continuing to hold negative thoughts. Seeing this clearly written down helps the person to make a decision about how helpful these thoughts are.

Countertransference: the effect of the person receiving therapy on the therapist.

Creutzfeldt-Jakob disease (CJD): this rare type of dementia affects about one person in a million in the UK. 'Original' CJD usually occurs in middle age. 'New variant CJD' (vCJD) can be apparent in younger people and progresses rapidly, often to death within one year. There has been much publicity about the link between vCJD and eating beef from cattle infected with bovine spongiform encephalopathy (BSE).

Criminal justice and court diversion teams: often experienced mental health nurses attend court and where necessary carry out mental health assessments of people appearing before magistrates. They also work on a short-term basis with people going through the court process who have a mental health problem.

Crisis intervention: when a person finds themselves much more dependent on external sources of support than at other times in their life. It has three distinct phases. Impact is where a threat is recognized. Then recoil occurs, which is an attempt to restore equilibrium, but failure can leave the person feeling stressed and defeated. Finally, adjustment/adaptation or breakdown occurs, where the person begins to move to a different level of functioning.

Crisis resolution teams: focus on managing crises in the community. Through being supported in the home environment the service user and their family avoid the trauma of being required to go into hospital.

Defence mechanisms: can be experienced as very powerful feelings triggered in response to painful memories and feelings to protect the person from the pain of those memories. Often the person is not aware of the connection between the defence mechanisms and the difficult memories and will interpret these feelings in different ways. Defence mechanisms perform a protective function for the person as they avoid the need to confront the source of their problems. A significant part of the work of psychotherapy involves understanding and overcoming defence mechanisms.

Delirium: an acute confusional state which is experienced at the extremes of life. People who have long-term physical conditions or are dependent on illicit drugs or alcohol are most at risk. Delirium can affect the individual in several ways and be terrifying for the person who is affected, especially if they experience symptoms such as visual hallucinations and misinterpreting the actions of others as threatening.

Dementia: an organic mental health problem which is not a single disease but group of different illnesses which all cause degenerative changes in brain tissue and a progressive decline in cognitive functioning. Typical symptoms are loss of memory, confusion and a change in personality, mood and behaviour. Examples of dementia-type illnesses are Alzheimer's disease, Lewy body disease, vascular disease and Pick's disease.

Denial: the refusal to acknowledge the existence of a real situation or the feelings associated with it.

Depression: a functional mental health problem which may manifest itself in four ways: low mood (e.g. a loss of interest in activities the person previously pursued); physical symptoms such as loss of sexual appetite (libido); cognitive changes (e.g. the person may have difficulty concentrating); and behavioural changes (e.g. a loss of interest in personal appearance).

Diabetes: there are two types of diabetes. Type I is where our production of insulin is affected and needs to be replaced. This usually occurs in people under 40 and has a rapid onset with readily evident signs and symptoms. Type II diabetes is when the body still produces insulin but it is not sufficient, or the insulin does not work effectively. Type II diabetes commonly occurs in adults over 40, however, childhood diabetes is increasing due to obesity.

Disability Discrimination Act: passed in 1995 and a revised Act was introduced in 2005 to outlaw discrimination in employment and education and permit access to public services and transport for people with disabilities, including mental health problems.

Disability Rights Commission: established to develop a code of conduct to provide practical guidance to employers on how to reduce discrimination and promote equality in the workplace and services for people with disability.

Discrimination: being treated negatively due to prejudice. A common example is people not being given jobs for which they are qualified and suited due to other personal attributes. Discrimination is apparent in the role and attitudes of other people rather than the person with a mental health problem. However, these have an impact on people with mental health problems, materially in the form of direct socioeconomic disadvantage but also in terms of loss of self-esteem, confidence and social exclusion, with the potential worsening of their mental health.

Dreams: Freud believed dreams to be essential in highlighting the differences between the (primary) process of the unconscious and the (secondary) process of the conscious. When we are dreaming our unconscious influences our thoughts and feelings. These may be represented as symbols or images which use our ideas and experiences to make a patchwork narrative reflecting our concerns or emotional traumas. When we are asleep we are engaged in a mental life which is distinct from our everyday conscious experience. Dreams offer an excellent source of access to the unconscious. A basic assumption of Freudian theory is that unconscious conflicts involve instinctual impulses or drives that originate in childhood. The patient, through analysis, recognizes these unconscious conflicts and his or her adult mind can find solutions that were unattainable to the immature mind of the child, such as resilience factors (e.g. self-esteem, sociability and autonomy, family compassion and warmth, absence of parental discord, social support systems and encouragement of personal effort and coping).

Early intervention teams: work with service users identified as being potential high users of services in the future. An advantage is the early identification of mental health problems; also, working with people when they are younger reduces the level and extent of service provision the person requires later in their life.

Eating disorder: a functional mental health problem which incorporates a range of problems characterized by dramatic fluctuations in weight which may be in the form of gain or loss, mistaken beliefs and perceptions by the person about their body size and shape, and maladaptive eating behaviour. In some cases the person does not eat because they mistakenly believe they are overweight and introduce a rigorous regime of dietary control and deprivation of food (anorexia nervosa). Alternatively the person binge eats large amounts of food and then purges through vomiting or by using laxatives (bulimia nervosa).

Empowerment: involves the active facilitation of choice, freedom, autonomy and control through encouragement, nurturance and fostering. Time is given freely by professionals with a view to talking, listening and engaging in joint activities.

Epilepsy: is a term which describes a range of disorders which are characterized by seizures or fits. The neurones in the brain work on electrical impulses and in epilepsy the electrical impulses are disrupted, causing the individual to have a seizure. This may appear as a momentary lapse in attention or a generalized seizure with tonic-clonic features.

Evidence-based interventions: interventions that have been systematically studied by researchers and proven to be effective in certain situations or with specific client groups.

Experimental learners: are keen to apply new ideas or learning in practice. They tend to be energetic and enthusiastic to solve problems in practice, yet become frustrated if the change takes a long time to implement or barriers are encountered.

Exposure: a technique where the feared stimulus is confronted either gradually in graded exposure or by confronting the most feared stimulus in 'flooding'. Often this means that people confront themselves with their feared situations one by one. The aim is to stay long enough in the feared situation to make the fear reduce or disappear.

Formative assessment: is student-centred and allows the identification of needs to reach learning goals, improve performance and identify potential opportunities through agreeing and negotiating the learning contract to assess the student's skills, knowledge and learning and to reflect on the students' performance.

Free association: the person is first encouraged to speak about anything that comes into their conscious mind, without giving any thought to the meaning. Then the therapist helps the person understand and make sense of these unconscious unwanted feelings. The therapist's main role therefore is to interpret the clues that are revealed through the person's free association.

Frontotemporal dementia (Pick's disease): striking changes in behaviour precede memory problems and there is a marked loss of the person's ability to express him or herself. Onset is typically in the forties or fifties.

Functional mental health problems: can be divided into psychotic disorders, which include schizophrenia, and mood disorders and other affective disorders (e.g. depression, anxiety, obsessive-compulsive disorder, phobias, anorexia nervosa and bulimia nervosa and personality disorders).

Graded task assignments: behaviours that are new to the person but which they wish to incorporate in their behavioural repertoire. They are placed in a hierarchical order and then practised from the least to the most difficult.

HIV/AIDS-related dementia: most people who are HIV-positive will not have dementia but many who progress to develop AIDS will experience severe dementia. The cause may be an HIV virus in the brain or due to tumours or infections resulting from reduced immunity.

Human Rights Act: the 1998 Act incorporates most of the provisions of the European Convention on Human Rights within English law. The Human Rights Act protects our basic human rights in a number of articles. There are four articles with particular relevance to the care and treatment of people with a mental health problem: Article 2, the right to life; Article 3, the prohibition of torture; Article 5, the right to liberty and security; and Article 8, the right to respect for a private and family life.

Huntington's disease (Huntington's chorea): a fairly rare inherited disorder which manifests itself in middle age. It is characterized by jerky movements in addition to progressive dementia.

Interpersonal model: developed by Hildegard Peplau and concerned with the growth of the service user. The model is based on the idea that people have needs which can be physical, psychological and emotional, and it is necessary for the person to achieve satisfaction in all these areas to experience a rewarding and enjoyable life. The role of the mental health nurse is to first ensure survival of the person and to act as an agent of change by using their interpersonal skills to achieve a therapeutic goal. Second, they assist the person to understand their mental health problem(s) and develop, by promoting creative and innovative ways to work through experiences. The model consists of four stages: orientation, identification, exploitation and evaluation.

Investigating double standards: the person is invited to think about someone else in a similar position and asked whether they would apply the same standards to the other person as they believe are applicable to them. Through realizing that our beliefs are not always correct we can review whether our feelings and thoughts lead us to have realistic expectations.

Investigating evidence: the person learns to look for 'real' evidence in support of their thoughts and beliefs. People learn to become 'personal scientists' and to evaluate the evidence. By seeking objective evidence and facts the person can check their beliefs and feelings in relation to the evidence and develop a balanced view.

Lasting power of attorney (LPA): enables another nominated person to make decisions on behalf of the person when they lose mental capacity. These will include decisions regarding the person's health and welfare.

Learning contract: agreed activities the student will undertake to develop their understanding, meet the practice outcomes and achieve their own personal learning goals. The learning contract is a cohesive document which proceeds logically and has clear goals, actions and objectives.

Learning theory: considers how humans learn. The three most prominent learning theories are operant learning, respondent learning and modelling.

Mental capacity: a person lacks capacity if, in relation to a certain matter at the time, they are unable to make a decision because of an impairment or disturbance in the functioning of the mind or brain which may be temporary or permanent.

Mental Capacity Act 2005: a statutory framework intended to empower and protect people who may not be able to make their own decisions. The Act also enables people to plan ahead for a time when they may lose their capacity. The Act is based on five principles: that there should be a presumption of the person having mental capacity unless we are aware of evidence to the contrary; individuals should be supported to make independent decisions; people retain the right to make eccentric or unwise decisions; the law operates in the person's best interests; where the person is not able to make a choice the least restrictive intervention should be chosen.

Mental health: there are many different definitions. However, it can be described as a capacity to enter into and sustain mutually satisfying personal relationships, a continuing progression of psychological development, an ability to play and to learn so that attainments are appropriate for age and intellectual level, and also the development of a moral sense of right and wrong.

Mental Health Act 1983: provided four criteria for determining mental illness, which were: incomplete development of the mind; psychopathic disorder; disturbance which prevents normal development; and a mental disturbance which interferes with normal behaviour and daily life. This definition of mental health has been superseded by the revised Mental Health Act 2007 which has introduced just one definition of mental health.

Mental Health Act 2007: a revision of the 1983 Act following a lengthy review of stakeholders in, and providers of, mental health services. The new Act provided a single definition of mental illness that simply states that it is: 'any disorder or disability of mind'. It introduced a new 'treatability test' that created a principle of 'appropriate treatment' based not necessarily on improving health but on preventing the disorder worsening. The new Act introduced supervised Community Treatment Orders (CTOs) which make it possible to manage the care of people with mental health problems living in the community. Within the provisions of a CTO the person can be subject to recall to hospital if it is deemed necessary for treatment of their mental illness. However, if the person's mental health improves sufficiently the order can be revoked. The range of practitioners who can implement mental health legislation has been broadened from psychiatrists and approved social workers (ASWs) to include any mental health care professional with appropriate training.

Mental Health Bill (2006): revised the legislation to use just one definition of mental health which focuses on the problem(s) the service user is experiencing, rather than diagnosis.

Mental health disorder: either a severe mental health problem which is persistent or the simultaneous occurrence of a number of problems also in the presence of a number of risk factors.

Mental health forums: give service users and carers the opportunity to express their concerns, learn about new mental health policies and interventions and gain increased influence and social inclusion within communities for people with mental health problems. The forums are run by service users and carer organizations, and their meetings are also usually open to mental health workers and members of the public.

Mental health promotion: any action to enhance the mental well-being of individuals, families, organizations and communities, and a set of principles which recognize that how people feel is not an abstract and elusive concept, but a significant influence on health.

Mental illness: an 'umbrella' term which covers a range of disorders with varied causes. A person is said to be mentally ill if their responses are prolonged; are triggered by inappropriate events; or where the person's quality of life is impeded and they experience significant distress over a sustained period of time.

Mental illness prevention: Primary prevention targets the 'non-clinical' population to prevent the occurrence of illness (e.g. relaxation methods to reduce anxiety and stress). Secondary prevention is focused on people who are already unwell and aims to reduce the length, frequency or intensity of the illness (e.g. CBT-based 'self-help' books). Tertiary prevention aims to reduce or prevent the negative consequences associated with illness (e.g. development of an occupational and leisure programme for someone with a severe and enduring illness such as bipolar disorder or schizophrenia).

Mentors: nurses who are on the professional registration in the same discipline of nursing as the students they are mentoring, have been on the professional register for at least one year, have continued to develop their skills and knowledge during this time, have successfully completed a recognized mentor training programme, are capable of fulfilling the requirements of the role of student mentor and assessor and who receive regular updates on the mentor role.

Metaphor: identification of an image or symbol which visually represents what a person is feeling. This technique allows the feelings to be appreciated in the specific way in which they affect the person.

Modelling: involves the therapist demonstrating the desired response to the person or demonstrating assertive responses in other people. Modelling works on the basis that people learn not only from their own actions but from seeing those of other people. An example is of parents who smoke. A child may see the parent frequently smoke and be influenced to participate in the same behaviour.

Modernising Mental Health Services: Safe, Sound and Supportive: a government policy initiated in 1998 to promote social inclusion. People with mental health problems and their carers should be involved in their care and services should communicate with them and seek to promote empowerment.

National Service Framework (NSF) for mental health: this 1999 initiative was the result of a major review of the mental health services and the first national strategy for mental health services. It was significantly supported with a commitment of funding and resources to implement the changes it proposed.

Negative automatic thoughts: the person monitors their thoughts when they feel depressed, anxious or are experiencing other strong negative emotions. There are a number of variations of irrational thinking strategies which can be identified through monitoring negative automatic thoughts.

Nursing and Midwifery Council (NMC): regulatory body of nursing, to protect the public through maintaining standards of practice. Standards of accountability, responsibility and competence are set out in the code of conduct.

Obsessive-compulsive disorder (OCD): a functional mental health problem, where the person experiences persistent obtrusive negative thoughts (obsessions), and strong urges to carry out specific actions or rituals (compulsions) to prevent feared outcomes from occurring (e.g. hand-washing, checking, collecting, hoarding, touching and counting rituals).

Old age: there is some dispute as to when this phase of life begins. The increasing lifespan of adults in modern society and the growing numbers of older adults, especially those aged 80 and older, have resulted in a redefining of later adulthood into two distinct life stages or age groups, with the 'younger-old' being those between 65 and 75.

Operant learning: works on the premise that we learn from the consequences of our actions. Behaviours which are followed by positive or enjoyable consequences are inclined to happen more often, while behaviour followed by negative consequences tends to be avoided.

Organic mental health problems: are caused by the effects of physical illnesses on the functioning of the brain. They include dementia-type illnesses, infectious causes and can also result from alcohol and substance misuse.

Personality disorder: a functional mental health problem where established patterns of maladaptive thinking, feeling and behaving differ significantly from the expectations of the person's culture and produce detrimental outcomes. Characteristics include repeated chaotic interpersonal relationships and behaviour and the person's inner conflicts being expressed through the way in which they relate to others.

Placing events in perspective: an especially useful method where the person is catastrophizing, which is a tendency to think of the 'worst case scenario' and often a feature of anxiety-related problems. The person is asked to rate the event that triggered the catastrophizing on a continuum from 0 to 100 with 100 being a catastrophe. The idea is then considered from the perspective of: 'How bad would it be if that happened?'

Postmodernism and recovery: rather than having a single cause and there being a 'correct' way to treat mental illness, it is in fact the result of many causes and has many possible treatments. In this view, mental illness is not a health problem but just a different way of being.

Practice document: while on your practice placement you will be expected to complete pre-set outcomes in a practice document. These correspond with the standards of the NMC code of conduct and the requirements for entry to the professional register on achievement of competence at the end of the course. There will be different expectations of the level of skill, competence and autonomy as you progress through the course.

Practice placements: specialist clinical areas where students will be based for a period of time in order to gain experience of nursing care.

Problem-based learning (PBL) or inquiry-based learning (IBL): the current method of nurse training with an increased focus on the acquisition of practice-based skills and knowledge, which bridges the gaps highlighted by Project 2000. Students are still supernumerary in practice and learn proficiencies and technical competencies in skills laboratories at the university. Practice-based scenarios form part of theoretical study to integrate theory and practice. The course involves 50 per cent theory and 50 per cent practice.

Professional portfolio: a collection of evidence supporting personal and professional development and learning. It is not possible to state definitively what ought to be included in a portfolio other than it should summarize learning to date. The portfolio should comprise more than simply a collection of certificates and achievements but reflect the personal meaning and value of the learning to the individual and what it has contributed to their growth and understanding.

Project 2000: method of nursing introduced in the 1980s to increase recruitment and professionalism in nursing. It was a more academic approach with the emphasis on theoretical learning. Students still had placements in practice but they were supernumerary, with a significant amount of time devoted to theoretical study in the classroom.

Projection: where unwanted feelings are displaced onto another person who appears to be a threat.

Psychoanalysis: a long-term therapeutic relationship between a therapist and a client. The therapy is based on an interpersonal relationship and the same therapist works with the same person for the duration. There are three phases of the psychotherapeutic process. First, the introduction involves setting and establishing the boundaries and assessing the person's problems and needs. The working phrase involves 'working through' the person's issues to arrive at a resolution to their problems and a sense of 'personal growth', and to develop adaptive defence mechanisms to cope in the future. The third phase, termination, refers to the ending of the therapeutic relationship which is negotiated after a successful 'working through' and the achievement of 'personal growth'. Freud developed a model to understand how the mind worked, and in order to do this he developed three mechanisms called the id, the ego and the super-ego. These are not anatomical structures or physical parts of the brain but concepts to help explain how the psyche works.

Psychoanalytic therapy: a 'talking treatment' that aims to repair the mind (psyche) by uncovering unconscious forces, drives and impulses and making these accessible to the client. Psychoanalysis is a therapy which assists the person to develop an insight into the unconscious motivations and impulses by which they are driven. Freud was the founder of psychoanalysis. He believed there was a structure to the psyche which comprised differing levels of consciousness: unconscious, pre-conscious and conscious.

Psychodynamic approach: term used to describe the newer approaches and developments in psychoanalytic theory.

Psychodynamic practice: this model offers a concept of the mind and the mechanisms by which it works and helps us to understand why people behave in seemingly repetitive, destructive ways. It is the essential 'one-to-one' helping relationship involving advanced listening and communication skills. The psychodynamic model provides a framework to address profound disturbances and inner conflicts concerning issues of loss, attachment, anxiety, and personal development.

Psychological effects of ageing: Erikson's model of psychosocial development is an influential concept and helps us make sense of the issues we confront at various stages or the lifespan. Each of Erikson's life stages has a relevant challenge which must be overcome in order to proceed to the next. The challenge in the mature life stage requires that we develop 'integrity' rather than succumb to 'despair'. By reaching integrity we come to terms with our life and are able to look back and accept events and the choices we have made as having been a necessary part of our life. Despair involves unresolved feelings over the past and emotions such as anger and resentment.

Psychomotor learning: relates to actions or practical tasks.

Psychosis: a functional mental health problem which leads the person to lose touch with reality and attribute personalized or unusual meanings to events or phenomena. It is an acute mental illness and frequently people can experience an episode of psychosis and fully recover.

Pulse: the number of rhythmic expansions of arteries in response to the contractions of the heart over one minute. It indicates the rate and strength of the heartbeat. A fast pulse is referred to as tachycardia, while a slow pulse is called bradychardia. The average pulse varies between 60 and 80 beats per minute for adults and is more rapid in children.

Rating negative thoughts: when the person has identified the negative emotion the therapist asks how strong this feeling is on a scale of 0 to 100 per cent. The person indicates which thoughts were associated with each of the negative feelings. Then all the thoughts are listed according to how much the person believed the thought at the time the feeling was present.

Rationalization: when we justify our own behaviour to avoid criticism.

Reaction formation: the fixation in consciousness of an idea, affect or desire that is opposite to a feared unconscious impulse.

Reality orientation (RO): a therapeutic approach that can be used by practitioners, care workers and carers who are supporting people with dementia. RO is concerned with taking regular opportunities to sensitively orientate the person, for example, to tactfully inform them of the time of day and the location. There are a range of RO strategies that can be utilized on an individual or group basis including charts and orientation aids and prompts.

Reattribution of negative automatic thoughts (NATs) and beliefs: after the person has disputed the NATs or irrational beliefs another thought or belief needs to be formulated. The goal of reattribution is not to change the person's emotional state from depressed to happy but from feeling overwhelmed to being able to make a realistic appraisal.

Recovery maximizes a person's quality of life and social inclusion while managing risk effectively by encouraging their skills and promoting their independence and autonomy. The intention is to foster hope for the future and successful integration into the community.

Recovery-focused approach: a modern approach to care, influenced by people who have actually experienced mental health problems. It requires that we accept different explanations, viewpoints and positions about the experience of mental illness so as to be able to work with people rather than challenging them – or even worse, seeking to impose our own explanation and understanding on the person's experience.

Recovery model: the role of the mental health nurse and other multidisciplinary health care professionals in secure and forensic services is to support the person in retaining a sense of hope and identity in often challenging circumstances.

Reflection: the method by which experience is transformed into knowledge. It is a process of focusing carefully, thoughtfully and in detail on beliefs or knowledge, the ideas and logic on which these are based, and considering the consequences and implications which might arise.

Reflective journal: while there are no rules about keeping a reflective journal, if the document is to be a useful learning tool it is important that you find it enjoyable to produce, and that it is an honest account of how you feel about practice. The reflective journal has a number of uses, providing an account of significant events in practice experience, a method of evaluating the placement and of appreciating personal and professional development.

Reflective learners: watch and observe others completing a task before attempting it themselves. In arriving at a decision reflective learners will consider all of the consequences. While reflectors seek out all of the information before proceeding and are well prepared they can be indecisive where there is no clear guidance and reluctant to initiate new experiences.

Regression: a return to an earlier stage of development when confronted by a challenge.

Relaxation training: the person learns a specific strategy to relax. There are two techniques used to teach this method. The progressive muscle relaxation technique teaches the person to relax major muscle groups in the body and acquire the skill to bring the relaxation response under voluntary control. It is mainly focused on helping people to distinguish between tension and relaxation. The second strategy is called suggestive relaxation and is based on undertaking guided imagery with the client and by doing so creating a state of relaxation.

Reminiscence therapy: is concerned with stimulating the recall of past memories or events by utilizing music, video, photographs and images (e.g. recordings of popular musicals, viewing film clips, listening to music and viewing pictures from the past).

Repression: the withdrawal from consciousness of an unwanted idea, affect or desire by pushing it down or repressing it into the unconscious part of the mind.

Resistance: the person receiving therapy can become defensive and display resistance by unconsciously attempting to halt further insight by censoring their true feelings.

Respiration: an autonomic act under the control of the nervous system and sensitive to the amount of carbon dioxide in the blood. It is a two-way process where we breathe in by inhaling oxygen from the air which then enters the bloodstream and is transferred from the blood to the tissues. We then exhale carbon dioxide which is a byproduct of energy production from the bloodstream though the lungs. The normal range for adults when at rest is 16 to 18 breaths per minute.

Respondent learning: when we make a connection between two events that originally were unconnected. A famous example is of Pavlov's experiments with his dogs.

Response/stimulus hierarchy: involves constructing a list of the most to the least feared situations or responses. The list can be used in exposure and systematic desensitization. Each of the situations/behaviours is rated for discomfort/anxiety on a 0–100 scale with 100 being the most uncomfortable or anxiety-provoking. These ratings are called subjective units of discomfort, or SUDs.

Risk: in mental health risk can be grouped into a number of specific categories. These include suicide, violence and/or aggression, self-harm and neglect.

Risk assessment: a specific and focused appraisal of all potential sources of threat, danger and harm at a particular time. The assessment should be comprehensive in scope and consider all of the relevant facts and history which are available and focus on the person with the mental health problem. Risk assessments should be regularly repeated and reviewed in order to be useful and responsive to changing circumstances.

Risk management: actions taken to address and minimize risk based on the information emerging from a risk assessment. Types of risk management are preventative risk, interventionist and post-incident responses.

Schizophrenia: a functional mental health problem which is often mistakenly thought to be a split personality. Instead it is a fragmentation of the person's perception and grasp of objective reality, which affects their mood, thinking and behaviour, and makes it difficult for them to be able to separate their own thoughts and perceptions from what occurs outside of them.

Self-harm: a functional mental health problem often regarded as the same as attempted suicide. However, in practice it is not so easy to clearly place a person's motive in one or other category. Self-harming actions include tattooing, piercing, plastic surgery or other cultural acts, for example, tribal scars. People frequently self-harm to relieve pent up feelings of emotion or anger or to express pain and feelings of self-loathing or worthlessness.

Setting behavioural targets: specific behaviours that the person wants to change are highlighted. This is helpful as it specifically points in the direction of what needs to be done.

'Sign off' mentors: mentors or practice educators who have undergone additional training and are responsible for 'signing off' students as proficient at the end of their training.

Social exclusion: often experienced as a combination of interrelated factors, including the inability to engage in the social life around a person, which most people take for granted. Contributing factors are low income, unemployment and lack of a social network.

Social theory of ageing: also known as disengagement theory, this relates to the way in which older people may 'naturally' start to disengage from societal contacts and spend more time alone, pursuing solitary activities.

Stigma: can be defined as evident where an individual is devalued, or possesses an attribute which is deeply discrediting. Often stigma is based on a misconception or exaggeration of certain characteristics with little resemblance to reality. Through emphasizing differences between groups of people in a shared community, stigma leads to increasing divisions and social exclusion of the stigmatized group.

Sublimation: the diversion or deflection of instinctual drives, usually sexual, into areas of activity that are not linked to the instincts.

Substance misuse: within mental health this is defined as dependence, either psychological, physical or both, on a substance which alters the person's psychological functioning. Substances which can be misused include nicotine, caffeine, alcohol, amphetamines and associated compounds, cannabis, cocaine, opioids, hallucinogens, inhalants, sedatives, hypnotics, and anxiolytics. The effects vary depending on the choice, amount taken, frequency of use, individual susceptibility to the effects, and the combination of substances used. Frequently people experience low mood and personality changes, become more impulsive when under the influence, or have impaired judgement.

Substance misuse teams: The revised Mental Health Act has widened the definition of mental illness to include substance misuse. Traditionally substance misuse teams have regarded their work as separate from mental health services and a distinct specialism.

Summative assessment: involves identifying a certain level of competence and evaluating the student and teacher's performance.

Supervised Community Treatment Orders (CTOs): the Mental Health Act 2007 made it possible to manage the care of people with mental health problems in the community, but a person may be subject to recall to hospital if deemed necessary. However, if the person's mental health improves sufficiently, the order can be revoked.

Systematic desensitization (SD): relaxation training is a vital element of SD. SD is used in the treatment of anxiety problems and the person first learns to relax. The second step is for the therapist to create a 'fear hierarchy'. The person's fear is analysed and a list of stimuli created, ranging from being a little fearful to very anxiety-provoking. Then the person is asked to relax and the therapist asks them to imagine the situation that is lowest in the fear hierarchy. If the person can imagine the anxiety-provoking situation without losing the relaxation state, then the next step in the fear hierarchy is taken. Often SD is combined with exposure. When the person has overcome certain feared situations in their own imagination, the therapist will suggest testing them out in reality.

Systemic practice: is characterized by the key notion that young people have a social context which influences their behaviour to a greater or lesser extent and affects their perception of their problem. An important factor is the family and this has led to the practice of family therapy.

Task-centred practice: a popular base for contemporary assessment and intervention. It may be used as a set of activities rather than a theoretically-based approach from which a set of activities flows.

Temperature: measures the warmth of the body. The body's temperature is indicative of changes within the body and the environment. While the normal range is from 36 to 37.5°C there is a variation between the sites where the temperature is taken, with oral readings 0.2°C below those of rectal readings.

The Ten Essential Shared Capabilities: provided a framework of professional values and attitudes to promote socially inclusive practice within clinical settings as there were government concerns that the mental health workforce was not meeting the needs of service users. The key aspects of this document are: working in partnership; respecting diversity; practising ethically; challenging inequality; promoting recovery; identifying people's needs and strengths; providing service user-centred care; making a difference; promoting safety and positive risk; and personal development and learning.

Theorists: learners who consider problems logically and in sequential stages and seek to understand the broader picture. Individual cases which do not conform to an overall coherent picture can

be regarded as confusing. Often theorists therefore lack pragmatic skills.

Tidal model: the most prominent model in modern mental health nursing, developed by Phil Barker. It functions on the premise that people are defined by their experience. The model was developed within a practice-based setting and has four assumptions: mental health nursing relates to the person's future development, as opposed to the origins of distress and interpersonally involves the nurse and service user; only the person undergoing mental distress accurately experiences the problem; the correct function of nursing is for the practitioner to help the person rediscover their life through reconciling their past and present and to realize future opportunities and through working collaboratively in an interpersonal relationship; mental illness is experienced as a disturbance of living and the activity and focus of the mental health nurse, probably uniquely among other branches of nursing, is on the person's relationship with what is defined as mental health and illness.

Training in self-reinforcement: learning how to bring about change in problematic behaviours.

Transference: during psychotherapy the person can relive and revisit aspects of their past and childhood which can generate powerful feelings and lead to the person projecting these feelings onto the therapist.

Urinalysis: reagent strips are dipped into a sample pot of urine which has been collected and stored in a clean and dry container. Urinalysis is particularly important for identifying levels of substances which are normally not secreted and might indicate the presence of an underlying physical health problem. It is a non-invasive method of assessment which can identify a range of factors.

Validation therapy: attempts to enter the inner emotional and personal world of a individual with dementia and involves seeking to develop an awareness of their feelings and the underlying meaning of verbal communication. In validation therapy the therapist attempts to understand the world from the perception of the older person rather than interpreting the situation from their own. There is no attempt to impose a current reality in terms of dates and times; instead the practitioner explores the underlying meaning of the person's behaviour and speech.

Vascular (multi-infarct) dementia: brain damage is caused by tiny strokes arising from an insufficient supply of blood to the brain.

Weight: as part of a physical assessment on admission to hospital a person will be weighed as a baseline measurement in case there is later concern regarding their weight change during their time in hospital.

Index

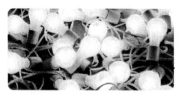
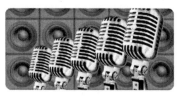
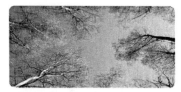
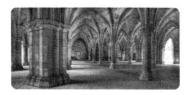
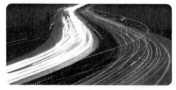
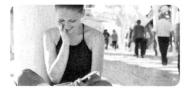
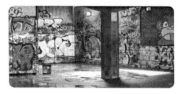
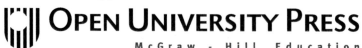